Cognitive Dysfunction in Bipolar Disorder

A Guide for Clinicians

Cognitive Dysfunction in Bipolar Disorder

A Guide for Clinicians

Edited by
Joseph F. Goldberg, M.D.
Katherine E. Burdick, Ph.D.

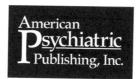

American Psychiatric Publishing, Inc.

Washington, DC
London, England

Copyright © 2008 American Psychiatric Publishing, Inc.
ALL RIGHTS RESERVED

Manufactured in the United States of America on acid-free paper
12 11 10 09 08   5 4 3 2 1
First Edition

Typeset in Adobe Galliard and Optima

American Psychiatric Publishing, Inc.
1000 Wilson Boulevard
Arlington, VA 22209-3901
www.appi.org

Library of Congress Cataloging-in-Publication Data
Cognitive dysfunction in bipolar disorder : a guide for clinicians / edited by Joseph F. Goldberg, Katherine E. Burdick.—1st ed.
    p. ; cm.
    Includes bibliographical references and index.
    ISBN 978-1-58562-258-0 (alk. paper)
    1. Manic-depressive illness. 2. Cognition disorders. I. Goldberg, Joseph F., 1963–II. Burdick, Katherine E., 1972–
    [DNLM: 1. Bipolar Disorder—complications. 2. Bipolar Disorder—physiopathology. 3. Cognition—physiology. 4. Cognition Disorders—etiology. WM 207 C6756 2008]
RC516.C62 2008
616.89′5—dc22   2008014109

British Library Cataloguing in Publication Data
A CIP record is available from the British Library.

For my wife and partner, Carrie L. Ernst, M.D.,
my children, Joshua and Brian Goldberg,
for their inspiration and energy,
and my parents, Daniel and Ethel Goldberg

J.F.G.

To my husband and colleague, Raphael J. Braga, M.D.,
and my father, Henry, and late mother, Bonnie,
for their lifelong encouragement
toward the pursuit of knowledge

K.E.B.

Contents

Contributors

Carrie E. Bearden, Ph.D.
Assistant Professor in Residence, Jane & Terry Semel Institute for Neuroscience and Human Behavior, Department of Psychiatry and Biobehavioral Sciences and Department of Psychology, University of California, Los Angeles, California

Katherine E. Burdick, Ph.D.
Assistant Professor of Psychiatry, Albert Einstein College of Medicine, the Bronx, New York; Director, Neurocognitive Assessment Unit, Division of Psychiatry Research, The Zucker Hillside Hospital, North Shore Long Island Jewish Health System, Glen Oaks, New York

Catherine M. Cahill, M.Sc., M.Psychol.
Clinical Psychologist, University of Sydney, Northern Clinical School, Royal North Shore Hospital; Clinical Psychologist, Traumatic Stress Clinic, Westmead Hospital, Sydney, Australia

Luke Clark, D.Phil.
University Lecturer, Department of Experimental Psychology, University of Cambridge, Cambridge, England

Colin M. DeFreitas, M.A.
Graduate Student, Department of Psychology, Simon Fraser University, Burnaby, British Columbia

Melissa P. DelBello, M.D.
Vice-Chair for Clinical Research and Associate Professor of Psychiatry and Pediatrics, University of Cincinnati College of Medicine, Cincinnati, Ohio

Safa Elgamal, M.D., M.Sc., Ph.D.
Schlegel Research Chair in Aging and Assistant Professor of Cognitive Neuroscience, University of Waterloo, Waterloo, Ontario, Canada

David C. Glahn, Ph.D.
Director of Neuroimaging Core in Psychiatry and Associate Professor, Department of Psychiatry and Research Imaging Center, University of Texas Health Science Center at San Antonio, San Antonio, Texas

Joseph F. Goldberg, M.D.
Associate Clinical Professor of Psychiatry, Mount Sinai School of Medicine, New York, New York; Director, Affective Disorders Research Program, Silver Hill Hospital, New Canaan, Connecticut

Terry E. Goldberg, Ph.D.
Professor of Psychiatry, Albert Einstein College of Medicine, Bronx, New York; Director of Research in Neurocognition, Division of Psychiatry Research, The Zucker Hillside Hospital, North Shore Long Island Jewish Health System, Glen Oaks, New York

Frederick K. Goodwin, M.D.
Director, Psychopharmacology Research Center, and Research Professor, Department of Psychiatry and Behavioral Sciences, The George Washington University School of Medicine and Health Sciences, Washington, D.C.

Guy Goodwin, M.D.
W.A. Handley Professor of Psychiatry, University of Oxford, Warneford Hospital, Oxford, England

Glenda MacQueen, M.D., Ph.D.
Head, Mood Disorders Program; Associate Professor, Department of Psychiatry and Behavioral Neurosciences; Adjunct Member, Intestinal Diseases Research Program, McMaster University, Toronto, Ontario, Canada.

Gin S. Malhi, M.B.Ch.B., B.Sc. (Hons), F.R.C.Psych., F.R.A.N.Z.C.P., M.D.
Professor and Head, Discipline of Psychological Medicine, University of Sydney, Sydney, Australia

Anabel Martinez-Aran, Ph.D.
Head of the Neuropsychology Bipolar Disorders Program, Hospital Clinic, Institut d'Investigacions Biomèdiques August Pi i Sunyer, Centro de Investigación Biomédica en Red de Salud Mental, University of Barcelona, Barcelona, Spain

David J. Miklowitz, Ph.D.
Professor of Psychology and Psychiatry, Department of Psychology, University of Colorado, Boulder, Colorado

Philip Mitchell, M.B., B.S., M.D., F.R.A.N.Z.C.P., F.R.C.Psych.
Professor and Head, School of Psychiatry, University of New South Wales, New South Wales, New Zealand

Cory F. Newman, Ph.D.
Director, Center for Cognitive Therapy, Associate Professor of Psychology, Department of Psychiatry, University of Pennsylvania School of Medicine, Philadelphia, Pennsylvania

Paula K. Shear, Ph.D.
Professor of Psychology and Psychiatry, Director of Clinical Training, and Codirector of Graduate Studies, Department of Psychology, University of Cincinnati, Cincinnati, Ohio

Marta Sokolowska, Ph.D.
Research Scientist, Department of Clinical Pharmacology, DecisionLine Clinical Research Corporation, Toronto, Ontario, Canada

Ivan J. Torres, Ph.D.
Associate Professor L.T., Department of Psychology, Simon Fraser University, Burnaby, British Columbia; Clinical Neuropsychologist, Riverview Hospital, Coquitlam, British Columbia; Research Scientist, BC Mental Health and Addiction Services; Research Consultant, Mood Disorders Centre, University of British Columbia, Vancouver, British Columbia, Canada

Eduard Vieta, M.D., Ph.D.
Professor of Psychiatry, University of Barcelona; Director of the Bipolar Disorders Program, Clinical Institute of Neuroscience, Hospital Clinic, Institut d'Investigacions Biomèdiques August Pi i Sunyer, Centro de Investigación Biomédica en Red de Salud Mental, University of Barcelona, Barcelona, Spain

Lakshmi N. Yatham, M.B.B.S., F.R.C.P.C., M.R.C.Psych.
Professor of Psychiatry and Associate Head of Research and International Affairs, Department of Psychiatry, University of British Columbia, Vancouver, British Columbia, Canada

L. Trevor Young, M.D., Ph.D.
Professor and Head, Department of Psychiatry, University of British Columbia, Vancouver, British Columbia, Canada

Disclosure of Competing Interests

The following contributors to this book have indicated a financial interest in or other affiliation with a commercial supporter, a manufacturer of a commercial product, a provider of a commercial service, a nongovernmental organization, and/or a government agency, as listed below:

Luke Clark, D.Phil.—*Consultant:* Cambridge Cognition, GlaxoSmith-Kline.

Melissa P. DelBello, M.D.—*Consulting/Advisory board:* AstraZeneca, Eli Lilly, GlaxoSmithKline, Pfizer, France Foundation; *Research support:* AstraZeneca, Eli Lilly, Shire, Janssen, Pfizer, Somerset Pharmaceuticals; *Speaker's bureau:* AstraZeneca, GlaxoSmithKline, Pfizer, France Foundation, Bristol Myers Squibb.

Joseph F. Goldberg, M.D.—*Consultant:* AstraZeneca, Cephalon, Eli Lilly, GlaxoSmithKline; *Speaker's bureau:* Abbott Laboratories, Astra-Zeneca, Eli Lilly, GlaxoSmithKline, Pfizer.

Frederick K. Goodwin, M.D.—*Consultant:* GlaxoSmithKline, Lilly, Pfizer, Wyeth, AstraZeneca; *Research support:* GlaxoSmithKline; *Speaker's bureau:* GlaxoSmithKline, Pfizer, Eli Lilly.

Guy Goodwin, M.D.—*Advisory board:* AstraZeneca, BMS, Eli Lilly, Lundbeck, P1Vital, Sanofi-Aventis, Servier, Wyeth; *Grant support:* Sanofi-Aventis, Servier; *Honoraria:* AstraZeneca, BMS, Eisai, Lundbeck, Sanofi-Aventis, Servier.

Philip Mitchell, M.D.—*Consultant:* Alphapharm; *Honoraria:* AstraZeneca, Eli Lilly, Janssen-Cilag.

Marta Sokolowska, Ph.D.—*Employer:* DecisionLine Clinical Research Corporation.

Eduard Vieta, M.D., Ph.D.—*Grant support:* Instituto Carlos III, CIBER-SAM, Spain; *Grant support/Consultant:* AstraZeneca, Bristol Myers Squibb, Eli Lilly, GlaxoSmithKline, Janssen-Cilag, Merck Sharp & Dohme, Novartis, Organon, Otsuka, Pfizer, Sanofi, Servier.

The following authors have no competing interests to report:

Carrie E. Bearden, Ph.D.
Katherine E. Burdick, Ph.D.
Catherine M. Cahill, M.Sc., M.Psychol.
Colin M. DeFreitas, M.A.
Safa Elgamal, M.D., M.Sc., Ph.D.
David C. Glahn, Ph.D.
Terry E. Goldberg, Ph.D.
Glenda MacQueen, M.D., Ph.D.

Gin S. Malhi, M.B.Ch.B, B.Sc. (Hons), M.R.C.Psych., F.R.A.N.Z.C.P., M.D.
Anabel Martinez-Aran, Ph.D.
David J. Miklowitz, Ph.D.
Cory F. Newman, Ph.D.
Paula K. Shear, Ph.D.
Ivan J. Torres, Ph.D.
Lakshmi N. Yatham, M.B.B.S., F.R.C.P.C., M.R.C.Psych.
L. Trevor Young, M.D., Ph.D.

Foreword

This volume represents an ambitious, even bold, undertaking. The editors express it succinctly in the preface when they describe the book as both "timely" and "premature." It is timely in that those of us who study and treat patients with bipolar disorder have only recently begun to appreciate that the symptoms, the functional deficits, and ultimately the pathophysiology of the major "mood" disorders involve a great deal more than mood. In contrast, neurologists and "schizophrenologists" have long appreciated the relevance of neuropsychology and the cognitive sciences.

My personal experience reflects this recent awakening of bipolar experts to the cognitive dimensions of the illness. For example, in my own clinical practice, I am finding that my evaluation of patients' progress has increasingly focused on where they are cognitively, particularly with respect to the so-called executive functions. For another personal window to the emergence of a neuropsychology of bipolar disorder, one has only to note that the neuropsychology chapter in the second edition of *Manic-Depressive Illness* is twice as long as the equivalent chapter in the first edition (Goodwin and Jamison 1990, 2007).

So this book is indeed timely—that is, it is time for all of us who treat bipolar patients to enlarge our focus and give the cognitive dimensions their due. But by pairing *timely* with *premature* in their preface, the editors give emphasis to the reality that, despite rapid progress, there are still many questions about cognitive function in bipolar disorder that remain unanswered.

This carefully edited, balanced, and comprehensive book is an important contribution to our field precisely because it plows new ground, carefully identifying the major gaps in knowledge while, nevertheless, outlining with clarity and readability the astounding amount of new information that continues to accumulate at an accelerating pace from the increasingly intertwined disciplines of neuropsychology, neuroimaging, neurogenetics, and the new field of functional outcomes research. This book is aimed at clinicians, and its aim is on target. Complex neuropsychological data and concepts are laid out in clear, largely jargon-free language, further enlightened by well-chosen examples and case histories. Equally important to its being on target is that the authors manage to achieve clarity without talking down

Cognitive Dysfunction in Bipolar Disorder

to clinicians. The introductory and summary chapters by Drs. Goldberg and Dr. Burdick are especially noteworthy examples of clarity undistorted by oversimplification.

Given the relative youth of the research in this field, many readers will be surprised by the number of areas in which a consensus is already emerging. This is testimony to the vitality of this new field, which includes seasoned neuropsychologists who, having cut their teeth in schizophrenia, are applying their experience and creativity to bipolar disorder. At the same time, developments in the neuropsychology of bipolar disorder have also been facilitated by the rapid development of increasingly sophisticated functional neuroimaging technologies.

One area of consensus has to do with attention: it is disturbed in bipolar disorder across all phases, including remission. It is quite conceivable that many of the learning and memory problems experienced by patients with bipolar disorder may be secondary to this underlying deficit in attention. The importance of this deficit is highlighted in Chapter 6, "Improving Psychotherapy Practice and Technique for Bipolar Disorder: Lessons From Cognitive Neuroscience," wherein Goldberg and colleagues cite therapeutic techniques for enhancing attention.

That bipolar patients have apparently "state-independent" deficits in some executive functions represents another area of consensus. State-independent findings are intriguing because they may be markers of some preexisting, underlying vulnerability, perhaps genetic. But to reemphasize and expand on a point made in this book, considerable caution must be exercised in the interpretation of state-independent (or so-called well-state) findings. For one thing, the ethics of clinical investigation requires that patients whose current well state has been achieved with the help of medications not be withdrawn from those medications for research purposes. On the other hand, when a patient is in an acute episode of mania or depression (the ill state), it is permissible to allow a brief drug-free washout period before a medication trial is initiated. Thus, state-independent findings almost invariably involve a treatment confound. A further problem is that most of the ill versus well comparisons are cross-sectional; there is a dearth of longitudinal studies in which well and ill periods can be compared in the same patient. Likewise, there are very few data on individuals at high risk for bipolar disorder studied before the onset of their first episode.

Finally, let me extract from this rich stew a few additional morsels that I found to be especially thought provoking:

- Poor adherence to treatment, which characterizes more than half of all bipolar patients and which is probably the largest single factor contributing to poor response, in some cases derives from cognitive dysfunction; that is, poor insight into the illness and failure to remember or appreciate the consequences of not treating it.

- Following the lead of the schizophrenia field, cognitive function has recently been getting some attention at the U.S. Food and Drug Administration (FDA), and some measures of cognition may be required for registration trials of new agents for bipolar disorder.
- Specific cognitive functions are substantially heritable and are emerging as endophenotypes in the study of risk factors for bipolar disorder.
- Anxiety symptoms in bipolar patients (which are common) can significantly impair cognitive function. Given that anxiety symptoms are treatable, this association is of considerable clinical importance.
- Assessment of functional outcomes in drug trials is now being required by the FDA, and it is clear that neurocognition is the major determinant of the extent of functional recovery.
- The cognitive effects of the medications used in bipolar disorder may well go in either direction, even with the same drug. For example, lithium at higher doses can interfere with some cognitive functions, while at the same time its neuroprotective effects might well be expected to translate into some positive cognitive effects over time.
- When comparing cognitive measures in bipolar and unipolar patients, it is critical to match both groups for total number of episodes; unfortunately, this is rarely done.

I predict that this book will have considerable impact, both on clinical research and on clinical care. It will be a shame if it does not. It may be both timely and premature, but for me, timely carries the day.

Frederick K. Goodwin, M.D.

References

Goodwin FK, Jamison KR: Manic-Depressive Illness. New York, Oxford University Press, 1990

Goodwin FK, Jamison KR: Manic-Depressive Illness: Bipolar Disorders and Recurrent Depression, 2nd Edition. New York, Oxford University Press, 2007

Preface

The presence of prominent affective symptoms has classically been viewed as the hallmark feature of bipolar disorder and as a fundamental characteristic that discriminates bipolar illness from primary psychotic disorders. Although mood disturbances are the sine qua non of bipolar disorder, contemporary research has pointed increasingly to nonaffective elements of psychopathology associated with the diagnosis. Problems with work and social functioning persist for lengthy periods in many individuals with bipolar disorder after the resolution of manic or depressive episodes, even in the absence of subsyndromal affective symptoms. These problems point to other factors that likely mediate functional recovery, including the ability to plan and think clearly, exercise reasonable judgment, solve problems with novelty and creativity, remember important information, recognize alternative points of view, and appreciate the ramifications of decisions made in everyday life—processes that lie at the heart of all functional human endeavors.

Cognition spans a wide range of mental operations that bear on numerous aspects of bipolar disorder. For example, the loss of insight contributes to the ability to recognize signs of affective relapse, maintain treatment adherence, and exercise financial, medical, social, and professional decision making. Another example is executive function, which is a prerequisite for the capacity to understand and consent to treatment, whether routine or experimental. Confusion about the diagnosis of bipolar disorder itself stems in part from an overlap between symptoms of bipolar disorder and those of other conditions that involve problems with distractibility and sustained attention (e.g., attention-deficit/hyperactivity disorder) and disorders of planning and impulse control (e.g., impulse control disorders and Cluster B personality disorders). Cognitive problems may be misconstrued by patients or clinicians as signs of psychopathology, or vice versa. Prescribers are often challenged when attempting to differentiate medication side effects from primary depressive or other illness symptoms, such as cognitive disorganization or trouble concentrating. Psychotherapists can become frustrated when patients with bipolar disorder have persistent trouble incorporating new insights and perspectives, or when they perseverate on distorted attitudes and beliefs and fail to change maladaptive behaviors, leaving all parties confused about volitional resistance versus frank cognitive inflexibility and problems in emotional learning. Most importantly, the potential for impulsive aggression and suicidal behavior represents perhaps the most extreme and catastrophic instance in which limbic system overactivity disengages from executive control.

Although cognitive impairment was once regarded as a disturbance relevant mainly to schizophrenia, there has emerged a growing body of evidence—both clinical and experimental—that identifies neurocognitive dysfunction as a fundamental yet frequently ignored or misidentified illness dimension in bipolar disorder. Scientific strides toward understanding basic elements of central nervous system disturbance in bipolar disorder have drawn on this awareness, as evidenced by neuroimaging studies that focus heavily on functional brain activity during tasks that engage prefrontal and subcortical structures. Efforts to identify genetic correlates of disease have paid growing attention to trait phenomena that may not be readily apparent (i.e., endophenotypes) and exist independent of fluctuating mood symptoms, such as impulsivity, sensation seeking, formal thought disorder, and cognitive function.

Our purpose in developing this book has been to provide a scientifically based, clinically relevant overview of the major dimensions of neurocognition as they pertain to individuals with bipolar disorder. Chapter 1 includes an overview of basic concepts and definitions related to neurocognition, as well as a reader-friendly review of neurocognitive domains (e.g., attention, working memory, processing speed), examples of their operation in everyday life, the neuroanatomical regions with which they are associated, and common tests used to assess their function. Chapters 2 and 3 focus in greater depth on attention and memory, respectively, incorporating findings from the research literature. Chapter 4 considers the genetic underpinnings of cognition and describes the concepts of attention, memory, and executive function as heritable (or endophenotypic) traits, with examples that link genetic markers with neuroimaging and, strikingly, evidence of cognitive deficits in the unaffected relatives of individuals with bipolar disorder. Chapter 5 addresses the impact of affective, anxiety, and psychotic symptoms on cognition, with clinical examples depicting the differentiation of psychopathology signs from cognitive deficits. Pertinent findings on affective and anxiety symptoms, as well as antidepressant use in bipolar disorder, are included from the National Institute of Mental Health Systematic Treatment Enhancement Program for Bipolar Disorder (NIMH STEP-BD). Chapter 6 describes ways in which core concepts from cognitive neuroscience can be adapted to tailor psychotherapy practice and technique. It addresses the question, How might psychotherapists incorporate knowledge of neurocognitive function in order to better understand and treat common problems that arise for patients with bipolar disorder? Chapters 7 and 8 undertake a review and discussion of cognitive effects that are associated with psychotropic agents used for bipolar disorder. Chapter 8 summarizes pertinent data from large-scale clinical trials, including the National Institute of Mental Health Clinical Antipsychotic Trials of Intervention Effectiveness (CATIE), and discusses pharmacological strategies that may help to minimize cognitive deficits and potentially improve cognitive functioning. Chapter 9 provides an overview of cognitive function in children and adolescents with bipolar disorder and suggests ways to help clinicians look beyond attentional deficits when distinguishing juvenile bipolar disorder from attention-deficit/hyperactivity disorder. Chapter 10 describes the impact of cognition on functional outcome in bipolar disorder—a key relationship in the explanation of psychosocial or occupational disability. Chapter 11 discusses the impact of cognition across the life span of individuals with bipolar disorder, tackling questions such as whether repeated episodes of bipolar disorder cause cognitive deterioration and how cognitive deficits differ between younger and older adult patients with bipolar disorder. Finally, Chapter 12 provides a summary of main concepts and take-home points from the book as a whole, along with guidance for practitioners in the approach to cognitive assessment and management. Our hope is that the information contained in this volume will have immediate and broad clinical applicability to all mental health professionals involved in the assessment and treatment of individuals with bipolar disorder, whether one's work focuses predominantly on psychopharmacology, psychotherapy, occupational adjustment, family or organizational systems, or clinical research.

It is difficult to estimate the extent to which this book is more timely or premature—likely some of both, inasmuch as clinical research specific to neurocognitive function in bipolar disorder is in its relative infancy. Interest in cognitive function in bipolar disorder represents an area of rapid scientific growth. At present, however, many key studies relevant to cognition in bipolar disorder have been conducted in other psychiatric or neuropsychiatric disorders—such as studies of the cognitive effects of anticonvulsants in epilepsy or of neurocognitive changes when antipsychotics are used in schizophrenia—prompting the need for cautious extrapolation from other disease states. The scarcity of studies focusing on cognition specifically in bipolar disorder stems from faulty assumptions that cognitive dysfunction occupies a relatively minor role (if any) in bipolar disorder and that the cognitive profiles of psychotropic drugs (both adverse and beneficial) generalize across disorders. Our hope is that this book will be a first step toward correcting such distortions and that it will lay groundwork for future clinical and research efforts in this nascent but exciting area.

We each owe immeasurable thanks and gratitude to our spouses—Carrie L. Ernst, M.D., and Raphael Braga, M.D., respectively—and our families (especially Joshua and Brian Goldberg, whose entreaties for more of their father's time spent on the baseball fields of Fox Meadow than on the computer have not gone unheard) for their never-ending understanding, support, encouragement, and insights that helped foster our efforts. This book could not have been completed without the dedicated efforts of our colleagues who have generously provided their time, knowledge, and expertise in writing chapters. Edited books often carry the risk of appearing disjointed. If we have succeeded in failing to allow such an outcome, it likely reflects not so much our own neurocognitive mettle but, more accurately, the cohesion with which investigators in this field know one another's work (it is a small, but growing, community) and have produced largely convergent and complementary findings.

Finally, a debt of gratitude also must be extended to our and our collaborators' innumerable patients and their families, without whom the observations and ideas that inspired this text would not have been possible.

Joseph F. Goldberg, M.D.
Katherine E. Burdick, Ph.D.

1

Overview and Introduction

Dimensions of Cognition and Measures of Cognitive Function

Katherine E. Burdick, Ph.D.
Terry E. Goldberg, Ph.D.

Cognition can be defined as the mental process of knowing and includes aspects such as awareness, perception, reasoning, and judgment. The field of neuropsychology focuses primarily on assessing aspects of cognition via a variety of computerized and pencil-and-paper tests to assay brain function. Because cognition is a complex trait, we start this chapter by reviewing some common terminology for basic neuropsychological constructs and then discuss what is known about the underlying factor structure of cognition, acknowledging that these seemingly individual processes are inherently interdependent. Throughout this book, the terms *neurocognition* and *cognition* are used interchangeably to denote objective, performance-based operations related to the uptake and manipulation of information, as contrasted with subjective or self-reported complaints related to problems with thinking. It is also important to note the distinction between *cognition* as used in this text to describe neuroanatomically based functions related to information processing in the brain and *cognition* as it is used to reflect core patterns of beliefs and attitudes relevant to the practice of cognitive psychotherapy. As discussed in later chapters, cognitively oriented psychotherapies may be of substantial benefit to individuals with bipolar disorder and may rest heavily on principles described in this text as a means to deliver more effective treatment.

1

A Cognitive Pocket Dictionary: Brain Processes From Basic to Complex

The fundamental neuroanatomical substrates that subserve distinct neurocognitive functions are summarized in Table 1–1. Broad neurocognitive concepts and terminology are described more fully here in the context of normal and abnormal domains in individuals with bipolar disorder. Descriptions of domains and tests described below are derived from Spreen and Strauss (1998).

TABLE 1–1. Neurocognitive domains and associated neuroanatomical structures

Neurocognitive domain	Neuroanatomical structure
Attention	
Vigilance	Locus coeruleus
Alerting	Posterior parietal lobe
	Superior colliculus
Detection/conflict	Anterior cingulate
	Ventral prefrontal cortex
Inhibition/decision making	Orbitofrontal cortex
	Anterior cingulate
Spatial/verbal working memory	Superior parietal lobe
	Dorsolateral prefrontal cortex
Verbal fluency	Prefrontal cortex
Facial affect discrimination	Amygdala
	Dorsolateral prefrontal cortex
Motor speed/skill	Subcortical ganglia
	Basal ganglia
Memory	
Encoding	Hippocampus
	Prefrontal cortex
Storage	Hippocampus
Retrieval	Ventromedial prefrontal cortex
	Temporoparietal junction
Executive function	
Logical reasoning	Left frontal cortex
	Temporal cortex
Cognitive control	Ventrolateral and dorsolateral prefrontal cortex
	Anterior cingulate
Set shifting	Cerebellum
	Left dorsolateral prefrontal cortex
	Basal ganglia

- *Sensation.* Sensation is the initial sensory stimulation that results in the physiological arousal necessary to register information entering the cognitive processing system. Sensation is a passive activity, in that an organism merely receives a sensory signal, such as a loud noise, a flashing light, or a sharp prick of pain. Sensory deficits are primary deficits with regard to the adequate processing of information; however, they are generally not the focus of neuropsychological evaluation, with the exception of ensuring intact sensory capacity from the outset (i.e., ensuring adequate hearing and visual acuity).

- *Perception.* Perception is the process of using the senses to acquire information about the surrounding environment or situation, which involves an active processing of a nearly constant stream of incoming data. Perception includes functions that range from simple (e.g., noticing the color of a traffic light) to more complex interpretations that take into account both simple feature detection (e.g., "The light is red") and past experience from learning (e.g., "When the light is red, I stop the car"). Perceptual deficits can be striking when seen in a clinical setting, such as when a person has prosopagnosia (the inability to recognize human faces despite normal visual acuity and an intact capacity to identify common objects). Similarly, various disorders of body awareness can result, for example, in an inability to recognize one's own arm as belonging to oneself despite the ability to name the body part accurately as an arm. Of note, aberrant perceptions (e.g., hallucinations) that arise in psychotic affective disorders have not been shown to have a direct impact on performance during neurocognitive testing, as described further in Chapter 5 of this volume, "Impact of Mood, Anxiety, and Psychotic Symptoms on Cognition in Patients With Bipolar Disorder."

- *Attention.* Attention is believed by many to be the most basic cognitive construct to reflect *conscious* processing of information. It involves alertness, mental focus, serious consideration, and concentration. Several different types of attention that are commonly discussed in clinical neuropsychological assessment are believed to be subserved by separate neural networks acting in concert to achieve normal consciousness and filtering of irrelevant stimuli (Posner and Petersen 1990). In the context of this model of attention, psychotherapeutic interventions bears on the redirection of thoughts and emotions (e.g., mindfulness training) and is discussed in Chapter 6 of this volume, "Improving Psychotherapy Practice and Technique for Bipolar Disorder: Lessons From Cognitive Neuroscience."

  Attention can be broken down into three systems: arousal (vigilance), orienting, and detection.

- *Arousal.* Arousal is believed to be an automatic process (i.e., acting very early in information processing and not under conscious control), involving the ability to achieve and maintain an alert state. For example, a person who is sleeping is in a very low arousal state, whereas a soldier on a battlefield is in a highly vigilant state (high arousal). A person's ability to sustain attention is most frequently assessed using a purposefully boring task that requires the maintenance of attention to a repeating stimulus (target). For example, a subject may be asked to press a button on the computer pad each time a letter (flashing on the screen) is immediately followed by the same letter, with the total task time running approximately 10–15 minutes (Continuous Performance Test—Identical Pairs Version [Cornblatt et al. 1988]). Subjects who have sustained attention deficits will make more errors, particularly during later stages of the task as their interest and attention have drifted.
- *Orienting.* Also known as *attentional shifting,* orienting is an automatic process involved in target detection that allows the subject to localize a target for analysis. Orienting occurs as a normal response in the proper deployment of attention in space. For example, if a person is intensely interested in a book when a baseball rapidly approaches from his or her visual periphery, the person's attention is appropriately drawn very rapidly away from the book and toward the baseball. Specific measures used in cognitive neuroscience paradigms (e.g., Attention Network Test [Fan et al. 2002]) can differentiate this type of attention from sustained attention and detection, although this aspect of attention is not frequently assessed in clinical evaluations.
- *Detection.* Detection is a complex attentional construct involving multiple overlapping concepts. Generally referred to as the *executive attention network,* this construct is not to be confused with the larger construct of executive function, described below. Detection involves conscious processing by cortical areas, often referred to as *selective attention,* and includes such skills as inhibition of automated responses, filtering of irrelevant competing information (conflict), and dividing attention to process more than one stimulus at a time. One of the most classic neuropsychological measures, the Stroop Test (Stroop 1935), taps this attentional domain. In this test, the subject is first asked to read a page of color words (e.g., *red, blue,* and *green*) as quickly as possible. Then, a second page is presented to the subject with a similar setup, but instead of words, it contains rows of *X*s, printed in different colored inks that correspond to the previous color words, and the subject is asked to name the color of the ink as

quickly as possible. Finally, the third page presents color words written in incongruent ink (e.g., the word *blue* written in green ink), and the subject is asked to name the color of the ink. Because reading words is such an automatic response, it requires a conscious effort to stop oneself from reading and to instead name the ink color. This is known as the "Stroop effect" and is a classic example of inhibition of automated response, which activates prefrontal brain regions that are otherwise not activated during attentional tasks that do not require conscious processing.

- *Working memory.* Prior to the 1960s, the functions now attributed to working memory were referred to as belonging to short-term memory. This construct has since been refined to include any mental process that entails temporary storage and manipulation of data, implying an active process as opposed to passive maintenance of information. Some theorists consider working memory to be the first stages of memory; however, recent literature tends to deal with working memory as its own, unique domain. There are many standardized measures that tap the working memory construct and capture a wide range of task difficulty. One example of a working memory measure in the auditory/verbal domain is Digit Span Backward, from both the Wechsler Adult Intelligence Scale, Third Edition (WAIS-III; Wechsler 1997a) and the Wechsler Memory Scale, Third Edition (Wechsler 1997b). This task requires the subject to listen to the examiner read a string of numbers (e.g., 1-4-6-2) and then repeat the numbers aloud to the examiner but in the reverse order (correct response: 2-6-4-1). The length of the number string increases as the task progresses, and discontinuation occurs when a subject is no longer able to accurately complete the task, thus testing the limits of the subject's working memory capacity. This task and similar measures of working memory require the subject to first store the information presented and then subsequently perform some type of mental operation on the information. Another measure of working memory is the n-back task, in which information in a series is presented to a subject, who must compare a given stimulus to a prior stimulus that was presented *n* steps previously. Working memory, which is primarily linked to prefrontal cortical function, is discussed in Chapter 3 of this volume, "Memory Deficits Associated With Bipolar Disorder," and Chapter 4, "The Endophenotype Concept: Examples from Neuropsychological and Neuroimaging Studies of Bipolar Disorder."
- *Memory.* Memory is the ability of the mind or of an individual or organism to retain learned information and knowledge of past events and experiences and to retrieve them. As noted in Chapter 3 of this volume,

memory problems are among the most commonly encountered cognitive complaints of individuals with bipolar disorder. However, patients'
subjective experience of memory impairment may also reflect deficits in
other cognitive domains, such as attentional problems.

There are multiple models of memory, which we do not describe in
detail in this chapter. Generally, from an information processing perspective, there are three stages of memory: encoding, storage, and retrieval.

- *Encoding.* Also referred to as *registration*, endcoding is the stage
  in which an organism takes in and combines information for storage.
  This initial stage of memory formation is also frequently considered
  the earliest stage of learning. Sensory memory processes are contained within this stage and consist of the formation of very brief and
  immediate representations of stimuli presented (approximately 200-
  to 300-ms poststimulus presentation). Humans are capable of stor-
  ing relatively large quantities of information in this way; however,
  the representation degrades very quickly (also within a few hundred
  milliseconds, unless the information is rehearsed or prepped in some
  other way for storage).
- *Storage.* Storage is the stage in which a permanent record of the
  perceived information is formed. Short-term memory will allow a
  person to recall information for up to about 1 minute without rehearsal, but capacity is believed to be around seven ($\pm$ two) items
  (Lezak 1995). For example, a typical phone number (555–1212)
  would be relatively easily recalled within 1 minute without rehearsal,
  but recall of longer strings of information or of the 7-digit phone
  number at greater duration from presentation would require some
  form of memory strategy, such as mentally repeating the number
  multiple times to lay down a stronger representation. Long-term
  memory is also a part of the storage process, but unlike sensory and
  short-term memory, it represents the capacity to store large quantities of information over much longer periods of time, sometimes
  even indefinitely. Whereas short-term memory is carried out by neural connectivity between temporal/parietal regions and the prefrontal cortex, long-term memory formation results in more stable and
  enduring changes to neural structures across multiple brain regions.
  The hippocampus is particularly critical in the initial transfer of information from short-term to long-term memory but is not believed
  to be the location of permanent memory representations beyond a
  few months postconsolidation. The immediate recall of a new phone
  number utilizes sensory memory capacity (and at longer durations,

short-term memory), but the memory can also be stored more permanently and retained over very long periods of time given proper consolidation. For example, due to the frequency with which a person repeats his or her own phone number (rehearsal), very often the person will be able to recall his or her childhood phone number, despite not having used it in many years.

– *Retrieval.* Retrieval is the recall, or calling back, of information that was encoded and stored, typically in response to some cue or query. Commonly, memory tasks assess an individual's ability to recall information (such as a list of 12 words read aloud) immediately and then again at some delayed interval, typically 20–30 minutes after presentation. Retrieval processes, when intact, allow an individual to readily access previously stored information; however, specific deficits may arise in retrieval when encoding and memory storage are adequate. For example, one may see impairment in free recall ("How many words do you remember from the list of 12 that were presented to you?") but intact recognition performance ("From the following list of words, which were previously presented?"). Patterns of performance on memory tests such as these can indicate whether or not presented material was adequately learned in the first place and at which point in the memory process a breakdown may have occurred.

• *Executive function.* This domain encompasses an array of capacities that are generally believed to engage and control the other cognitive processes of attention, working memory, learning, and memory. Although there is wide debate in the field of neuropsychology as to which processes fall within the executive function domain, Norman and Shallice (1986) described several situations in which an executive control mechanism would be required. These include 1) situations requiring planning and decision making (e.g., mapping a travel route from home to a particular destination); 2) error detection and troubleshooting (e.g., reviewing one's answers to a test); 3) processes that are not well learned or that require a novel response (e.g., when first learning a new language); 4) situations that are technically difficult (e.g., any complex multitasking activity); and 5) tasks that require an individual to overcome a highly learned (habitual) response in favor of a novel response (e.g., learning to operate a stick-shift vehicle after previously having learned to operate an automatic vehicle).

A multitude of executive function measures are available to tap a very wide range of skills (some of the most common measures are listed in Table 1–2). One such task that has been used extensively in studies and is described commonly in the literature is the Wisconsin Card Sorting Test (Grant and Berg 1993). This test requires an individual to deduce, with very little initial instruction, the rules for sorting cards that are categorized with multiple attributes (color, number, and form). The examiner provides feedback only by responding "correct" or "incorrect" to each attempt to sort cards; the respondent then either continues with a successful approach or alters his or her approach to achieve success. Further, at given intervals, the examiner changes the rules of assortment without notifying the respondent, again requiring the individual to demonstrate flexibility in response and a capacity to shift sets in order to succeed. Frontal lobe damage is most commonly linked to executive dysfunction and not only can result in impaired performance on these types of tests but can also lead to noticeable changes in personality and social behavior (e.g., hypersexuality in a previously conservative individual or anger outbursts in a normally relaxed individual). Although deficits in other cognitive domains can result in specific functional impairments that can be overcome using compensatory strategies, it is more likely that executive dysfunction will result in considerable functional disability, given its importance in social interactions and activities of daily living.

- *Intelligence.* Cognition was once believed to be a unitary construct that most closely resembled the notion of intelligence, or intellectual capacity. Standardized tests of intelligence, initially developed to assess capacity for service in the military, are now commonly used to measure general cognitive ability and to predict a person's potential in an academic setting. Although it is not uncommon for performance on specific subtests of intelligence scales, such as the WAIS, to be used to describe a person's neuropsychological profile in modern-day clinical assessment, these tests were not designed to localize lesions or to measure the extent of damage to the brain, as were more classic neuropsychological measures. In fact, normal intellectual function, as defined by an average intelligence quotient (IQ), does not necessarily imply normal neuropsychological function. The majority of this book deals with constructs (e.g., attention, working memory) that are more specific in terms of cognitive functioning and are thought to be subserved by more discrete brain areas than is intelligence. Particularly with regard to patients with bipolar disorder, measures of gross intellectual capacity or general cognitive ability alone are not especially useful in describing the cognitive dysfunction common to the illness. Deficits in patients with bipolar disorder are typically more specific to some of the cognitive domains that we have described above.

Cognitive Architecture

Cognitive architecture refers to the delineation of domains of cognitive function and the relationships among them. Approaches have generally involved lesion studies that indicate double dissociations among different cognitive functions; functional neuroimaging studies that use tasks to deconstruct the neural systems engaged; and perhaps most widely, factor analysis and its variants, including principal components analysis and structural equation modeling. Of course, the cognitive architecture that is found ultimately depends on the specific tests administered. When a battery of commonly used clinical neuropsychological tests is administered to patients and healthy controls, several distinct domains of function typically emerge, including but not limited to those listed previously in this chapter. Table 1–2 lists some of the tests commonly associated with each domain.

Delineating domains of function is thought to have pragmatic, as well as theoretical, utility. First, doing so can decrease the number of variables (because factor scores or composites are usually calculated) and thus reduce multiple comparisons for data analysis. Second, delineation of domains can be used to shape test batteries and ensure that they cover multiple but relatively independent domains. This strategy was used in the MATRICS (Measurement and Treatment Research to Improve Cognition in Schizophrenia) process (Nuechterlein et al. 2004), in which a battery of tests was selected on the basis of their loading on presumptive factors. This battery will likely come into wide use in clinical studies of cognitive enhancing agents for all psychiatric disorders, because the U.S. Food and Drug Administration has given its imprimatur for using the battery in registration trials.

Finally, we would be remiss if we did not note that there are usually unexpected findings in this work. For instance, two measures of executive function—the n-back task and the Wisconsin Card Sorting Test (Grant and Berg 1993)—generally load on different factors. Conversely, superficially very different tests, such as verbal fluency (a measure of verbal production) and the Trail Making Test (a measure of complex attention) (Spreen and Strauss 1998), both load on a speed factor (presumably because both tests are timed). Perhaps most interestingly, data resulting from direct comparisons between the cognitive architecture of clinical samples (most commonly patients with schizophrenia) and that of controls suggest strong similarities in the modular organization of cognitive function regardless of affected status and despite large effect size differences noted in level of performance on neurocognitive measures. Less is known about the factor structure of cognition in bipolar disorder; however, recent data have begun to characterize deficits common to this illness (Genderson et al. 2007).

TABLE 1–2. Commonly utilized neuropsychological tests and processes assayed

Domain/Test	Processes assayed
Attention/Working memory/Processing speed	
Continuous Performance Test[a]	Target detection, reaction time, sustained attention, impulsivity
Cancellation tests (e.g., d2 Test of Attention[b])	Visual scanning, sustained attention, processing/motor speed
WAIS-III Digit Symbol	Visual scanning, tracking, processing/motor speed
Trail Making Test—Parts A and B[b]	Rapid visual scanning, sequencing, mental flexibility, processing/motor speed
WAIS-III Digit Span Forward	Immediate auditory attention, attention span capacity (untimed)
WAIS-III Digit Span Backward	Auditory attention, verbal working memory (untimed)
WAIS-III Spatial Span Forward	Visual attention span capacity (untimed)
WAIS-III Spatial Span Backward	Visual working memory capacity (untimed)
Memory	
List learning (e.g., California Verbal Learning Test[b])	Episodic memory, learning strategies, immediate and delayed free recall, cued recall
Story recall (e.g., WMS-III Logical Memory)	Episodic memory, memory for stories presented verbally, gist memory
WMS-III Visual Reproduction	Memory for visual designs, visuospatial construction abilities
Rey-Osterrieth Complex Figure[b]	Memory for complex visual designs, visuospatial construction abilities
Benton Visual Retention Test[b]	Visual memory, visual perception, visual construction abilities
WMS-III Faces and Family Pictures	Visual memory for social information, visual recall of location
Executive functions	
Wisconsin Card Sorting Test[c]	Abstraction, concept formation, mental flexibility, set shifting and maintenance, capacity to learn from experience/feedback
Design fluency[d]	Production of novel abstract designs under timed constraints
Stroop Test[b]	Set shifting, cognitive control, inhibition of a prepotent response in favor of a novel one
N-back task	Updating of information, resistance to interference

TABLE 1–2. Commonly utilized neuropsychological tests and processes assayed *(continued)*

Domain/Test	Processes assayed
Intelligence/General capacity	
Wechsler Intelligence Scales (WAIS-III, WISC, WPPSI)	General intellectual capacity, verbal capacity, nonverbal capacity
Raven's Progressive Matrices[b]	Reasoning in the visual modality
Wide Range Achievement Test—Reading[b] or National Adult Reading Test[b]	Estimated premorbid intellectual capacity

Note. WAIS-III=Wechsler Adult Intelligence Scale, Third Edition (Wechsler 1997a); WISC=Wechsler Intelligence Scale for Children; WMS-III=Wechsler Memory Scale, Third Edition (Wechsler 1997b); WPPSI=Wechsler Preschool and Primary Scale of Intelligence.
[a]Cornblatt et al. 1988.
[b]To see this measure and learn how it can be used, see Spreen and Strauss 1998.
[c]Grant and Berg 1993.
[d]Ruff 1996.

These are discussed in great detail in the coming chapters and are reviewed briefly in the following section.

Cognition in Bipolar Disorder

Bipolar disorder afflicts at least 2% of the population and remains a leading worldwide cause of disability, morbidity, and mortality from suicide (Goodwin and Jamison 2007; Murray and Lopez 1996). Although its precise etiologies are unknown, bipolar illness is characterized by its recurrent and episodic nature involving disturbances of mood, sleep, behavior, perception, and cognition (Goodwin and Jamison 2007). Bipolar disorder has a spectrum presentation, with major subtypes of bipolar I and bipolar II, which presumably fall along a continuum of severity. Patients with bipolar I disorder by definition experience full mania, which commonly includes concurrent symptoms of psychosis, such as delusional thinking and hallucinations. Patients with bipolar II disorder have milder symptoms of mania, which do not involve psychosis, are typically shorter in duration, and do not significantly interfere with daily functioning.

During acute episodes of both depression and mania, patients with both subtypes of bipolar illness demonstrate significant cognitive impairment, which until recently has been largely overlooked. Over the past decade, researchers have converged on the clear finding that performance on neurocognitive tasks in nearly every major domain is disrupted during manic, depressed, or mixed phases of bipolar illness (Basso et al. 2002; Martinez-Aran et al. 2000). Of even greater interest is the finding that some of these neurocognitive deficits do not completely remit during periods of euthymia (Martinez-Aran et al. 2004a, 2004b; see also Chapter 4 of this volume). Studies that focused on periods during affective symptom remission found significant ongoing neurocognitive impairment, including deficits in attention, memory, and executive function (Clark et al. 2002; Ferrier et al. 1999; Harmer et al. 2002; Liu et al. 2002; Martinez-Aran et al. 2002, 2004b; Rubinsztein et al. 2000; Thompson et al. 2005; van Gorp et al. 1998; Zubieta et al. 2001). The impact of persistent neurocognitive impairment during periods of euthymia profoundly influences the lives of patients with bipolar disorder, with a direct influence on clinical course, functional outcome (Martinez-Aran et al. 2004b), and psychosocial functioning (Martinez-Aran et al. 2004a), making this an important target for treatment.

Cognitive Dysfunction as a Trait in Bipolar Disorder

As elaborated in Chapter 5 of this volume, the considerable effects of mood state on neurocognitive performance can confound data indicating neurocognitive impairment in acutely ill patients. However, the persistence of neurocognitive impairment during periods of symptom remission suggests that it may be a traitlike feature of bipolar disorder. In euthymic bipolar disorder patients, domain-specific deficits have been demonstrated in attention (Clark et al. 2002, 2005; Ferrier et al. 1999; Liu et al. 2002; Thompson et al. 2005), verbal learning and memory (Clark et al. 2002; Ferrier et al. 1999; Martinez-Aran et al. 2002, 2004b, and executive function (Clark et al. 2002; Ferrier et al. 1999; Martinez-Aran et al. 2002, 2004b; Mur et al. 2007; Thompson et al. 2005). We focus this brief review on the domains that have provided the most consistent evidence thus far for traitlike impairment in bipolar patients: attention, verbal learning and memory, and executive function. Subsequent chapters focus specifically on these deficits and their neuroanatomical and clinical correlates.

Attention

Impaired performance on attentional measures has been described in patients with bipolar disorder across mood states. Attention is a complex neurocognitive domain with several subcomponents and represents an important area of focus, because intact attentional capacity is essential to all higher cognitive skills. Sustained attention, or vigilance, is impaired in patients with bipolar disorder regardless of whether they are studied during periods of mania or depression (Najt et al. 2005; Rund et al. 1992; Sereno and Holzman 1996), and the observed impairments do not remit completely during euthymia (Clark et al. 2002, 2005; Liu et al. 2002). In addition, selective attention deficits during acute episodes do not normalize during euthymia (McGrath et al. 1997; Zalla et al. 2004).

Thompson et al. (2005) reported a broad pattern of attentional impairment in a large cohort ($n=63$) of euthymic bipolar disorder patients compared with healthy controls ($n=63$), with deficits noted on Stroop Test performance and vigilance measures that were both statistically ($P<0.002$) and clinically (>26% of euthymic patients fell below the fifth percentile on these measures) significant. These deficits were not causally related to residual symptomatology, further supporting their traitlike characteristics.

Verbal Learning and Memory

Several aspects of memory are reportedly impaired in euthymic bipolar disorder patients. Performance on verbal measures of immediate and delayed recall is impaired in remitted bipolar disorder patients who have low levels of affective symptoms (Clark et al. 2002; Ferrier et al. 1999) and in patients with strictly defined euthymic bipolar disorder (Martinez-Aran et al. 2004b). Visual memory performance has received little attention in euthymic bipolar disorder patients; however, Rubinsztein et al. (2000) reported deficits on a measure of visuospatial recognition in a group of euthymic patients compared with healthy controls.

It is important to reiterate that memory is hierarchically subserved by multiple cognitive processes that occur earlier in processing, including attention. Hence, memory may not be reliably assessable in patients with attentional problems unless formal neurocognitive testing is undertaken. Patients themselves may also report memory difficulties when in fact they may more accurately have deficits in other domains of information processing (e.g., impaired attention or executive function). They also may misattribute signs of psychopathology (e.g., depression or anxiety) to problems with memory per se (see Chapter 5 of this volume).

Executive Function

Recent studies indicate that impaired executive function is the most consistently reported neurocognitive deficit in euthymic bipolar disorder patients. After controlling for variables such as age, estimated intellectual function, and subsyndromal affective symptoms, several studies have demonstrated deficits in components of executive function, including planning (Ferrier et al. 1999; Thompson et al. 2005), set shifting (Clark et al. 2002; Coffman et al. 1990; Ferrier et al. 1999; Martinez-Aran et al. 2004b), cognitive control (Martinez-Aran et al. 2004b; Thompson et al. 2005; Zalla et al. 2004), and verbal fluency (Atre-Vaidya et al. 1998; Ferrier et al. 1999). A study by Dixon et al. (2004) assessed the relationship between cognitive function and symptomatology in bipolar disorder by comparing patients during mania ($n=15$), depression ($n=15$), and remission ($n=15$). Results support the prevalence of executive deficits, including cognitive control (response initiation, strategic thinking, and inhibitory control) across mood states, which persist during euthymia.

Larson et al. (2005) allowed for the parsing of executive dysfunction in euthymic bipolar disorder patients by using two experimental measures: the Object Alternation Task, which assesses a component of cognitive control or inhibition, and the Delayed Response Task, which measures spatial delayed working memory. Data from this study indicate that working memory capacity is spared in euthymia, whereas cognitive control (behavioral self-regulation) is impaired.

Comparisons With Schizophrenia

Although research investigating cognition in bipolar disorder is in its relative infancy, there is an abundance of evidence for significant and diffuse neurocognitive impairment in schizophrenia (Keefe and Fenton 2007). Because these two illnesses share a number of clinical characteristics (i.e., psychosis, depressive symptoms, medications), several studies have directly compared cognitive function in patients with bipolar disorder and in patients with schizophrenia, typically in the context of acute symptomatology. Because this book's focus is restricted to bipolar disorder, we do not conduct an exhaustive review of these comparative studies; rather, we briefly summarize the handful of existing studies that have included relatively large samples of patients with bipolar disorder ($n > 30$), keeping in mind that several additional, smaller studies have also been conducted (for a full review, see Daban et al. 2006).

In general, patients with bipolar disorder consistently perform better than patients with schizophrenia on measures of current intellectual function (intelligence quotient [IQ]) (for a review of works for all findings discussed in this paragraph, see Daban et al. 2006). However, results on tests designed to assay premorbid IQ have been less consistent, with some studies indicating comparable premorbid intellectual functioning for the two groups (both lower than that of healthy individuals) and other studies reporting lower premorbid IQ in patients with schizophrenia than in patients with bipolar disorder. Performance on measures of sustained and selective attention is impaired to the same extent in patients with schizophrenia and patients with bipolar disorder, but only during acute mood episodes. Nonetheless, although attention appears to improve with remission of acute affective symptomatology, several studies have demonstrated the persistence of attention deficits in patients with schizophrenia or bipolar disorder during periods of euthymia relative to healthy controls. Likewise, verbal memory deficits are notable in patients with schizophrenia and in those with bipolar illness; however, patients with bipolar disorder generally perform somewhat better than patients with schizophrenia on most memory measures, despite significant impairment when compared with healthy controls. Finally, in the executive function domain, patients with bipolar disorder who are acutely ill frequently perform qualitatively and quantitatively similarly to patients with schizophrenia on a variety of executive measures. However, upon clinical recovery, performance significantly improves in the group with bipolar disorder for many of these tasks, whereas executive deficits persist in patients with schizophrenia. Table 1–3 summarizes studies involving at least 30 subjects per diagnostic group that directly compare cognitive profiles of patients with schizophrenia and patients with bipolar disorder. Nonetheless, this remains an area of interest deserving of additional study with regard to state versus trait manifestations, prodromal or pre-illness characteristics, the impact of illness course on cognition, and the potential to intervene and treat the cognitive symptoms of these devastating disorders.

TABLE 1–3. Studies comparing neurocognitive performance of subjects with bipolar disorder and subjects with schizophrenia

Authors	Subjects	Cognitive domains	Findings	Comments
Hoff et al. 1990	35 BP vs. 30 SZ	Verbal IQ, memory	BP=SZ both domains	Acute mania vs. SZ; no HC
Jones et al. 1993	49 BP vs. 100 SZ vs. 46 CC	Premorbid IQ	BP>SZ	Clinical controls used in lieu of healthy comparison sample; limited measures
Green et al. 1994	31 BP vs. 63 SZ vs. 48 HC	Visual backward masking	BP=SZ<HC	All patients were chronically ill
Addington and Addington 1997	40 BP vs. 59 SZ vs. 40 HC	Sustained attention	SZ<BP<HC	Patients were partially remitted
Mojtabai et al. 2000	72 BP vs. 102 SZ vs. 49 UP	Verbal IQ, attention, memory, executive function	BP=UP>SZ all domains	First episode partial remission
Verdoux and Liraud 2000	33 BP vs. 20 SZ vs. 48 CC	Attention, verbal memory, executive function	BP>SZ verbal memory; BP=SZ attention and executive function	Clinical controls used in lieu of healthy comparison sample
Rossi et al. 2000	40 BP vs. 66 SZ vs. 64 HC	Executive function	BP=SZ perseverative errors on WCST; WCST categories completed BP>SZ	Patients were remitted at the time of testing
Altshuler et al. 2004	49 BP vs. 20 SZ vs. 22 HC	Premorbid IQ, verbal IQ, attention, memory, executive function	BP=HC>SZ premorbid IQ, verbal IQ, Trails B; BP=SZ<HC memory, WCST; BP=SZ=HC Stroop, fluency	Subjects were all male
Zalla et al. 2004	37 BP vs. 25 SZ	IQ, attention, executive function	BP=SZ all measures except verbal fluency (BP>SZ)	First-degree relatives were also included

Note. BP=bipolar; CC=clinical controls; HC=healthy controls; IQ=intelligence quotient; SZ=schizophrenia; UP=unipolar depression; WCST=Wisconsin Card Sorting Test.

Functional Neuroanatomy

Chapter 4 of this volume addresses genetic and neuroimaging findings related to cognitive dysfunction in bipolar disorder. As a prelude to this material, we briefly summarize current neuroimaging findings with regard to the primary neural circuitry model proposed by several leading bipolar disorder research groups (Drevets et al. 1997; Mayberg et al. 1999; Strakowski et al. 2005).

It has been hypothesized that the interplay between cortical regions responsible for cognitive control and the limbic areas that are critical to emotional response is compromised in patients with bipolar disorder and may be responsible for the core symptoms of the disease (Strakowski et al. 2005). Dysregulation of various nodes in the cortical-limbic circuitry is thought to produce affective symptoms, including depression and mania (Strakowski et al. 2005). Cortical-limbic system structures include the amygdala, hippocampus and parahippocampal gyrus, ventral striatum, insula, cingulate cortex, and orbitofrontal cortex (Ongur and Price 2000). These structures are involved in response to or appraisal of threat (amygdala); the integration of affectively valenced information and behavioral response, particularly related to anticipated social outcome (ventral prefrontal cortex); and affective and conflict monitoring (subgenual and dorsal cingulate). Because of reciprocal connectivity between these areas, it is likely that dysfunction within the system brings about both the emotional dysregulation that characterizes the illness and the concomitant neurocognitive impairment that is common in bipolar disorder (see Figure 1–1). There is substantial evidence from recent neuroimaging studies to suggest that this circuitry is abnormal in patients with bipolar disorder (Strakowski et al. 2005); however, the exact nature and course of the abnormalities are not yet known, thereby raising the question as to whether these changes occur as a result of the disease or whether they represent potential markers of genetic risk for the illness. We believe this model is critical to an understanding of the core symptoms of bipolar illness and the related neurocognitive impairment, making it an important frame of reference for the topics discussed throughout this book.

Conclusions

A growing body of evidence suggests that cognitive dysfunction is a central phenomenological component of bipolar disorder. Not only has this become an area of intense research, but the reported functional implications of cognitive impairment in individuals with bipolar disorder have drawn clinical attention to the imminent need to identify its correlates, clarify its etiology, and ultimately prevent its occurrence. The chapters that follow address a range of topics related to cognition in bipolar disorder that are of

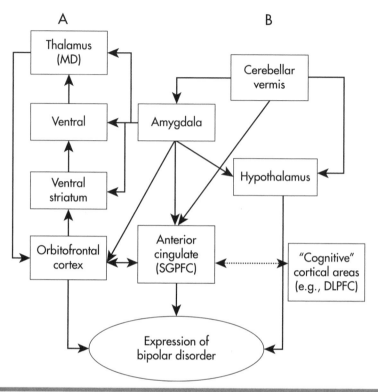

FIGURE 1–1.   Schematic of the anterior limbic network as a model of the expression of bipolar symptoms.

(A) "Iterative" prefrontal subcortical network that samples inputs from other brain regions to modulate appropriate behavioral responses. (B) Limbic areas that modulate (e.g., amygdala) or express the response (e.g., hypothalamus). DLPFC=dorsolateral prefrontal cortex; MD=mediodorsal nucleus; SGPFC=subgenual prefrontal cortex.

Source.   Reprinted from Strakowski SM, DelBello MP, Adler CM: "The Functional Neuroanatomy of Bipolar Disorder: A Review of Neuroimaging Findings." *Molecular Psychiatry* 10:105–116, 2005. Used by permission from Macmillan Publishers, Ltd.

direct utility to practicing clinicians and are of increasing importance to the quality of life of patients with bipolar disorder.

Take-Home Points

• The term *cognition* refers to the act of attending to stimuli in the environment and processing the information on several hierarchical levels. The field of neuropsychology has sought to measure and quantify an individual's performance in a number of discrete cognitive domains via paper-and-pencil and computer-based tasks that are designed to tap functions of specific brain regions or neural networks.

- Attention, working memory, processing speed, learning and memory, and executive functions are among the individual cognitive domains that are important to a person's intellectual and functional capacity. These domains are inherently interconnected and act in concert to provide for fluid conscious thought.

- Cognitive dysfunction has become a primary area of clinical and research interest in patients with bipolar disorder, despite previous, erroneous assumptions that cognition is largely uncompromised in these patients. Although cognition has been a focus of research in schizophrenia for many years, it has only recently gained attention as an important aspect of bipolar illness. Indeed, emerging evidence suggests that patients with bipolar disorder endure significant cognitive impairment during acute affective episodes, as well as persistent, traitlike cognitive impairment in the domains of attention, verbal learning and memory, and executive function during periods of remission or euthymia. Further, these persistent deficits have been shown to be directly related to functional disability and quality of life in patients with bipolar disorder.

- Cognitive impairment in patients with bipolar disorder is thought to be related to disrupted brain circuitry in neural networks, which primarily include regions of the prefrontal cortex and the limbic system (see Figure 1–1). This aberrant neural circuitry may serve as the basis for both the cardinal symptoms of affective dysregulation and the cognitive impairment that is common in patients with bipolar disorder.

References

Addington J, Addington D: Attentional vulnerability indicators in schizophrenia and bipolar disorder. Schizophr Res 23:197–204, 1997

Altshuler LL, Ventura J, van Gorp WG, et al: Neurocognitive function in clinically stable men with bipolar I disorder or schizophrenia and normal control subjects. Biol Psychiatry 56:560–569, 2004

Atre-Vaidya N, Taylor MA, Seidenberg M, et al: Cognitive deficits, psychopathology, and psychosocial functioning in bipolar mood disorder. Neuropsychiatry Neuropsychol Behav Neurol 11:120–126, 1998

Basso MR, Lowery N, Neel J, et al: Neuropsychological impairment among manic, depressed, and mixed-episode inpatients with bipolar disorder. Neuropsychology 16:84–91, 2002

Clark L, Iversen SD, Goodwin GM: Sustained attention deficit in bipolar disorder. Br J Psychiatry 180:313–319, 2002

Clark L, Kempton MJ, Scarnà A, et al: Sustained attention-deficit confirmed in euthymic bipolar disorder but not in first-degree relatives of bipolar patients or euthymic unipolar depression. Biol Psychiatry 57:183–187, 2005

Coffman JA, Bornstein RA, Olson SC, et al: Cognitive impairment and cerebral structure by MRI in bipolar disorder. Biol Psychiatry 27:1188–1196, 1990

Cornblatt BA, Risch NJ, Faris G, et al: The Continuous Performance Test, Identical Pairs Version (CPT-IP), I: new findings about sustained attention in normal families. Psychiatry Res 26:223–238, 1988

Daban C, Martinez-Aran A, Torrent C, et al: Specificity of cognitive deficits in bipolar disorder versus schizophrenia: a systematic review. Psychother Psychosom 75:72–84, 2006

Dixon T, Kravariti E, Frith C, et al: Effect of symptoms on executive function in bipolar illness. Psychol Med 34:811–821, 2004

Drevets WC, Price JL, Simpson JR Jr, et al: Subgenual prefrontal cortex abnormalities in mood disorders. Nature 386:824–827, 1997

Fan J, McCandliss BD, Sommer T, et al: Testing the efficiency and independence of attentional networks. J Cogn Neurosci 14:340–347, 2002

Ferrier IN, Stanton BR, Kelly TP, et al: Neuropsychological function in euthymic patients with bipolar disorder. Br J Psychiatry 175:246–251, 1999

Genderson MR, Dickinson D, Diaz-Asper CM, et al: Factor analysis of neurocognitive tests in a large sample of schizophrenic probands, their siblings, and healthy controls. Schizophr Res 94:231–239, 2007

Goodwin FK, Jamison KR: Manic-Depressive Illness: Bipolar Disorder and Recurrent Depression, 2nd Edition. New York, Oxford University Press, 2007

Grant DA, Berg EA: Wisconsin Card Sorting Test. Lutz, FL, Psychological Assessment Resources, 1993

Green MF, Nuechterlein KH, Mintz J: Backward masking in schizophrenia and mania, I: specifying a mechanism. Arch Gen Psychiatry 51:939–944, 1994

Harmer CJ, Clark L, Grayson L, et al: Sustained attention deficit in bipolar disorder is not a working memory impairment in disguise. Neuropsychologia 40:1586–1590, 2002

Hoff AL, Shukla S, Aronson T, et al: Failure to differentiate bipolar disorder from schizophrenia on measures of neuropsychological function. Schizophr Res 3:253–260, 1990

Jones PB, Bebbington P, Foerster A, et al: Premorbid social underachievement in schizophrenia: results from the Camberwell Collaborative Psychosis Study. Br J Psychiatry 162:65–71, 1993

Keefe RS, Fenton WS: How should DSM-V criteria for schizophrenia include cognitive impairment? Schizophr Bull 33:912–920, 2007

Larson ER, Shear PK, Krikorian R, et al: Working memory and inhibitory control among manic and euthymic patients with bipolar disorder. J Int Neuropsychol Soc 11:163–172, 2005

Lezak MD: Neuropsychological Assessment, 3rd Edition. New York, Oxford University Press, 1995

Liu SK, Chiu CH, Chang CJ, et al: Deficits in sustained attention in schizophrenia and affective disorders: stable versus state-dependent markers. Am J Psychiatry 159:975–982, 2002

Martinez-Aran A, Vieta E, Colom F, et al: Cognitive dysfunctions in bipolar disorder: evidence of neuropsychological disturbances. Psychother Psychosom 69:2–18, 2000

Martinez-Aran A, Vieta E, Colom F, et al: Neuropsychological performance in depressed and euthymic bipolar patients. Neuropsychobiology 46 (suppl 1):16–21, 2002

Martinez-Aran A, Vieta E, Colom F, et al: Cognitive impairment in euthymic bipolar patients: implications for clinical and functional outcome. Bipolar Disord 6:224–232, 2004a

Martinez-Aran A, Vieta E, Reinares M, et al: Cognitive function across manic or hypomanic, depressed, and euthymic states in bipolar disorder. Am J Psychiatry 161:262–270, 2004b

Mayberg HS, Liotti M, Brannan SK, et al: Reciprocal limbic-cortical function and negative mood: converging PET findings in depression and normal sadness. Am J Psychiatry 156:675–682, 1999

McGrath J, Scheldt S, Welham J, et al: Performance on tests sensitive to impaired executive ability in schizophrenia, mania and well controls: acute and subacute phases. Schizophr Res 26:127–137, 1997

Mojtabai R, Bromet EJ, Harvey PD, et al: Neuropsychological differences between first-admission schizophrenia and psychotic affective disorders. Am J Psychiatry 157:1453–1460, 2000

Mur M, Portella MJ, Martinez-Aran A, et al: Persistent neuropsychological deficit in euthymic bipolar patients: executive function as a core deficit. J Clin Psychiatry 68:1078–1086, 2007

Murray CJ, Lopez AD: Evidence-based health policy: lessons from the Global Burden of Disease Study. Science 274:740–743, 1996

Najt P, Glahn D, Bearden CE, et al: Attention deficits in bipolar disorder: a comparison based on the Continuous Performance Test. Neurosci Lett 379:122–126, 2005

Norman DA, Shallice T: Attention to action: willed and automatic control of behavior, in Consciousness and Self-Regulation (Advances in Research, Vol 4). Edited by Davidson RJ, Schwartz GE, Shapiro D. New York, Plenum, 1986, pp 1–18

Nuechterlein KH, Barch DM, Gold JM, et al: Identification of separable cognitive factors in schizophrenia. Schizophr Res 72:29–39, 2004

Ongur D, Price JL: The organization of networks within the orbital and medial prefrontal cortex of rats, monkeys and humans. Cereb Cortex 10:206–219, 2000

Posner MI, Petersen SE: The attention system of the human brain. Annu Rev Neurosci 13:25–42, 1990

Rossi A, Arduini L, Daneluzzo E, et al: Cognitive function in euthymic bipolar patients, stabilized schizophrenic patients, and healthy controls. J Psychiatr Res 34:333–339, 2000

Rubinsztein JS, Michael A, Paykel ES, et al: Cognitive impairment in remission in bipolar affective disorder. Psychol Med 30:1025–1036, 2000

Ruff RM: Ruff Figural Fluency Test. Odessa, FL, Psychological Assessment Resources, Inc., 1996

Rund BR, Orbeck AL, Landro NI: Vigilance deficits in schizophrenics and affectively disturbed patients. Acta Psychiatr Scand 86:207–212, 1992

Sereno AB, Holzman PS: Spatial selective attention in schizophrenic, affective disorder, and normal subjects. Schizophr Res 20:33–50, 1996

Spreen O, Strauss E: A Compendium of Neurological Tests: Administration, Norms, and Commentary, 2nd Edition. New York, Oxford University Press, 1998

Strakowski SM, Delbello MP, Adler CM: The functional neuroanatomy of bipolar disorder: a review of neuroimaging findings. Mol Psychiatry 10:105–116, 2005

Stroop JR: Studies of interference in serial verbal reactions. J Exp Psychol 18:643–662, 1935

Thompson JM, Gallagher P, Hughes JH, et al: Neurocognitive impairment in euthymic patients with bipolar affective disorder. Br J Psychiatry 186:32–40, 2005

van Gorp WG, Altshuler L, Theberge DC, et al: Cognitive impairment in euthymic bipolar patients with and without prior alcohol dependence: a preliminary study. Arch Gen Psychiatry 55:41–46, 1998

Verdoux H, Liraud F: Neuropsychological function in subjects with psychotic and affective disorders: relationship to diagnostic category and duration of illness. Eur Psychiatry 15:236–243, 2000

Wechsler D: Wechsler Adult Intelligence Scale, 3rd Edition (WAIS-III): Administration and Scoring Manual. San Antonio, TX, The Psychological Corporation, 1997b

Wechsler D: Wechsler Memory Scale, 3rd Edition (WMS-III): Administration and Scoring Manual. San Antonio, TX, The Psychological Corporation, 1997b

Zalla T, Joyce C, Szoke A, et al: Executive dysfunctions as potential markers of familial vulnerability to bipolar disorder and schizophrenia. Psychiatry Res 121:207–217, 2004

Zubieta JK, Huguelet P, O'Neil RL, et al: Cognitive function in euthymic bipolar I disorder. Psychiatry Res 102:9–20, 2001

2

Attentional and Executive Functioning in Bipolar Disorder

Luke Clark, D.Phil.
Guy Goodwin, M.D.

Bipolar disorder is characterized by intermittent and recurrent episodes of mania and depression. These pathological mood states have a clear impact on cognitive function. Mania is in part distinguished by distractibility, inappropriate speech and behavior, increased goal-directed behavior, and a tendency to make decisions associated with potentially painful consequences. Depression is characterized by a lack of concentration, difficulty making decisions, motor slowing, and changes in memory. Neuropsychological testing aims to determine the pattern of cognitive dysfunction in a disorder via the use of standardized quantitative assessment. The information gained through neuropsychological assessment can be applied at the level of the individual patient to guide psychological intervention and monitor treatment. Neuropsychological testing can also provide insights into the underlying neuropathological processes in bipolar disorder. Further details regarding neuropsychological testing and assessment procedures are provided in Chapter 12 of this volume, "Summary and Assessment Recommendations for Practitioners."

Support for this work was provided through a graduate scholarship (Clark) from the Medical Research Council of the United Kingdom.

Characterization of the neuropsychological profile in bipolar disorder has proved challenging for a number of reasons. First, several domains of cognitive function are disrupted, including attention, executive function, emotional processing, and memory (Bearden et al. 2001; Quraishi and Frangou 2002).

Second, bipolar disorder appears to be characterized by both transient (state-related) and enduring (trait-related) changes in cognition (Clark and Goodwin 2004). A state-related deficit is manifested during episodes of mania and/or depression and recovers markedly if not entirely during symptom remission. State effects should covary with ratings of symptom severity. In contrast, a trait-related marker is present during periods of illness remission and persists independently of symptom status. Trait markers may be genetic in origin and may represent potential endophenotypes for bipolar and related disorders (see Chapter 4 of this volume, "The Endophenotype Concept: Examples From Neuropsychological and Neuroimaging Studies of Bipolar Disorder"). Alternatively, a trait marker may be acquired during the illness course and hence reflect the length of illness and the number of previous episodes (Cavanagh et al. 2002; Kessing 1998). Phenomenologically, enduring deficits may relate to structural brain abnormalities in bipolar disorder (Strakowski et al. 2005) and may be associated with psychosocial difficulties that can persist in remitted patients relative to their premorbid status (Abood et al. 2002; Coryell et al. 1993; Scott 1995).

A third difficulty with descriptions of the cognitive profile is that the manic and depressive states of bipolar disorder have some neuropsychological similarities but also some important differences. Understanding of these differences has been hampered by the paucity of research comparing bipolar depression with major depressive disorder.

Finally, a wide range of clinical factors may have an impact on cognitive function in bipolar disorder. These include medications (Frangou et al. 2005), the presence of comorbid conditions such as substance use disorders (van Gorp et al. 1998), and the presence of suicidal symptoms (Swann et al. 2005).

In this chapter, we examine two domains of cognitive function in relation to bipolar disorder: attention and executive function. Although these domains are often considered separately, they have considerable theoretical overlap. As defined in the previous chapter, *attention* refers to the ability to selectively and flexibly process some information in the environment at the expense of other information. For example, if you are at a dinner party, how do you focus on a discussion with your host while ignoring the conversation behind you? How do you maintain your attention when the conversation becomes boring? How do you shift your attention when an old friend arrives? The attentional system of the human brain appears to comprise several processes that are mediated by independent, albeit interacting, neurobiological systems. Separate mechanisms may be responsible for selective attention, divided attention, sustained attention, and shifting attention (Desimone and Duncan 1995; Posner and Petersen 1990). In this chapter, we focus mainly on the processes of selective attention, sustained attention, and shifting attention, which have been the objects of most serious investigation in bipolar disorder.

Executive function is a broad term that refers to a collection of higher-level cognitive processes, including planning, working memory, strategy deployment, inhibitory control, and cognitive flexibility (Stuss and Levine 2002). Some commonly used tests of executive function are described in Table 2–1. Executive processes may enable humans to deviate from a "default mode" of stereotyped behavior locked to environmental stimuli (Mesulam 2002). Based on a large corpus of research in patients with lesions to the prefrontal cortex (PFC) (e.g., due to penetrating head injury or tumor resection), executive function is considered to be intrinsically related to the integrity of the PFC. Patients with lesions in the dorsal and lateral aspects of the PFC often present with a frontal "dysexecutive" syndrome (Shallice and Burgess 1991). A common example of dysexecutive behavior is difficulty organizing everyday activities (e.g., given a simple shopping list of 10 items from four different shops, the patient may choose an inefficient route around the shops and may need to return to one shop several times to buy different items).

Damage to the more ventral aspects of the PFC is associated with a distinct profile in which patients' behavior becomes socially inappropriate, impulsive, and emotionally labile. Another symptom is the tendency to make risky decisions associated with long-term negative repercussions (Bechara et al. 1994). This syndrome, sometimes called *frontal disinhibition syndrome* or *acquired sociopathy* (Damasio et al. 1990; Malloy et al. 1993), was described in the famous case of Phineas Gage and in more recent case studies with circumscribed ventral PFC lesions (Cato et al. 2004; Eslinger and Damasio 1985). The notable parallels between a number of these behavioral changes and the symptoms of mania have generated considerable interest in the role of ventral PFC in bipolar disorder.

Two examples highlight the overlap between executive function and attention. First, cognitive flexibility is typically assessed with tasks of attentional shifting, in which the subject must adapt his or her responding from one dimension (or "set") to another. Imagine that you are looking for a friend on a railway platform. You know that your friend will be wearing a black jacket and a red scarf. You start by screening the crowd for the black jacket ("sort by jacket color"), but you realize too many people are wearing

TABLE 2–1. Some common neuropsychological tests used to assess executive function, attention, and decision making

Domain	Test[a]	Function measured	Description	Associated frontal region
Executive function	Verbal fluency	Volition; response initiation	Subject is asked to name words beginning with F, A, and S in 1 minute.	Dorsolateral prefrontal cortex
	Tower of London	Forward planning	Subject is asked to plan a complex series of moves to match two arrangements of balls and hoops.	Dorsolateral prefrontal cortex
	N-back	Working memory	Subject is asked to respond if the stimulus matches the stimulus presented n trials ago.	Dorsolateral prefrontal cortex
	Wisconsin Card Sorting Test	Attentional set shifting; perseveration	Subject sorts cards according to the shape, color, or number of stimuli on each card. The rule occasionally changes without warning, and the subject must shift set using trial-by-trial feedback.	Dorsolateral prefrontal cortex
Attention	Trail Making Test—Part B	Attentional shifting; psychomotor speed	Subject is presented with a page containing the numbers 1–12 and letters A–L. Time taken to join circles in the alternating order 1-A-2-B-3-C…is recorded.	Frontal cortex
	Stroop Test	Selective attention; interference control.	Subject is asked to name ink color of incongruent color words.	Anterior cingulate cortex
	Continuous Performance Test	Sustained attention; impulse control	Subject must monitor a stream of digits or letters for prespecified target stimuli, which occur unpredictably and infrequently over several minutes.	(Right) frontal cortex
Decision making	Iowa Gambling Task	Risk-taking; reinforcement learning	Subject must learn the profile of wins and losses on four card decks; two decks are associated with higher wins but occasional high losses, and result in overall debt.	Ventromedial prefrontal cortex

[a]To see these tests and learn how they can be used, see Lezak et al. 2004.

black jackets. You shift your attention to searching for the red scarf ("sort by scarf color"). An inflexible (or cognitively rigid) individual may carry on searching by jacket color despite the inefficiency of this tactic. Second, tests of selective attention typically assess the subject's ability to make a response while suppressing a more natural (or prepotent) response driven by the stimulus array. Selective attention is commonly assessed with the Stroop Test, in which the subject is presented with color words presented in the same or an incongruous ink color as the word describes. When the subject is asked to say aloud the ink color, he or she must inhibit the more natural tendency to read the word. Functional imaging studies have consistently demonstrated greater activity in the anterior cingulate cortex in incongruent Stroop trials (when there is a mismatch between word identity and ink color) than in congruent trials (when word identity and ink color indicate the same response) (Bush et al. 2000; Pardo et al. 1990).

Several lines of evidence indicate pathophysiological mechanisms in the PFC and anterior cingulate cortex in bipolar disorder. Studies of patients with secondary mood disorder (i.e., affective disturbance due to a primary organic pathology) have found that the prevalence of depressed mood is disproportionately increased following damage to the left frontal cortex and left subcortical structures (Robinson et al. 1983; Starkstein et al. 1987). Although this association remains controversial (Carson et al. 2000; Singh et al. 1998), a study of a large number of cases substantiated the link between poststroke depression and infarcts affecting prefrontal and subcortical regions in the left hemisphere (Vataja et al. 2001). Cases of secondary mania are considerably more unusual than secondary depression but are typically associated with right hemisphere damage to the frontal cortex and basal ganglia (Robinson et al. 1988). This difference in laterality is consistent with Davidson's model of emotional processing, which proposes that the right frontal lobe specializes in avoidance behavior and the left frontal lobe specializes in approach behavior (Davidson 1992; Davidson and Irwin 1999). By this reasoning, when a person has a lesion to one hemisphere, the contralateral frontal cortex comes to dominate behavior.

The data in secondary mood disorders also highlight the important connectivity between the frontal cortex and basal ganglia—connectivity that is pertinent to executive function and attentional function. A series of parallel, segregated loops connect sectors of the frontal lobe (motor cortex, frontal eye fields, dorsolateral PFC, ventrolateral PFC, and orbital-medial PFC) with discrete stations in the basal ganglia and thalamus (Alexander et al. 1986). As a result of this connectivity, patients with specific basal ganglia pathology (e.g., Parkinson's or Huntington's disease) also show impaired performance on tasks associated with frontal lobe integrity, including attentional shifting, forward planning, and working memory (Cools 2006).

These neurological disorders are also associated with elevated levels of depression, which are increased compared with nonneurological disorders that are nonetheless matched for level of disability (Ehmann et al. 1990). Several neuropsychiatric disorders and symptoms have been suggested to relate to specific frontal-striatal loops (Mega and Cummings 1994). The "affective loop" linking the orbitofrontal cortex and anterior cingulate cortex with the ventral striatum is implicated in mood disorders (as illustrated schematically in Chapter 1 of this volume, "Overview and Introduction: Dimensions of Cognition and Measures of Cognitive Function," Figure 1–1).

Structural brain abnormalities in the PFC have been confirmed in patients with bipolar disorder. Histological examination of postmortem tissue has confirmed neuropathology in the anterior cingulate cortex and dorsolateral prefrontal cortex. Using magnetic resonance imaging to measure regional brain volumes, Drevets et al. (1997) showed that the subgenual subregion of the anterior cingulate cortex (lying below the genu of the corpus callosum) was reduced in volume in patients with bipolar disorder with a family history of affective disorder. A similar effect was seen in subjects with major depressive disorder, and this effect has been replicated in first-episode cases of psychotic mood disorder (Hirayasu et al. 1999). Studies using voxel-based morphometry to characterize structural differences across the whole brain have confirmed gray matter reductions in the PFC (Lochhead et al. 2004; Lopez-Larson et al. 2002; Lyoo et al. 2004).

Attentional and Executive Function in Mania

Patients with mania display widespread neuropsychological deficits in domains, including executive function, attention, impulse control, and decision making (Clark et al. 2001; McGrath et al. 1997; Mur et al. 2007; Murphy et al. 1999, 2001; Swann et al. 2003). Deficits in sustained attention among patients with euthymic bipolar disorder appear to be independent of problems with working memory, or holding ideas in mind (Harmer et al. 2002). We recruited a group of 15 manic patients with bipolar I diagnoses from inpatient facilities in Oxford, England (Clark et al. 2001). Patients showed high symptom ratings on the Young Mania Scale (YMS; mean = 21.1, indicating moderately severe levels of mania) and minimal evidence of depressive symptoms based on the Hamilton Rating Scale for Depression (Ham-D; mean = 5.7), indicating that they were mainly in manic episodes rather than mixed episodes. Most patients were receiving neuroleptic medications, often in combination with a benzodiazepine. Patients were compared with 30 healthy controls matched for age, gender, and years of education. The manic group showed statistically significant impairments across the majority of tasks in a thorough neuropsychological assessment, but measures of sustained attention (a Rapid Visual Information

Processing [RVIP] test) and verbal learning (the California Verbal Learning Test) detected much stronger effect sizes (Cohen's $d \approx 2.0$) than did the other tasks. A multivariate discriminant function analysis showed that these two tests alone correctly classified 87% of manic subjects and 91% of subjects overall, indicating that sustained attention and verbal learning deficits may be closely associated with the manic syndrome.

The RVIP task used in our study is a traditional continuous performance test in which the subject monitors a stream of digits for prespecified target sequences (e.g., 3-5-7 in a consecutive sequence). The subject responds on a button box whenever a target sequence is presented. Targets are presented infrequently and unpredictably over a total task duration of 7 minutes, such that the subject must maintain attentional focus for a lengthy period in order to perform well. Manic participants showed two effects on this task: Perhaps unsurprisingly, they detected a much smaller proportion of the target sequences than did healthy controls (50.2% vs. 75.7%). In addition, they made many more false responses—that is, inappropriate, impulsive button presses to nontarget stimuli (see Figure 2–1). This pattern has been confirmed in studies using similar tasks by Sax et al. (1995, 1998, 1999) and by Swann et al. (2003).

In addition to having problems with focusing and sustaining attention, manic patients have difficulties shifting attention. Manic patients resemble patients with frontal lobe damage on attentional shifting tasks such as the Wisconsin Card Sorting Test (see test description in Table 2–1). Both groups of patients perseverate in that they continue to select stimuli in accordance with a previously reinforced rule that has been changed by the experimenter and thus become incorrect (Clark et al. 2001; McGrath et al. 1997; Morice 1990; Tam et al. 1998). There is accumulating evidence that different kinds of attentional shift may be anatomically segregated within the PFC. The intradimensional-extradimensional (ID-ED) task is a two-choice visual discrimination test in which the subject progresses through a series of stages involving different kinds of attentional shift (Downes et al. 1989). Reversal shifts involve shifting from one stimulus to the other, on the basis of changing response feedback. An ID shift requires generalization of a learned rule to some novel stimuli, whereas an ED shift requires a switch from one stimulus dimension to another. In human subjects, the majority of the errors committed on the ID-ED task occur at either the reversal stages or the extradimensional shift stage. Studies using an ID-ED analogue task in marmosets have demonstrated a neuropsychological double dissociation in that lesions to the orbitofrontal cortex impaired reversal shifting, whereas lesions to the dorsolateral PFC impaired extradimensional shifting (Dias et al. 1996). Studies using functional neuroimaging in human patients with lesions and in healthy controls have confirmed orb-

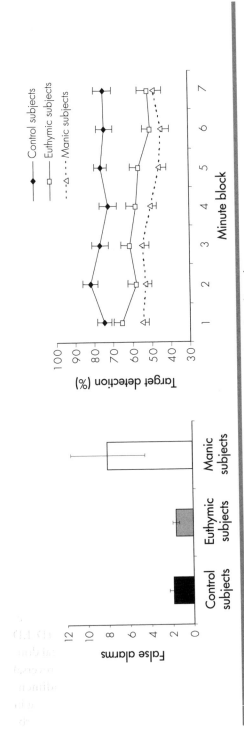

FIGURE 2–1. Sustained attention performance in patients with bipolar disorder.

Testing conditions occurred either during a manic episode ($n=15$) or during euthymic phase ($n=30$). Healthy controls ($n=30$) were group-matched for age, gender, and years of education. The Rapid Visual Information Processing lasted 7 minutes. Manic patients made more false alarms than controls and euthymic patients. Both bipolar groups displayed reduced target detection. The manic patients detected fewer targets for the duration of the task, whereas the euthymic group showed an increased vigilance decrement.

Source. Reprinted from Clark L, Goodwin GM: "State- and Trait-Related Deficits in Sustained Attention in Bipolar Disorder." *European Archives of Psychiatry and Clinical Neuroscience* 254:61–68, 2004. Used with permission from Springer Science and Business Media. See also Clark et al. 2001, 2002.

itofrontal and/or ventrolateral PFC (Brodmann area 11/47) involvement in reversal learning (Cools et al. 2002; Fellows and Farah 2003; Hornak et al. 2004; Rolls et al. 1994) coupled with dorsolateral prefrontal involvement in higher-level dimensional shifts (Monchi et al. 2001; R.D. Rogers et al. 2000). Our study in patients with mania demonstrated increased error rates at both the reversal and the extradimensional stages of the ID-ED task (Clark et al. 2001) (see Figure 2–2). This implies quite a widely distributed disturbance of processing in the frontal cortex.

Impaired judgment in mania can also be measured objectively using laboratory tests of decision making. The Iowa Gambling Task (Bechara et al. 1994) is sensitive to impaired judgment in patients with lesions to the ventromedial PFC and has been widely used in neuropsychiatric populations (Dunn et al. 2006). In this task, subjects make a series of 100 card choices from four decks of cards. Each card choice wins the subject a number of points, but occasional choices additionally result in a penalty. The four decks differ in the profile of wins and losses: Decks A and B are the risky decks, associated with higher immediate wins but occasional dramatic losses that result in net loss over time. Decks C and D are the safe decks, associated with smaller wins but also negligible losses so that subjects accumulate a profit over time. Healthy subjects overcome an initial preference for the risky decks and learn to choose the safe decks over the 100 choices. The classic profile associated with ventromedial PFC lesions is that patients maintain their preference for the risky decks for the duration of the task, despite accruing substantial losses (Bechara et al. 1994, 2000). In our initial study of mania (Clark et al. 2001), patients with mania, compared with healthy controls, had lower total net scores (total safe choices minus total risky choices) on the Iowa Gambling Task. However, on average, the manic patients did not significantly prefer the safe decks over the risky decks, and thus did not fully resemble the profile for patients with ventromedial damage to the PFC. It is possible that the poor performance of patients with mania resulted from a failure to learn the reward and punishment contingencies of the four decks, consistent with deficits generally related to learning new information (e.g., as measured on the California Verbal Learning Test).

On a related test, the Cambridge Gamble Task, manic patients showed impaired probability judgment and increased deliberation times (Murphy et al. 2001). This test aimed to remove the learning elements from the Iowa Gambling Task, so as to isolate behavioral changes specifically related to risk-taking behavior. Although the manic patients did not show an overall increase in betting behavior on the task, they were less able to moderate their bets by the odds that were available. Moreover, their deficit in probability judgment correlated with mania symptom ratings on the YMS. Pa-

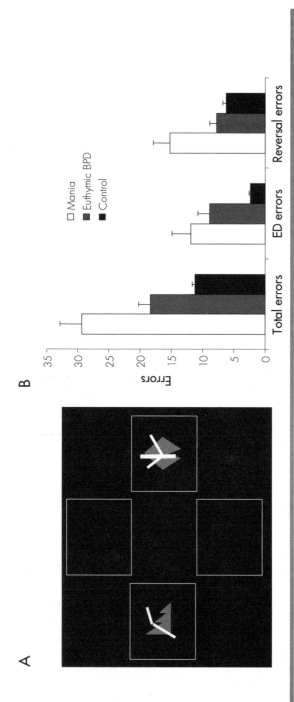

FIGURE 2–2.   Shifting of attention in patients with bipolar disorder.

The Cambridge Neuropsychological Test Automated Battery (CANTAB) Intradimensional-Extradimensional Shift ID-ED task (http://www.cantab.com) is a two-choice visual discrimination task using compound stimuli (in this example, overlapping gray shapes and white lines). The subject performs a series of attentional shifts based on trial-by-trial feedback. (A) In reversal stages, the subject shifts from one stimulus (e.g., the gray jagged stimulus on the left in view A to the other (the gray shape on the right in view A), ignoring the alternative dimension (the white lines). At the extradimensional (ED) shift stage, the subject is presented with novel stimuli and must shift responding from the gray shapes to the white lines. (B) Subjects with mania (*n*=15) make more errors than controls at both the ED shift and reversal stages. Patients with euthymic bipolar disorder (BPD) (*n*=30) make more errors at the ED shift stage.

Source.   (A) Used with permission from Clark et al. 2002. (B) From Clark et al. 2001. Copyright 2007 Cambridge Cognition Limited. All rights reserved.

tients with euthymic bipolar disorder and patients with major depressive disorder showed intact performance on the task (Rubinsztein et al. 2000). Therefore, decision-making deficits seem to be closely related to the manic state. A subsequent functional imaging experiment measured regional cerebral blood flow in patients with mania during performance of a similar gambling task that presented a choice between a small likely reward and a larger but less likely reward (Rubinsztein et al. 2001). In these patients, brain activations associated with decision making were increased in the anterior cingulate cortex (Brodmann area 32) but reduced in the inferior frontal gyrus (Brodmann area 47), suggesting a dysregulation of medial and ventral prefrontal circuitry.

Subsequent work has shown impaired judgment of patients on other objective measures of decision making. On a two-choice guessing task, manic patients were more likely to switch responding in a condition with a large proportion of errors (Minassian et al. 2004). On an advice-taking task, bipolar patients in whom a positive mood had been induced by a psychological manipulation tended to make decisions that opposed the advice of a collaborator (Mansell and Lam 2006). This effect was not seen in patients in the negative mood condition or in healthy controls under positive (or negative) mood inductions (Mansell and Lam 2006) but is yet to be confirmed in patients who are currently in a manic episode.

These findings clearly indicate widespread impairments in executive and attentional function during the manic phase of bipolar disorder. In addition to demonstrating impairment on tasks traditionally associated with the dorsolateral PFC, such as planning and attentional set shifting, manic patients have displayed marked impairment on measures associated with the orbitofrontal region, including laboratory tests of decision making, reversal learning, and impulse control. Functional imaging studies that have scanned manic patients in the resting state have also indicated changes in orbitofrontal cortex blood flow and metabolism. Blumberg et al. (1999) reported a 22% reduction in blood flow in the orbitofrontal cortex in a group of five manic patients. Goodwin et al. (1997) scanned a group of 14 patients before and after voluntary withdrawal of lithium medication. Half the patients developed manic symptoms by the time of the second off-lithium scan, and the increase in mania ratings correlated with increased perfusion in the orbitofrontal cortex and anterior cingulate cortex. Drevets et al. (1997) also found that patients during manic episodes showed increased resting state blood flow in the subgenual cingulate region, the same region that was reduced in volume in the patients with bipolar disorder. The disadvantage of these resting state studies is that it is not possible to control for thought content during scanning, and increased activity may relate simply to aspects of the manic state, such as rapid thoughts.

Some studies have begun to examine functional response during task performance in patients with mania (e.g., Rubinsztein et al. 2001). During performance of a Go–No Go task requiring the suppression of impulsive responses, as indicated by functional magnetic resonance imaging, a group of 11 manic patients showed blunted responses in the right lateral orbito-frontal cortex (Brodmann area 47) (Altshuler et al. 2005), a region that is known to be critical for inhibitory control (Aron et al. 2003). A compara-ble finding in the right orbitofrontal cortex was reported by Blumberg et al. (2003) during performance of the Stroop Test by manic patients. (This study revealed an interesting pattern of state- and trait-related changes and is discussed in the following section, "Function in Remitted [Euthymic] Bipolar Disorder.") In conclusion, these preliminary activation studies in manic patients appear to demonstrate a more consistent pattern of orbito-frontal cortex dysfunction during mania, which may give rise to the symp-toms of disinhibition and poor decision making.

Function in Remitted (Euthymic) Bipolar Disorder

In the Kraepelinian distinction between bipolar disorder and schizophrenia (dementia praecox), a defining feature of bipolar disorder was the apparent recovery of function between episodes, in contrast with the deteriorating course of dementia praecox. However, in recent years, there has been in-creasing recognition that some degree of neurocognitive impairment may persist in patients with bipolar disorder outside of acute illness episodes. These enduring deficits may be amenable to pharmacological or psycho-logical treatment to improve functional outcome in patients with bipolar disorder.

To assess neurocognitive function in remitted bipolar patients, we re-cruited a group of 30 outpatients with bipolar I disorder who were defined as euthymic (neutral mood), based on a Ham-D score of less than 9 and a YMS score of less than 9. The patients were mainly receiving mood-stabi-lizing medication (19 were receiving lithium), and one-third of the patients were receiving a selective serotonin reuptake inhibitor. We administered the same neuropsychological assessment used in our mania study and com-pared the patients against 30 healthy controls (Clark et al. 2002). The eu-thymic patients performed at the level of controls on several measures of executive function, including verbal fluency, the Stroop Test, a strategic working memory task, and the Tower of London test of forward planning. They also performed at normal levels on the Iowa Gambling Task of risky decision making. These results show that the patients were not globally im-paired (global impairment is a common finding in schizophrenia and some bipolar samples) and serve to highlight those domains in which impairment was measurable and hence are likely most typical of the bipolar cognitive profile during remission. The euthymic group differed significantly from controls on only three measures: the RVIP test of sustained attention, the California Verbal Learning Test memory task, and the ID-ED shifting task (specifically at the extradimensional shift stage; see Figure 2–2). On the RVIP, the euthymic group showed an increased vigilance decrement compared with controls: they performed at the levels of control subjects in the first minute of the test, but their target detection deteriorated at a steeper rate than that of controls (see Figure 1–1). Their response latencies to detect target stimuli were also slowed, but they did not show the increase in false responding that we saw in the patients with mania.

Mild affective symptoms were present in the euthymic patients. The patients scored significantly higher than controls on the Ham-D and YMS despite scoring below our cutoffs for euthymia. This observation, which is common in such samples, poses a conceptual question: Is it a confound of the recovered state when thinking about neuropsychological impairment or is it a defining feature of the recovered state? Practically speaking, when we controlled for these residual mood symptoms, the only neuropsychological measure that remained significantly impaired was target detection on the RVIP.

Several other studies have reported intact executive function in euthymic bipolar patients (Pirkola et al. 2005; Rubinsztein et al. 2000; van Gorp et al. 1998). In the van Gorp et al. (1998) study, only patients with comorbid alcohol dependency showed perseverative impairment on the Wisconsin Card Sorting Test. Intact decision making on the Cambridge Gamble Task was also seen in the Rubinsztein et al. (2000) study. Moreover, the sustained attention profile of impaired target detection coupled with intact false responding has been replicated in two further studies. In a longitudinal design, Liu et al. (2002) tested 15 bipolar patients at inpatient admission (clinical state not specified) and a second time within a few days of discharge. Upon admission, patients were severely impaired on the degraded-stimulus continuous performance test, in terms of both target detection and rate of false responding (analyzed using signal detection analysis). At discharge, the bipolar patients remained impaired on target detection but showed normal rates of false responding. In a between-groups study, Swann et al. (2003) tested 25 euthymic and 14 manic patients on a version of the Continuous Performance Test that included "catch" trials to elicit more impulsive responses. Both euthymic and manic patients detected significantly fewer targets than did controls (the manic patients were more impaired, albeit not significantly). Only the manic patients made more impulsive false responses on the task. Coupled with the data reviewed in the previous section, "Attentional and Executive Function in Mania," these studies suggest that orbitofrontal cortex dysfunction, measured by tests of decision making, reversal learning, and false responding, may be a state-related deficit in bipolar disorder that is associated with the manic syndrome.

The extent to which more general aspects of executive dysfunction recover during remission remains controversial. A number of studies, including our own, have suggested that executive deficits are not an invariable feature of the recovered state, although these studies may not have been sufficiently powered to detect small effects, and trend deficits were present in a number of domains (Clark et al. 2002; Harmer et al. 2002; Rubinsztein et al. 2000). However, a number of studies have detected executive deficits in remitted patients. Although some, primarily early, studies did not control adequately for residual symptoms (Atre-Vaidya et al. 1998; Coffman et al. 1990; Krabbendam et al. 2000; Tham et al. 1997; Zubieta et al. 2001), other, generally more recent, studies have shown significant executive dysfunction (e.g., on verbal fluency, forward planning, and working memory) even after controlling for residual mood symptoms (Ferrier et al. 1999; Frangou et al. 2005; Martinez-Aran et al. 2004; Mur et al. 2007; Thompson et al. 2005). Deficits on selective attention and attentional shifting (revealed via the Stroop Test, Trail Making Test—Part B, and Wisconsin Card Sorting Test) may also persist in carefully defined groups of euthymic patients (Altshuler et al. 2004; Ferrier et al. 1999). The magnitude of case-control differences may depend very critically on cohort selection, medication, and the size of the battery (i.e., results in very long batteries may be confounded by attentional fatigue). Our own experience is compatible with the explanation that sustained attention is an unusually sensitive domain for patients with bipolar disorder, even when all other tests indicate that the patients are very well recovered. This interpretation has important theoretical and practical significance. However, we do not dispute that there are bipolar patients who have poorer outcomes with regard to cognitive function and who, therefore, may perform more like patients with schizophrenia. The proportion of patients with severe impairments will depend heavily on the sample and from where it is drawn. The disability of individual patients must be seen in this light.

Further insights into cognitive function during remission have been gained from studies combining neuropsychological testing with functional imaging. Several of these studies have used the Stroop Test, which has been widely validated for use in neuroimaging and yields a robust signal in the anterior cingulate cortex. Gruber et al. (2002) reported reduced anterior cingulate activity in remitted bipolar patients compared with controls, which may indicate a failure to activate task-relevant neural circuitry in the bipolar group (see also Matsuo et al. [2002], who studied verbal fluency, and Monks et al. [2004], who studied n-back working memory). A subsequent study using a variation of the Stroop Test, in which the subject was required to name the ink color of rows of *X*s, found that bipolar patients showed reduced activation in the dorsolateral and ventrolateral regions of the PFC during incongruent blocks compared with baseline blocks (Kronhaus et al. 2006). In addition, the bipolar group appeared to show deactivation in orbital and medial regions of the PFC during the incongruent Stroop blocks. Relative deactivation of the orbitofrontal region was seen in Blumberg et al.'s (2003) study in euthymic patients, where the same effect was apparent in manic and depressed bipolar groups, suggesting a trait marker of pathophysiology in the orbitofrontal cortex. Task-related deactivations may be explained by relative hyperactivation of orbitofrontal circuitry during nonemotional or undemanding baseline task conditions (Kronhaus et al. 2006). Limbic hyperactivity during relatively nonemotional tasks has also been reported in patients with remitted bipolar disorder using other cognitive activation tasks, including a sustained attention task (Strakowski et al. 2004) and a serial reaction time task with implicit sequences (Berns et al. 2002). Put simply, these findings indicate that patients with bipolar disorder appear to recruit emotional networks in the brain to process nonemotional material. These findings are consistent with studies showing elevated emotionality in bipolar patients undergoing psychological mood manipulations (Kruger et al. 2006; Mansell and Lam 2006).

Several clinical and demographic factors accompany and may even mediate the persistent executive and attentional impairments in patients with bipolar disorder. Our own data indicate that some executive and memory dysfunction correlates with the presence of subclinical mood symptoms (Clark et al. 2002; Ferrier et al. 1999). Altshuler et al. (2004) reported that performance on the Wisconsin Card Sorting Test was bimodally distributed in euthymic patients, with a subgroup that was indistinguishable from controls and a subgroup that displayed pronounced impairment that was indistinguishable from patients with schizophrenia. Several studies have reported correlations between the level of executive dysfunction and the duration of bipolar illness and/or the number of illness episodes (Clark et al. 2002; Frangou et al. 2005; Thompson et al. 2005).

Function in Depression

In contrast to the literature on bipolar depression, there is a substantial literature assessing neurocognitive function in major depressive (unipolar) disorder (M.A. Rogers et al. 2004). Studies that have measured verbal fluency, selective attention (using the Stroop Test), forward planning, and working memory reveal inconsistent findings among subjects with major depressive disorder (Channon et al. 1993; Elliott et al. 1996; Franke et al. 1993; Grant et al. 2001; Purcell et al. 1997; Trichard et al. 1995). The most

reliable impairments have been shown in attentional shifting (Degl'Innocenti et al. 1998; Franke et al. 1993; Ilonen et al. 2000; Merriam et al.
1999), which has also been reported in dysphoric college students (Channon and Green 1999), suggesting a link to depressed mood as well as the
clinical syndrome of depression. Given the heterogeneous presentation of
unipolar depression, these mixed findings are perhaps unsurprising. Several
studies have failed to find any correlation between overall ratings of symptom severity and the degree of executive dysfunction (Degl'Innocenti et al.
1998; Porter et al. 2003; Trichard et al. 1995). However, executive impairment was particularly associated with melancholic features in cases of major
depressive disorder (Austin et al. 1999), and melancholic symptoms may be
especially prevalent in bipolar depression (Mitchell et al. 2001). Psychotic
features are also associated with a greater degree of impairment on the
Stroop Test (Schatzberg et al. 2000). Greater levels of apathy, often linked
to anterior cingulate damage and the neurological condition of akinetic
mutism, have also been correlated with performance on the Stroop Test, a
verbal fluency measure, and the Wisconsin Card Sorting Test (Feil et al.
2003).

At least some of the attentional and executive deficits that have been reported in major depressive disorder appear to recover fully upon symptom
remission. Sustained attention deficits (on target detection) seen during
acute depression (Hart et al. 1998; van den Bosch et al. 1996) were not
present in a group of remitted outpatients with at least two previous episodes of major depressive disorder (Clark et al. 2005b), and Liu et al. (2002)
showed intact performance on the degraded-stimulus continuous performance test in 22 outpatients with nonpsychotic major depression (Ham-D
mean = 5.8, indicating no clinically significant levels of depression).

In contrast to this wealth of data about unipolar depression, there is a
paucity of neuropsychological research on the depressed phase of bipolar
disorder. Sweeney et al. (2000) compared depressed bipolar, depressed unipolar, and manic bipolar patients on a number of tasks from the Cambridge
Neuropsychological Test Automated Battery (CANTAB) neuropsychological assessment. Although the manic patients showed severe executive impairment, the two depressed groups showed similar levels of unimpaired
performance on Tower of London planning and the ID-ED attentional
shifting task. However, the depressed groups showed only moderate symptom scores on the Ham-D. A recent study has reported impaired extradimensional set–shifting on the ID-ED task in a bipolar group with more
severe depression (Rubinsztein et al. 2006). Basso et al. (2002) tested depressed, manic, and mixed-state patients with bipolar disorder and reported
significant executive and attentional impairments on verbal fluency and on
the Trail Making Test—Part B in all three groups, with no significant dif-

ferences between groups. A further study by Borkowska and Rybakowski (2001) did not include a control group, but reported significantly worse performance on the Wisconsin Card Sorting Test, Trail Making Test, and Stroop Test by a group of unmedicated bipolar depressed patients than by a group of unipolar depressed patients who were matched for duration and severity of illness. The consensus from these studies is that executive and attentional impairments also occur in the depressed state of bipolar disorder. There is little evidence to indicate whether bipolar depression is characterized by cognitive changes indicative of orbitofrontal cortical dysfunction, such as impulsive false responding and impaired decision making, which are seen in mania.

Executive Function as an Endophenotype

Chapter 4 of this volume considers in detail the potential for neurocognitive function to serve as an endophenotype for bipolar disorder. Our own experience is limited but instructive. We have compared both sustained attention and attentional shifting in first-degree relatives of probands with bipolar I disorder and in subjects with recovered depression (Clark et al. 2005a, 2005b). We reasoned that because depression was quite common in relatives, we needed the latter group as a control. In fact, both the first-degree relatives and the recovered unipolar subjects showed increased errors when asked to shift set (Clark et al. 2005b). Therefore, such a pattern of response may contribute nonspecifically to the risk of mood disorder— for example, by contributing to an inflexible problem-solving style; it is not specific to bipolar illness. (See Chapter 6 of this volume, "Improving Psychotherapy Practice and Technique for Bipolar Disorder: Lessons From Cognitive Neuroscience," for further discussion of impaired capacity for set shifting and cognitive inflexibility as pertaining to interventions during psychotherapy.)

Clinical Implications

The clinical implications of attentional dysfunction may be profound. We know that patients with bipolar disorder tend to be well educated yet underachieving in their careers, as demonstrated in the following case vignette. Although poorly controlled symptoms can obviously contribute to this tendency, they are unlikely to be the whole story.

Case Vignette 1

A 29-year-old graduate student had his first episode of mania after beginning university studies, but he recovered and completed his undergraduate studies. After receiving his baccalaureate, he developed a persistent pattern of chronic unstable hypomania, which proved difficult to treat. He eventually responded to a combination of divalproex and an antipsychotic and was euthymic for 2 years. Over that time, he worked as a research officer for a charity, but he found great difficulty sustaining attention at a computer and disliked the pressure from other people in the post. He became manic again when working increased overtime to try to clear a backlog. He gave up his employment and his mood stabilized over a few months. At this stage in his life, he had not experienced depressive symptoms of significant intensity. When tested formally, he had very poor sustained attention and found the task subjectively more difficult than the rest of the battery. He subsequently experienced typical depressive episodes and did not work in paid employment for almost 6 years. Even when off all medication, his cognitive function remained limiting to his work aspirations.

Conclusions

Attentional and executive functions are critical to academic and professional success. Most of what is currently known about the relevant neuropsychology in patients with bipolar disorder is limited to work on the more severe forms of the disorder. Thus, in bipolar I disorder, sustained attention appears to be impaired as a function of illness progression. Researchers do not yet know whether this impairment can be prevented by effective treatment, but sustained attention could provide a worthwhile end point for long-term interventions. A relative failure to switch attention (perseveration) is also consistently seen in patients with bipolar disorder. However, this apparent variation in function is not confined to patients, but is also seen in unaffected relatives and in subjects with recurrent unipolar depression. Assessment of attention switching may provide a behavioral endophenotype that is associated with the risk of mood disorder of all types. Whether such assessment can shed light on mechanisms of cognition that contribute directly to the risk of depression is not certain, but it might do so. Enduring deficits of cognitive function are compounded by the effects of chronic symptoms, even when of a subsyndromal intensity, and possibly by the actions of the individual or combined medicines used to treat the disorder. The cognitive deficits we have described are an important part of the disability associated with bipolar disorder. They merit more attention as outcome measures in relation to clinical trials or as naturalistic outcomes under ordinary clinical conditions.

Take-Home Points

- Cognitive dysfunction in bipolar disorder involves both transient (state) and enduring (trait) characteristics.
- Neuroimaging studies reveal abnormal reductions in prefrontal cortical gray matter volume in patients with bipolar disorder, a finding that is consistent with executive dysfunction.

- When manic, patients with bipolar disorder show widespread difficulties in executive and attentional functions, including perseveration of thought and impaired capacity for sustained attention. These deficits, especially impaired capacity for sustained attention, largely persist during euthymia.

- When manic, patients with bipolar disorder show impulsive responding, impaired decision making, poor judgment when gauging probabilities, and difficulty moderating risk-taking behavior. These deficits largely *remit* during euthymia.

- Remitted bipolar patients show limbic hyperactivity when processing nonemotional information, consistent with observations of "trait emotionality."

- Recovered bipolar patients may have persistent deficits in selective attention, attentional shifting, and verbal planning (functions of the dorsolateral prefrontal cortex), and in decision making, reversal learning, and impulse control (functions of the orbitofrontal cortex).

- Some executive dysfunction, such as cognitive inflexibility during problem solving, is evident in both bipolar and unipolar patients—and their relatives—and may be a function of depression more than diagnostic polarity.

- Deficits in attention and executive functioning are notably related to functional impairment in patients with bipolar disorder, often resulting in failure to reach optimal levels of psychosocial functioning.

References

Abood Z, Sharkey A, Webb M, et al: Are patients with bipolar affective disorder socially disadvantaged? a comparison with a control group. Bipolar Disord 4:243–248, 2002

Alexander GE, DeLong MR, Strick PL: Parallel organization of functionally segregated circuits linking basal ganglia and cortex. Annu Rev Neurosci 9:357–381, 1986

Altshuler LL, Ventura J, van Gorp WG, et al: Neurocognitive function in clinically stable men with bipolar I disorder or schizophrenia and normal control subjects. Biol Psychiatry 56:560–569, 2004

Altshuler LL, Bookheimer SY, Townsend J, et al: Blunted activation in orbitofrontal cortex during mania: a functional magnetic resonance imaging study. Biol Psychiatry 58:763–769, 2005

Aron AR, Fletcher PC, Bullmore ET, et al: Stop-signal inhibition disrupted by damage to right inferior frontal gyrus in humans. Nat Neurosci 6:115–116, 2003

Atre-Vaidya N, Taylor MA, Seidenberg M, et al: Cognitive deficits, psychopathology, and psychosocial functioning in bipolar mood disorder. Neuropsychiatry Neuropsychol Behav Neurol 11:120–126, 1998

Austin MP, Mitchell P, Wilhelm K, et al: Cognitive function in depression: a distinct pattern of frontal impairment in melancholia? Psychol Med 29:73–85, 1999

Basso MR, Lowery N, Neel J, et al: Neuropsychological impairment among manic, depressed, and mixed-episode inpatients with bipolar disorder. Neuropsychology 16:84–91, 2002

Bearden CE, Hoffman KM, Cannon TD: The neuropsychology and neuroanatomy of bipolar affective disorder: a critical review. Bipolar Disord 3:106–150; discussion 151–153, 2001

Bechara A, Damasio AR, Damasio H, et al: Insensitivity to future consequences following damage to human prefrontal cortex. Cognition 50:7–15, 1994

Bechara A, Tranel D, Damasio H: Characterization of the decision-making deficit of patients with ventromedial prefrontal cortex lesions. Brain 123:2189–2202, 2000

Berns GS, Martin M, Proper SM: Limbic hyperreactivity in bipolar II disorder. Am J Psychiatry 159:304–306, 2002

Blumberg HP, Stern E, Ricketts S, et al: Rostral and orbital prefrontal cortex dysfunction in the manic state of bipolar disorder. Am J Psychiatry 156:1986–1988, 1999

Blumberg HP, Leung HC, Skudlarski P, et al: A functional magnetic resonance imaging study of bipolar disorder: state- and trait-related dysfunction in ventral prefrontal cortices. Arch Gen Psychiatry 60:601–609, 2003

Borkowska A, Rybakowski JK: Neuropsychological frontal lobe tests indicate that bipolar depressed patients are more impaired than unipolar. Bipolar Disord 3:88–94, 2001

Bush G, Luu P, Posner MI: Cognitive and emotional influences in anterior cingulate cortex. Trends Cogn Sci 4:215–222, 2000

Carson AJ, MacHale S, Allen K, et al: Depression after stroke and lesion location: a systematic review. Lancet 356:122–126, 2000

Cato MA, Delis DC, Abildskov TJ, et al: Assessing the elusive cognitive deficits associated with ventromedial prefrontal damage: a case of a modern-day Phineas Gage. J Int Neuropsychol Soc 10:453–465, 2004

Cavanagh JT, van Beck M, Muir W, et al: Case-control study of neurocognitive function in euthymic patients with bipolar disorder: an association with mania. Br J Psychiatry 180:320–326, 2002

Channon S, Green PS: Executive function in depression: the role of performance strategies in aiding depressed and non-depressed participants. J Neurol Neurosurg Psychiatry 66:162–171, 1999

Channon S, Baker JE, Robertson MM: Working memory in clinical depression: an experimental study. Psychol Med 23:87–91, 1993

Clark L, Goodwin GM: State- and trait-related deficits in sustained attention in bipolar disorder. Eur Arch Psychiatry Clin Neurosci 254:61–68, 2004

Clark L, Iversen SD, Goodwin GM: A neuropsychological investigation of prefrontal cortex involvement in acute mania. Am J Psychiatry 158:1605–1611, 2001

Clark L, Iversen SD, Goodwin GM: Sustained attention deficit in bipolar disorder. Br J Psychiatry 180:313–319, 2002

Clark L, Kempton MJ, Scarna A, et al: Sustained attention deficit confirmed in euthymic bipolar disorder, but not in first-degree relatives of bipolar patients or euthymic unipolar depression. Biol Psychiatry 57:183–187, 2005a

Clark L, Scarna A, Goodwin GM: Impairment of executive function but not memory in first-degree relatives of patients with bipolar I disorder and in euthymic patients with unipolar depression. Am J Psychiatry 162:1980–1982, 2005b

Coffman JA, Bornstein RA, Olson SC, et al: Cognitive impairment and cerebral structure by MRI in bipolar disorder. Biol Psychiatry 27:1188–1196, 1990

Cools R: Dopaminergic modulation of cognitive function—implications for L-DOPA treatment in Parkinson's disease. Neurosci Biobehav Rev 30:1–23, 2006

Cools R, Clark L, Owen AM, et al: Defining the neural mechanisms of probabilistic reversal learning using event-related functional magnetic resonance imaging. J Neurosci 22:4563–4567, 2002

Coryell W, Scheftner W, Keller M, et al: The enduring psychosocial consequences of mania and depression. Am J Psychiatry 150:720–727, 1993

Damasio AR, Tranel D, Damasio H: Individuals with sociopathic behavior caused by frontal damage fail to respond autonomically to social stimuli. Behav Brain Res 41:81–94, 1990

Davidson RJ: Anterior cerebral asymmetry and the nature of emotion. Brain Cogn 20:125–151, 1992

Davidson RJ, Irwin W: The functional neuroanatomy of emotion and affective style. Trends Cogn Sci 3:11–21, 1999

Degl'Innocenti A, Agren H, Bäckman L: Executive deficits in major depression. Acta Psychiatr Scand 97:82–88, 1998

Desimone R, Duncan J: Neural mechanisms of selective visual attention. Annu Rev Neurosci 18:193–222, 1995

Dias R, Robbins TW, Roberts AC: Dissociation in prefrontal cortex of affective and attentional shifts. Nature 380:69–72, 1996

Downes JJ, Roberts AC, Sahakian BJ, et al: Impaired extra-dimensional shift performance in medicated and unmedicated Parkinson's disease: evidence for a specific attentional dysfunction. Neuropsychologia 27:1329–1343, 1989

Drevets WC, Price JL, Simpson JR Jr, et al: Subgenual prefrontal cortex abnormalities in mood disorders. Nature 386:824–827, 1997

Dunn BD, Dalgleish T, Lawrence AD: The somatic marker hypothesis: a critical evaluation. Neurosci Biobehav Rev 30:239–271, 2006

Ehmann TS, Beninger RJ, Gawel MJ, et al: Depressive symptoms in Parkinson's disease: a comparison with disabled control subjects. J Geriatr Psychiatry Neurol 3:3–9, 1990

Elliott R, Sahakian BJ, McKay AP, et al: Neuropsychological impairments in unipolar depression: the influence of perceived failure on subsequent performance. Psychol Med 26:975–989, 1996

Eslinger PJ, Damasio AR: Severe disturbance of higher cognition after bilateral frontal lobe ablation: patient EVR. Neurology 35:1731–1741, 1985

Feil D, Razani J, Boone K, et al: Apathy and cognitive performance in older adults with depression. Int J Geriatr Psychiatry 18:479–485, 2003

Fellows LK, Farah MJ: Ventromedial frontal cortex mediates affective shifting in humans: evidence from a reversal learning paradigm. Brain 126:1830–1837, 2003

Ferrier IN, Stanton BR, Kelly TP, et al: Neuropsychological function in euthymic patients with bipolar disorder. Br J Psychiatry 175:246–251, 1999

Frangou S, Donaldson S, Hadjulis M, et al: The Maudsley Bipolar Disorder Project: executive dysfunction in bipolar disorder I and its clinical correlates. Biol Psychiatry 58:859–864, 2005

Franke P, Maier W, Hardt J, et al: Assessment of frontal lobe functioning in schizophrenia and unipolar major depression. Psychopathology 26:76–84, 1993

Goodwin GM, Cavanagh JT, Glabus MF, et al: Uptake of 99mTc-exametazime shown by single photon emission computed tomography before and after lithium withdrawal in bipolar patients: associations with mania. Br J Psychiatry 170:426–430, 1997

Grant MM, Thase ME, Sweeney JA: Cognitive disturbance in outpatient depressed younger adults: evidence of modest impairment. Biol Psychiatry 50:35–43, 2001

Gruber SA, Rogowska J, Holcomb P, et al: Stroop performance in normal control subjects: an fMRI study. Neuroimage 16:349–360, 2002

Harmer CJ, Clark L, Grayson L, et al: Sustained attention deficit in bipolar disorder is not a working memory impairment in disguise. Neuropsychologia 40:1586–1590, 2002

Hart RP, Wade JB, Calabrese VP, et al: Vigilance performance in Parkinson's disease and depression. J Clin Exp Neuropsychol 20:111–117, 1998

Hirayasu Y, Shenton ME, Salisbury DF, et al: Subgenual cingulate cortex volume in first-episode psychosis. Am J Psychiatry 156:1091–1093, 1999

Hornak J, O'Doherty J, Bramham J, et al: Reward-related reversal learning after surgical excisions in orbito-frontal or dorsolateral prefrontal cortex in humans. J Cogn Neurosci 16:463–478, 2004

Ilonen T, Taiminen T, Lauerma H, et al: Impaired Wisconsin Card Sorting Test performance in first-episode schizophrenia: resource or motivation deficit? Compr Psychiatry 41:385–391, 2000

Kessing LV: Cognitive impairment in the euthymic phase of affective disorder. Psychol Med 28:1027–1038, 1998

Krabbendam L, Honig A, Wiersma J, et al: Cognitive dysfunctions and white matter lesions in patients with bipolar disorder in remission. Acta Psychiatr Scand 101:274–280, 2000

Kronhaus DM, Lawrence NS, Williams AM, et al: Stroop performance in bipolar disorder: further evidence for abnormalities in the ventral prefrontal cortex. Bipolar Disord 8:28–39, 2006

Kruger S, Alda M, Young LT, et al: Risk and resilience markers in bipolar disorder: brain responses to emotional challenge in bipolar patients and their healthy siblings. Am J Psychiatry 163:257–264, 2006

Lezak MD, Howieson DB, Loring DW: Neuropsychological Assessment, 4th Edition. New York, Oxford University Press, 2004

Liu SK, Chiu CH, Chang CJ, et al: Deficits in sustained attention in schizophrenia and affective disorders: stable versus state-dependent markers. Am J Psychiatry 159:975–982, 2002

Lochhead RA, Parsey RV, Oquendo MA, et al: Regional brain gray matter volume differences in patients with bipolar disorder as assessed by optimized voxel-based morphometry. Biol Psychiatry 55:1154–1162, 2004

Lopez-Larson MP, DelBello MP, Zimmerman ME, et al: Regional prefrontal gray and white matter abnormalities in bipolar disorder. Biol Psychiatry 52:93–100, 2002

Lyoo IK, Kim MJ, Stoll AL, et al: Frontal lobe gray matter density decreases in bipolar I disorder. Biol Psychiatry 55:648–651, 2004

Malloy P, Bihrle A, Duffy J, et al: The orbitomedial frontal syndrome. Arch Clin Neuropsychol 8:185–201, 1993

Mansell W, Lam D: "I won't do what you tell me!" Elevated mood and the assessment of advice-taking in euthymic bipolar I disorder. Behav Res Ther 44:1787–1801, 2006

Martinez-Aran A, Vieta E, Reinares M, et al: Cognitive function across manic or hypomanic, depressed, and euthymic states in bipolar disorder. Am J Psychiatry 161:262–270, 2004

Matsuo K, Kato N, Kato T: Decreased cerebral haemodynamic response to cognitive and physiological tasks in mood disorders as shown by near-infrared spectroscopy. Psychol Med 32:1029–1037, 2002

McGrath J, Scheldt S, Welham J, et al: Performance on tests sensitive to impaired executive ability in schizophrenia, mania and well controls: acute and subacute phases. Schizophr Res 26:127–137, 1997

Mega MS, Cummings JL: Frontal-subcortical circuits and neuropsychiatric disorders. J Neuropsychiatry Clin Neurosci 6:358–370, 1994

Merriam EP, Thase ME, Haas GL, et al: Prefrontal cortical dysfunction in depression determined by Wisconsin Card Sorting Test performance. Am J Psychiatry 156:780–782, 1999

Mesulam MM: The human frontal lobes: transcending the default mode through contingent processing, in Principles of Frontal Lobe Function. Edited by Stuss DT, Knight RT. New York, Oxford University Press, 2002, pp 8–30

Minassian A, Paulus MP, Perry W: Increased sensitivity to error during decision-making in bipolar disorder patients with acute mania. J Affect Disord 82:203–208, 2004

Mitchell PB, Wilhelm K, Parker G, et al: The clinical features of bipolar depression: a comparison with matched major depressive disorder patients. J Clin Psychiatry 62:212–216, 2001

Monchi O, Petrides M, Petre V, et al: Wisconsin Card Sorting revisited: distinct neural circuits participating in different stages of the task identified by event-related functional magnetic resonance imaging. J Neurosci 21:7733–7741, 2001

Monks PJ, Thompson JM, Bullmore ET, et al: A functional MRI study of working memory task in euthymic bipolar disorder: evidence for task-specific dysfunction. Bipolar Disord 6:550–564, 2004

Morice R: Cognitive inflexibility and pre-frontal dysfunction in schizophrenia and mania. Br J Psychiatry 157:50–54, 1990

Mur M, Portella MJ, Martinez-Aran A, et al: Persistent neuropsychological deficit in euthymic bipolar patients: executive function as a core deficit. J Clin Psychiatry 68:1078–1086, 2007

Murphy FC, Sahakian BJ, Rubinsztein JS, et al: Emotional bias and inhibitory control processes in mania and depression. Psychol Med 29:1307–1321, 1999

Murphy FC, Rubinsztein JS, Michael A, et al: Decision-making cognition in mania and depression. Psychol Med 31:679–693, 2001

Pardo JV, Pardo PJ, Janer KW, et al: The anterior cingulate cortex mediates processing selection in the Stroop attentional conflict paradigm. Proc Natl Acad Sci USA 87:256–259, 1990

Pirkola T, Tuulio-Henriksson A, Glahn D, et al: Spatial working memory function in twins with schizophrenia and bipolar disorder. Biol Psychiatry 58:930–936, 2005

Porter RJ, Gallagher P, Thompson JM, et al: Neurocognitive impairment in drug-free patients with major depressive disorder. Br J Psychiatry 182:214–220, 2003

Posner MI, Petersen SE: The attention system of the human brain. Annu Rev Neurosci 13:25–42, 1990

Purcell R, Maruff P, Kyrios M, et al: Neuropsychological function in young patients with unipolar major depression. Psychol Med 27:1277–1285, 1997

Quraishi S, Frangou S: Neuropsychology of bipolar disorder: a review. J Affect Disord 72:209–226, 2002

Robinson RG, Kubos KL, Starr LB, et al: Mood changes in stroke patients: relationship to lesion location. Compr Psychiatry 24:555–566, 1983

Robinson RG, Boston JD, Starkstein SE, et al: Comparison of mania and depression after brain injury: causal factors. Am J Psychiatry 145:172–178, 1988

Rogers MA, Kasai K, Koji M, et al: Executive and prefrontal dysfunction in unipolar depression: a review of neuropsychological and imaging evidence. Neurosci Res 50:1–11, 2004

Rogers RD, Andrews TC, Grasby PM, et al: Contrasting cortical and subcortical activations produced by attentional-set shifting and reversal learning in humans. J Cogn Neurosci 12:142–162, 2000

Rolls ET, Hornak J, Wade D, et al: Emotion-related learning in patients with social and emotional changes associated with frontal lobe damage. J Neurol Neurosurg Psychiatry 57:1518–1524, 1994

Rubinsztein JS, Michael A, Paykel ES, et al: Cognitive impairment in remission in bipolar affective disorder. Psychol Med 30:1025–1036, 2000

Rubinsztein JS, Fletcher PC, Rogers RD, et al: Decision-making in mania: a PET study. Brain 124 (part 12):2550–2563, 2001

Rubinsztein JS, Michael A, Underwood BR, et al: Impaired cognition and decision-making in bipolar depression but no "affective bias" evident. Psychol Med 36:629–639, 2006

Sax KW, Strakowski SM, McElroy SL, et al: Attention and formal thought disorder in mixed and pure mania. Biol Psychiatry 37:420–423, 1995

Sax KW, Strakowski SM, Keck PE Jr, et al: Symptom correlates of attentional improvement following hospitalization for a first episode of affective psychosis. Biol Psychiatry 44:784–786, 1998

Sax KW, Strakowski SM, Zimmerman ME, et al: Frontosubcortical neuroanatomy and the Continuous Performance Test in mania. Am J Psychiatry 156:139–141, 1999

Schatzberg AF, Posener JA, DeBattista C, et al: Neuropsychological deficits in psychotic versus nonpsychotic major depression and no mental illness. Am J Psychiatry 157:1095–1100, 2000

Scott J: Psychotherapy for bipolar disorder. Br J Psychiatry 167:581–588, 1995

Shallice T, Burgess PW: Deficits in strategy application following frontal lobe damage in man. Brain 114:727–741, 1991

Singh A, Herrmann N, Black SE: The importance of lesion location in poststroke depression: a critical review. Can J Psychiatry 43:921–927, 1998

Starkstein SE, Robinson RG, Price TR: Comparison of cortical and subcortical lesions in the production of poststroke mood disorders. Brain 110:1045–1059, 1987

Strakowski SM, Adler CM, Holland SK, et al: A preliminary fMRI study of sustained attention in euthymic, unmedicated bipolar disorder. Neuropsychopharmacology 29:1734–1740, 2004

Strakowski SM, Delbello MP, Adler CM: The functional neuroanatomy of bipolar disorder: a review of neuroimaging findings. Mol Psychiatry 10:105–116, 2005

Stuss DT, Levine B: Adult clinical neuropsychology: lessons from studies of the frontal lobes. Annu Rev Psychol 53:401–433, 2002

Swann AC, Pazzaglia P, Nicholls A, et al: Impulsivity and phase of illness in bipolar disorder. J Affect Disord 73:105–111, 2003

Swann AC, Dougherty DM, Pazzaglia PJ, et al: Increased impulsivity associated with severity of suicide attempt history in patients with bipolar disorder. Am J Psychiatry 162:1680–1687, 2005

Sweeney JA, Kmiec JA, Kupfer DJ: Neuropsychologic impairments in bipolar and unipolar mood disorders on the CANTAB neurocognitive battery. Biol Psychiatry 48:674–684, 2000

Tam WC, Sewell KW, Deng HC: Information processing in schizophrenia and bipolar disorder: a discriminant analysis. J Nerv Ment Dis 186:597–603, 1998

Tham A, Engelbrektson K, Mathe AA, et al: Impaired neuropsychological performance in euthymic patients with recurring mood disorders. J Clin Psychiatry 58:26–29, 1997

Thompson JM, Gallagher P, Hughes JH, et al: Neurocognitive impairment in euthymic patients with bipolar affective disorder. Br J Psychiatry 186:32–40, 2005

Trichard C, Martinot JL, Alagille M, et al: Time course of prefrontal lobe dysfunction in severely depressed in-patients: a longitudinal neuropsychological study. Psychol Med 25:79–85, 1995

van den Bosch RJ, Rombouts RP, van Asma MJ: What determines Continuous Performance Task performance? Schizophr Bull 22:643–651, 1996

van Gorp WG, Altshuler L, Theberge DC, et al: Cognitive impairment in euthymic bipolar patients with and without prior alcohol dependence. A preliminary study. Arch Gen Psychiatry 55:41–46, 1998

Vataja R, Pohjasvaara T, Leppavuori A, et al: Magnetic resonance imaging correlates of depression after ischemic stroke. Arch Gen Psychiatry 58:925–931, 2001

Zubieta JK, Huguelet P, O'Neil RL, et al: Cognitive function in euthymic bipolar I disorder. Psychiatry Res 102:9–20, 2001

3

Memory Deficits Associated With Bipolar Disorder

Safa Elgamal, M.D., M.Sc., Ph.D.
Marta Sokolowska, Ph.D.
Glenda MacQueen, M.D., Ph.D.

The first studies to demonstrate that patients with bipolar disorder have problems with aspects of memory function were generally focused on patients in the manic state; subsequently, verbal memory deficits have been suggested as a core cognitive deficit associated with acute mania (Clark et al. 2001). Given that acute mania is associated with the dysregulation of a multitude of brain systems, it is perhaps not surprising that memory is also impaired. Although the general assumption in the past was that memory recovered with resolution of the acute phase of illness, evidence suggests that functional recovery of all memory systems is not complete (Ferrier et al. 2004); the impact of bipolar disorder on certain aspects of memory is substantial, detectable even in the euthymic or asymptomatic phase of the disease (Ferrier et al. 1999; Kessing 1998; Thompson et al. 2005), and perhaps a function of total illness burden. Despite recognition that memory deficits may persist into the euthymic phase of illness, there is an unfortunate paucity of data examining the extent to which these deficits contribute to the ongoing functional impairment that is apparent in some people with bipolar disorder.

This work was supported by the Ontario Mental Health Foundation.

In this chapter, we summarize the literature examining memory deficits in patients with bipolar disorder, focusing on studies evaluating verbal and visual explicit memory, implicit memory, and working memory, with particular attention given to whether patients were assessed when symptomatic or euthymic. The term *memory* encompasses several relatively discrete neural systems (see Figure 3–1), and although a discussion of the neurobiological underpinnings of each system is beyond the scope of this chapter, we outline the commonly recognized memory systems and separately discuss the impairment associated with bipolar disorder for each system.

Explicit Memory

Explicit memory, which can also be called *declarative memory*, requires conscious and intentional recollection of information that can be assessed directly by measures of recall and recognition. Examples include the type of conscious memorization that occurs through deliberate practice, such as when committing a poem to memory or rehearsing lines for a play. Explicit memory includes both semantic and episodic forms: *Semantic memory* is related to factual knowledge and language acquisition and is generally resistant to decline until extensive neural damage occurs, such as in dementia. There is no reliable evidence that semantic memory is impaired in mood disorder. *Episodic memory*, which is the memory for past events, is more vulnerable, however, and is impaired in several psychiatric disorders, including bipolar disorder. Because explicit memory performance is dependent on the modality examined, we review verbal and visual episodic memory separately.

Verbal Memory

Patients With Symptomatic Bipolar Disorder

Verbal episodic memory is commonly assessed in the laboratory using verbal learning lists or paragraph recall. Most studies addressing verbal memory in mood disorder used the California Verbal Learning Test (CVLT) (Delis et al. 1987) or the Rey Auditory Verbal Learning Test (RAVLT) (Rey 1964), both of which include measures of immediate and delayed recall, free and cued recall, and recognition. The Wechsler Memory Scale—Revised (WMS-R) (Wechsler 1987) tests paragraph recall, measuring both the immediate and delayed components of verbal memory. Several studies have evaluated verbal memory function in bipolar patients across a range of mood states, and generally have reported that patients with bipolar disorder are impaired on tests of recall even in the euthymic state, whereas recognition is generally affected only in the symptomatic phase of illness (Basso et al. 2002; Fleck et al. 2003; Martinez-Aran et al. 2004a; Wolfe et al. 1987).

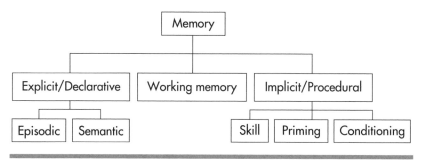

FIGURE 3–1. Memory subsystems.

When assessed on both recall and recognition using the RAVLT, de-pressed patients with bipolar disorder had impaired performance compared with healthy controls or patients with unipolar depression (Wolfe et al. 1987). The performance of affectively ill patients with recurrent episodes, whether bipolar or unipolar, was impaired when compared with that of controls on measures of free recall but not on measures of cued recall or recognition using Grober et al.'s (1988) free and cued selective reminding procedure (Fossati et al. 2002, 2004). Patients with bipolar disorder over-all appear to use a similar semantic clustering (i.e., organizational) strategy to that used by healthy controls but nevertheless show impaired encoding of verbal information (Bearden et al. 2006). Notably, however, recent data suggest that a subgroup of bipolar patients who carry an identified risk al-lele in the gene encoding catechol *O*-methyltransferase may utilize seman-tic clustering strategies less efficiently than do bipolar patients without the risk allele (Burdick et al. 2007).

After controlling for sex, education, and parental socioeconomic status, Seidman et al. (2002) found that patients with bipolar disorder (manic/ mixed subtype with psychotic features) performed poorly compared with controls on the Logical Memory subtest of the WMS-R (Wechsler 1987) as a measure of verbal memory. However, Coffman et al. (1990) reported no difference between manic psychotic patients and normal controls on the delayed recall trials of WMS and WMS-R.

Patients With Euthymic Bipolar Disorder

In general, most studies report that recall memory (a subtype of explicit/ declarative memory) remains impaired in patients with euthymic bipolar disorder (Depp et al. 2007; Goswami et al. 2006; Martinez-Aran et al. 2000; Quraishi and Frangou 2002). Several investigators found recall def-icits in these patients when assessed with the CVLT (Altshuler et al. 2004; Cavanagh et al. 2002; Depp et al. 2007; Doris et al. 2004; Martinez-Aran et al. 2004a; van Gorp et al. 1998, 1999) or the RAVLT (Krabbendam et al. 2000). Results of testing patients with first-episode mood disorder using the CVLT and the WMS-R suggested that only those patients who had psychotic features were impaired in recall relative to normal controls; in contrast to other studies, this may reflect a difference in the past illness burden between first- and multiple-episode patients (Albus et al. 1996).

Some investigators have found that the degree of recollection impairment diminishes when key variables are controlled. For example, Clark et al. (2002) observed that after they controlled for mood symptoms, the detected impairment in immediate recall on the CVLT dissipated. Others similarly found that the deficit observed on the RAVLT disappeared after controlling for age, intelligence quotient (IQ), and mood symptoms (Ferrier et al. 1999). Impaired learning of new verbal information in patients with bipolar disorder appears associated with blunted increases in regional cerebral blood flow in the left dorsolateral prefrontal cortex during encoding, as compared with that of healthy controls (Deckersbach et al. 2006).

Although recollection memory impairment is consistently reported in patients with bipolar disorder, few studies have demonstrated recognition impairment in euthymic patients (Smith et al. 2006; Watson et al. 2006). Watson et al. (2006) reported that the deficit in euthymic patients was significant for recognition but that verbal learning and delayed recall did not reach significance on the RAVLT. Patients with bipolar I or bipolar II disorder showed recall and recognition deficits when compared with healthy controls, but the deficits were more pronounced in patients with bipolar I diagnoses (Torrent et al. 2006). Both euthymic patients and healthy controls obtained nearly perfect scores on the recognition components of memory tasks, raising the possibility that the tests may not have detected subtle differences between groups if the sample sizes were not large enough (Clark et al. 2002; Fleck et al. 2003).

A summary of the results of studies examining verbal memory in patients with bipolar disorder is presented in Table 3–1.

Visual Memory

A variety of measures are used to assess explicit episodic visual memory, but the most commonly used are pattern and spatial recognition memory tasks using geometric patterns and spatial locations; the Visual Reproduction subtest of the WMS, including immediate and delayed design reproduction; the Rey-Osterrieth Complex Figure (ROCF) Test, which involves drawing complex figures from memory; and the delayed matching-to-sample task. A synopsis of the studies evaluating visual explicit memory in patients with bipolar disorder is presented in Table 3–2.

TABLE 3–1. Verbal memory in patients with bipolar disorder

Test	Study	Mood state	Finding(s)
CVLT	Smith et al. 2006	Euthymic	Recall and recognition: BD<HC and UD
	Altshuler et al. 2004	Euthymic, male	Recall: S=BD<HC
			Recognition: BD=S=HC
	Doris et al. 2004	Euthymic	Recall: BD<HC
	Martinez-Aran et al. 2004a	Euthymic	Recall and recognition: BD<HC
	Cavanagh et al. 2002	Euthymic	Immediate and delayed recall and recognition (false positives): BD<HC
	Clark et al. 2002	Euthymic	Verbal learning: BD<HC
	van Gorp et al. 1999	Euthymic (±alcohol dependence)	Free recall: BD+alcohol<HC
			Learning and cued recall: BD+alcohol<BD±alcohol<HC
	van Gorp et al. 1998	Euthymic (±alcohol dependence)	Total and cued recall: BD+alcohol and BD±alcohol<HC
			Free recall: BD+alcohol<HC
	Fleck et al. 2003	BD in mixed/manic or euthymic state	Free recall: E and M<HC
			Recognition: M<E and HC
	Basso et al. 2002	BD in manic, mixed, or depressed state	Standard scores: D, M, and mixed<HC
	Clark et al. 2001	Manic	Immediate recall: BD<HC
CVLT and WMS-R	Martinez-Aran et al. 2004b	BD in manic/depressed vs. euthymic state	Recall (CVLT): E, M, and D<HC
			Recognition: M and D<HC
			Recall (WMS-R): M, D<HC
CVLT and WMS-R	Albus et al. 1996	Euthymic, FE, BD, and UD±psychotic feature	Free recall: BD+UD<HC

TABLE 3–1. Verbal memory in patients with bipolar disorder *(continued)*

Test	Study	Mood state	Finding(s)
CVLT and selective reminding test	Ali et al. 2000	Mixed (euthymic, mildly hypomanic, and mildly depressed)	Immediate free and cued recall and total recall: BD<HC
CVLT, Brown-Peterson test, and WMS-R	Bora et al. 2005	Twins; mixed (euthymic, manic, and depressed)	BD twins<HC twins
RAVLT	Watson et al. 2006	Euthymic	Recognition: BD<HC
	Bora et al. 2005	Euthymic	Recall and recognition: BD<HC
	Krabbendam et al. 2000	Euthymic	Immediate and delayed recall: BD<HC
	Ferrier et al. 1999	Euthymic	BD<HC After controlling for age, IQ, and affective symptoms: BD=HC
	Wolfe et al. 1987	BD depressed	Recall: BD<UD<HC Recognition: BD<UD<HC
RAVLT and Digit Span Forward	Thompson et al. 2005	Euthymic BD	Learning and recall: BD=HC BD<HC
WMS-R logical memory	Seidman et al. 2002	Manic/mixed subtype with psychotic features	BD<HC
WMS-R	Mojtabai et al. 2000	BD with psychotic features	S<BD and S<BD+UD
WMS-R	Coffman et al. 1990	Not stated	BD=HC

TABLE 3–1. Verbal memory in patients with bipolar disorder *(continued)*

Test	Study	Mood state	Finding(s)
Free and cued selective reminding procedure	Fossati et al. 2004	FE depression, and multiple episodes UD and BD	First free recall: BD=UD<FE=HC Total free recall: BD=UD<HC
Free and cued selective reminding procedure	Fossati et al. 2002	BD depressed+major depression	Free recall: BD+UD<HC
Babcock Story Recall Test[a] and Buschke Selective Reminding Test[b]	Jones et al. 1994	Not stated	BD=HC

Note. BD=bipolar disorder; CVLT=California Verbal Learning Test (Delis et al. 1987); D=depressed state; E=euthymic state; FE=first episode; HC=healthy controls; IQ=intelligence quotient; M=manic state; RAVLT=Rey Auditory Verbal Learning Test (Rey 1964); S=schizophrenia; UD=unipolar depression); WMS-R=Wechsler Memory Scale—Revised (Wechsler 1987).
[a]Babcock and Levy 1940.
[b]Buschke and Fold 1974.

TABLE 3–2.   Visual explicit memory in patients with bipolar disorder

Mood state	Study	Method(s)	Finding(s)
Euthymic	Thompson et al. 2005	CANTAB Spatial Span	Immediate memory: BD<HC
	Deckersbach et al. 2004	ROCF	Immediate and delayed recall: BD<HC
	Sapin et al. 1987	Facial recognition tasks, Block Design of WAIS-R, and Benton Visual Retention Test	BD=HC
	van Gorp et al. 1998	ROCF and 3-minute delayed recall	BD=HC (regardless of alcohol dependence)
	Ferrier et al. 1999	ROCF	Recall: BD<HC
			After controlling for age, IQ, and affective symptoms: BD=HC
	Altshuler et al. 2004	ROCF	Male subjects: S<BD=HC
	Rubinsztein et al. 2000	Pattern and spatial recognition memory and delayed matching-to-sample test	Proportion correct: BD<HC
Manic	Murphy et al. 1999	Pattern and spatial recognition memory and simultaneous and delayed matching-to-sample test	Proportion correct and response latency: BD<HC
Depressed and manic/ mixed BD with psychotic features	Sweeney et al. 2000	Pattern and spatial recognition memory task	BD (manic/mixed)<UD and HC
BD in manic/depressed and euthymic state	Martinez-Aran et al. 2004b	WMS-R Visual Reproduction	Immediate recall: D<HC Delayed recall: D and M<HC
Twins; mixed (euthymic, manic, and depressed)	Gourovitch et al. 1999	WMS-R Visual Reproduction, ROCF, and facial recognition	Facial recognition: BD twin<unaffected twin Other tests: BD twin = unaffected twin

TABLE 3–2. Visual explicit memory in patients with bipolar disorder *(continued)*

Mood state	Study	Method(s)	Finding(s)
Manic/mixed and depressed	Goldberg et al. 1993	WMS-R Visual Reproduction	S<BD=UD
Euthymic, FE, BD, and UD patients ± psychotic feature	Albus et al. 1996	WMS-R Visual Reproduction	Mood disorders+psychotic features<HC
BD with psychotic features	Mojtabai et al. 2000	WMS-R Visual Reproduction	S<BD
Not stated (BD with psychotic features)	Coffman et al. 1990	WMS-R Visual Reproduction	BD<HC
Not stated	Jones et al. 1994	ROCF	BD=HC

Note. BD=bipolar disorder; CANTAB=Cambridge Neuropsychological Test Automated Battery; D=depressed state; FE=first episode; HC=healthy controls; IQ=intelligence quotient; M=manic state; ROCF: Rey-Osterrieth Complex Figure Test; S=schizophrenia; UD=unipolar depression; WAIS-R=Wechsler Adult Intelligence Scale—Revised (Wechsler 1981); WMS-R=Wechsler Memory Scale–Revised (Wechsler 1987).

Patients With Symptomatic Bipolar Disorder

In one study, the performance of patients was impaired relative to that of controls on delayed but not on simultaneous matching-to-sample tasks, and on mean proportions of correct responses and latency to respond for pattern and spatial recognition (Murphy et al. 1999). Using the same pattern and spatial recognition task used by Murphy et al. (1999), Sweeney et al. (2000) found that the proportion of correct responses produced by patients during mixed or manic states was lower than that of healthy controls and patients with major depression.

On the Visual Reproduction subtest of the WMS-R, delayed nonverbal recall was impaired in manic and depressed patients with bipolar disorder compared with controls, whereas immediate recall was impaired only in depressed patients with bipolar disorder (Martinez-Aran et al. 2004b). Using the same subtest, only bipolar patients with psychotic features had impaired performance compared with that of healthy controls (Albus et al. 1996; Coffman et al. 1990). Psychotic patients with bipolar disorder, however, performed better than those with schizophrenia on measures of immediate and delayed visual memory, suggesting that psychosis in people with bipolar disorder rendered them intermediate in performance compared with nonpsychotic patients with bipolar disorder and patients with both bipolar and psychotic disorders (Mojtabai et al. 2000). Consistent with this, Goldberg et al. (1993) found that in a comparison of patients with bipolar disorder, unipolar depression, or schizophrenia, those with mood disorders performed better than people with schizophrenia. Using a delayed non-matching-to-sample task, Glahn et al. (2006) observed that although both patients with bipolar disorder and patients with schizophrenia showed deficits in using contextual cues to detect novel visual stimuli (independent of symptom severity), bipolar patients also showed difficulty in holistic processing (i.e., forming a gestalt) when encoding information.

Patients With Euthymic Bipolar Disorder

Nonverbal organizational strategies during encoding, rather than deficits in retention, appear to differentiate patients with euthymic bipolar disorder from healthy controls (Deckersbach et al. 2004). Euthymic patients had a lower proportion of correct responses than healthy controls when pattern and spatial recognition were assessed in patients who had been in remission for at least 4 months (Rubinsztein et al. 2000). A similar deficit was also reported using the ROCF in euthymic patients (Ferrier et al. 1999). Moreover, clinically stable patients with psychotic features performed at levels equivalent to those of patients with schizophrenia and performed poorly compared with controls on copy and recall accuracy of the ROCF (Seidman et al. 2003). In contrast, however, other investigators reported that visual memory was not impaired in euthymic patients (Altshuler et al. 2004; Jones et al. 1994; van Gorp et al. 1998). Employing the Benton Visual Retention Test, the Wechsler Adult Intelligence Scale—Revised (WAIS-R) Block Design subtest, and two facial recognition tasks to examine visuospatial memory, Sapin et al. (1987) reported no difference between patients with euthymic bipolar disorder and controls, except that the patients with bipolar disorder had more difficulty in recognizing masked faces. Similarly, no significant immediate or delayed visual memory decline was observed in euthymic patients on the Visual Reproduction subtest of the WMS-R (Martinez-Aran et al. 2004b). Thus, it is apparent that studies of visual explicit memory in euthymic patients have generated conflicting findings; much of the discrepancy between studies may be accounted for by the variability in tasks that have been used to examine visual memory in this population.

In summary, symptomatic patients generally demonstrate impaired episodic memory function regardless of whether the verbal or visual domain is assessed. Results from euthymic patients are inconsistent; however, studies of verbal recall favor that the impairment extends into the euthymic phase, whereas studies of visual memory in euthymic patients have produced inconsistent findings.

Implicit Memory

Implicit memory, which is also identified as *nondeclarative* or *procedural memory*, includes the acquisition of skills, priming, and conditioning. In contrast to explicit memory, implicit memory does not require intentional and conscious recollection of learned material; examples include driving a car, playing a musical instrument, or correctly speaking one's native language. Retention and retrieval are exhibited without the awareness of remembering the event; thus, implicit memory is assessed using indirect measures such as word-fragment or word-stem completion, word identification priming, and picture naming priming.

Although explicit memory function in patients with bipolar disorder has been studied in some detail, only a few studies have evaluated implicit memory in these patients. Kwapil et al. (1990) found that performance of patients with bipolar disorder on recognition of semantic priming was similar to that of healthy controls and better than that of patients with schizophrenia. Implicit memory was examined in euthymic patients using the Star Mirror Tracing Task and the Pursuit Rotor Motor Learning Test. In this study, patients' performance was similar to that of controls, and a history of alcohol dependence did not affect the results (Altshuler et al. 2004; van Gorp et al. 1999). This is not surprising, given that implicit memory is not impaired in patients with Korsakoff syndrome (Kopelman and Corn 1988).

Working Memory

Working memory is a multicomponent system that requires the ability to temporarily store and simultaneously manipulate information (Baddeley 2001). According to Baddeley (1992), working memory involves a central executive system that modulates two main subsystems, the phonological and the visuospatial (for detailed explanation, see Baddeley 2001). Tasks may access different aspects of working memory or be dependent on other cognitive functions, such as attention, and in fact, there is no agreed-on border that delineates an attention task from a working memory task. The results of studies examining working memory in bipolar patients are summarized in Table 3–3.

The results of studies examining working memory in *symptomatic* bipolar disorder patients favor the existence of a working memory deficit, but this deficit may be a state marker of psychosis (McGrath et al. 2001). In one study, patients in a mixed/manic episode but not in a depressive episode performed poorly on a spatial working memory task, supporting the notion that this impairment is not related to a persistent neuropsychological deficit (Sweeney et al. 2000). In a more recent study, however, both symptomatic and euthymic patients performed equivalently to healthy controls on a Delayed Response Task as a measure of spatial delayed working memory (Larson et al. 2005). Another study of working memory indicated that independent of psychosis, nondepressed, first-episode bipolar patients performed comparably to healthy controls (Albus et al. 1996).

In contrast to studies of symptomatic patients, the majority of studies evaluating *euthymic* patients do not report problems with working memory. Euthymic patients were significantly impaired compared with controls on a visual memory span backward task, but the difference was not apparent when age, premorbid intelligence, and depressive symptoms were controlled; the deficit on a digit backward test remained significant even after controlling for such variables (Ferrier et al. 1999). The digit backward test is presumably a measure of working memory, executive functioning, and sustained attention; therefore, patients demonstrating a deficit on this task may not have a working memory deficit, because impaired sustained attention or executive functioning may contribute to the decline. Patients in another study performed at lower levels than controls on a non–working memory vigilance task (attention), although the groups performed similarly on a working memory vigilance task, supporting the notion of a deficit in sustained attention rather than working memory (Harmer et al. 2002).

In contrast to studies reporting intact working memory in euthymic patients, a recent study found that euthymic patients made more omission and commission errors than controls on the Sternberg paradigm as a measure of

TABLE 3–3. Working memory in patients with bipolar disorder

Mood state	Study	Method(s)	Finding(s)
Mania	Badcock et al. 2005	Spatial span task	Storage capacity: BD<HC
	Larson et al. 2005	Delayed Response Task	BD=HC
	McGrath et al. 2001	Visuospatial delayed response task	Percentage correct: BD<HC
	Sweeney et al. 2000	Spatial working memory test	Manic/mixed BD with psychotic features<HC
Euthymia	Watson et al. 2006	Sternberg paradigm	Errors of omission and commission: BD<HC
	Pirkola et al. 2005	WMS-R visual memory span and digit span	BD=HC
	Adler et al. 2004	Two-back working memory task	Percentage correct: BD<HC Trend: P=0.1 Reaction time: BD=HC
	Larson et al. 2005	Delayed Response Task	BD=HC
	Monks et al. 2004	Two-back working memory task	Male: BD=HC
	Harmer et al. 2002	Working memory vigilance test	BD=HC
	Gooding and Tallent 2001	Spatial working memory test	Reaction time: BD<HC Accuracy: BD=HC
	Ferrier et al. 1999	Digit span backward and visual memory span	BD<HC
FE mood disorder	Albus et al. 1996	WAIS-R (digit span) and reading span test	After covarying: BD=HC Mood disorders±psychotic feature=HC

Note. BD=bipolar disorder; FE=first episode; HC=healthy controls; WAIS-R=Wechsler Adult Intelligence Scale—Revised (Wechsler 1981); WMS-R=Wechsler Memory Scale—Revised (Wechsler 1987).

working memory (Watson et al. 2006). In another study, patients performed as accurately as matched controls on a spatial working memory task, but had significantly longer reaction times (Gooding and Tallent 2001). These studies suggest that working memory problems may be apparent on specific aspects of certain tasks, although the nature of the underlying deficit that would result in the specific patterns observed is unknown.

Factors Associated With Memory Problems in Bipolar Disorder

Several factors may contribute to memory performance in people with bipolar disorder. In addition to current illness state, there may be long-term effects of illness that accrue with repeated episodes and longer duration of illness. Medications may have either a salutary or negative effect on performance, as discussed in greater detail in Chapter 7 of this volume, "Adverse Cognitive Effects of Psychotropic Medications." Comorbid conditions, particularly substance use disorders, may have a detrimental effect. The results of a study of memory in euthymic bipolar disorder patients with and without a history of alcohol dependence suggest that patients with a positive history demonstrated more impaired CVLT performance than did patients with no history or healthy controls; several measures of cognitive function in patients were correlated with the age at onset of alcohol dependence (van Gorp et al. 1998).

Severity of memory impairment correlated with number of manic-depressive episodes in euthymic patients in many (Cavanagh et al. 2002; Clark et al. 2002; Denicoff et al. 1999; Fossati et al. 2002; Martinez-Aran et al. 2004b) but not all (Ferrier et al. 1999; Rubinsztein et al. 2000) studies. Most studies (Cavanagh et al. 2002; Clark et al. 2002; Denicoff et al. 1999; Martinez-Aran et al. 2004b; van Gorp et al. 1998) found that duration of illness has a negative effect on memory that is apparent in the euthymic state. However, Depp et al. (2007) suggested that the deficit is not related to the duration of illness or severity of mood symptoms.

Number of hospitalizations and months of hospitalization have been reported to negatively influence patients' performance on the delayed matching-to-sample test (Rubinsztein et al. 2000) and on the CVLT (Martinez-Aran et al. 2004b) but not on the pattern and spatial recognition test (Rubinsztein et al. 2000) or the Claeson-Dahl Verbal Learning Test, Retention Test, and Memory for Design Test (Tham et al. 1997).

Conclusions

Although studies evaluating memory in people with bipolar disorder have yielded conflicting results in some domains, consistent trends are apparent.

There is some agreement that verbal memory deficits are present even in the euthymic state and that visual memory is impaired in the symptomatic phase but not reliably found to be impaired in the euthymic phase. It remains to be definitively established whether much of the impairment observed for verbal memory is accounted for by residual symptoms, concurrent medication use, or other factors (e.g., past substance use). Within the confines of the very limited research available on implicit memory in patients with bipolar disorder, it appears that implicit memory is not impaired in patients with bipolar disorder, but priming may be impaired. The results of studies evaluating working memory in patients with euthymic bipolar disorder vary; some studies demonstrate working memory impairment whereas others do not. However, working memory appears to be reliably impaired in symptomatic patients.

Several factors that influence performance on tests of memory have been identified, including duration of illness, number of episodes, hospitalization, excessive alcohol consumption, and pharmacological treatments. Careful identification of the factors that might affect memory is essential for reliable assessment of memory in this clinical population. Tests must be reliable and valid without floor or ceiling effects. The sample sizes of studies examining patients with bipolar disorder should be large enough to ensure sufficient power in the study. Small sample sizes are associated with limited power and an increased possibility of type II errors. Thus, in many studies to date, the conclusion that no differences between groups exist may have been accepted when the clinical sample was, in fact, impaired. This is a particularly relevant possibility if researchers assume that only a portion of a clinical sample might have a significant degree of impairment, thereby increasing the risk of failing to recognize the valid impairment in this subgroup of patients. Future studies, therefore, will benefit from rigorous assessment of the patient and comparison groups, adequate sample sizes, and tests with strong psychometric properties.

Take-Home Points

- Verbal memory deficits in patients with bipolar disorder are evident in both euthymic and symptomatic phases of illness.
- Visual memory deficits are evident in patients only during affectively symptomatic phases of illness.
- Working memory deficits are evident in patients only during affectively symptomatic phases of illness.
- There is presently not sufficient evidence to indicate implicit or semantic memory dysfunction in patients with bipolar disorder.

- Multiple factors likely contribute to impaired memory performance in patients with bipolar disorder, although they are not presently well understood. Remedial strategies to help compensate for memory deficits may include writing lists and using written reminders for appointments.

- Patients with bipolar disorder as a whole may not necessarily benefit from memory strategies designed to overcome deficits in semantic clustering (e.g., "chunking" groups of semantically related concepts) or difficulties utilizing visual versus verbal or auditory modes of presentation (e.g., reviewing written notes vs. audiotaping a lecture), because these domains are generally intact for most patients with bipolar disorder. Nevertheless, mnemonic devices such as these could be potentially useful to a given patient based on his or her individual strengths and weaknesses.

References

Adler CM, Holland SK, Schmithorst V, et al: Changes in neuronal activation in patients with bipolar disorder during performance of a working memory task. Bipolar Disord 6:540–549, 2004

Albus M, Hubmann W, Wahlheim C, et al: Contrasts in neuropsychological test profile between patients with first-episode schizophrenia and first-episode affective disorders. Acta Psychiatr Scand 94:87–93, 1996

Ali SO, Denicoff KD, Altshuler LL, et al: A preliminary study of the relation of neuropsychological performance to neuroanatomic structures in bipolar disorder. Neuropsychiatry Neuropsychol Behav Neurol 13:20–28, 2000

Altshuler LL, Ventura J, van Gorp WG, et al: Neurocognitive function in clinically stable men with bipolar I disorder or schizophrenia and normal control subjects. Biol Psychiatry 56:560–569, 2004

Babcock H, Levy L: The Measurement of Efficiency of Mental Functioning (Revised Examination): Test and Manual of Directions. Chicago, IL, C.H. Stotling, 1940

Badcock JC, Michiel PT, Rock D: Spatial working memory and planning ability: contrasts between schizophrenia and bipolar I disorder. Cortex 41:753–763, 2005

Baddeley A: Working memory. Science 255:556–559, 1992

Baddeley AD: Is working memory still working? Am Psychol 56:851–864, 2001

Basso MR, Lowery N, Neel J, et al: Neuropsychological impairment among manic, depressed, and mixed-episode inpatients with bipolar disorder. Neuropsychology 16:84–91, 2002

Bearden CE, Glahn DC, Monkul ES, et al: Sources of declarative memory impairment in bipolar disorder: mnemonic processes and clinical features. J Psychiatr Res 40:47–58, 2006

Bora E, Vahip S, Gonul AS, et al: Evidence for theory of mind deficits in euthymic patients with bipolar disorder. Acta Psychiatr Scand 112:110–116, 2005

Burdick KE, Funke B, Goldberg JF, et al: COMT genotype increases risk for bipolar I disorder and influences neurocognitive performance. Bipolar Disord 9:370–376, 2007

Buschke H, Fold PA: Evaluating storage, retention, and retrieval in disordered memory and learning. Neurology 24:1019–1025, 1074

Cavanagh JT, Van BM, Muir W, et al: Case-control study of neurocognitive function in euthymic patients with bipolar disorder: an association with mania. Br J Psychiatry 180:320–326, 2002

Clark L, Iversen SD, Goodwin GM: A neuropsychological investigation of prefrontal cortex involvement in acute mania. Am J Psychiatry 158:1605–1611, 2001

Clark L, Iversen SD, Goodwin GM: Sustained attention deficit in bipolar disorder. Br J Psychiatry 180:313–319, 2002

Coffman JA, Bornstein RA, Olson SC, et al: Cognitive impairment and cerebral structure by MRI in bipolar disorder. Biol Psychiatry 27:1188–1196, 1990

Deckersbach T, McMurrich S, Oqutha J, et al: Characteristics of non-verbal memory impairment in bipolar disorder: the role of encoding strategies. Psychol Med 34:823–832, 2004

Deckersbach T, Dougherty DD, Savage C, et al: Impaired recruitment of the dorsolateral prefrontal cortex and hippocampus during encoding in bipolar disorder. Biol Psychiatry 59:138–146, 2006

Delis DC, Karmaer JH, Kaplan E, et al: California Verbal Learning Test, Adult Research Edition. New York, Psychological Corporation, 1987

Denicoff KD, Ali SO, Mirsky AF, et al: Relationship between prior course of illness and neuropsychological functioning in patients with bipolar disorder. J Affect Disord 56:67–73, 1999

Depp CA, Moore DJ, Sitzer D, et al: Neurocognitive impairment in middle-aged and older adults with bipolar disorder: comparison to schizophrenia and normal comparison subjects. J Affect Disord 101:201–209, 2007

Doris A, Belton E, Ebmeier KP, et al: Reduction of cingulate gray matter density in poor outcome bipolar illness. Psychiatry Res 130:153–159, 2004

Ferrier IN, Stanton BR, Kelly TP, et al: Neuropsychological function in euthymic patients with bipolar disorder. Br J Psychiatry 175:246–251, 1999

Ferrier IN, Chowdhury R, Thompson JM, et al: Neurocognitive function in unaffected first-degree relatives of patients with bipolar disorder: a preliminary report. Bipolar Disord 6:319–322, 2004

Fleck DE, Shear PK, Zimmerman ME, et al: Verbal memory in mania: effects of clinical state and task requirements. Bipolar Disord 5:375–380, 2003

Fossati P, Coyette F, Ergis AM, et al: Influence of age and executive functioning on verbal memory of inpatients with depression. J Affect Disord 68:261–271, 2002

Fossati P, Harvey PO, Le Bastard G, et al: Verbal memory performance of patients with a first depressive episode and patients with unipolar and bipolar recurrent depression. J Psychiatr Res 38:137–144, 2004

Glahn DC, Barrett J, Bearden CE, et al: Dissociable mechanisms for memory impairment in bipolar disorder and schizophrenia. Psychol Med 36:1085–1095, 2006

Goldberg TE, Gold JM, Greenberg R, et al: Contrasts between patients with affective disorders and patients with schizophrenia on a neuropsychological test battery. Am J Psychiatry 150:1355–1362, 1993

Gooding DC, Tallent KA: The association between antisaccade task and working memory task performance in schizophrenia and bipolar disorder. J Nerv Ment Dis 189:8–16, 2001

Goswami U, Sharma A, Khastigir U, et al: Neuropsychological dysfunction, soft neurological signs and social disability in euthymic patients with bipolar disorder. Br J Psychiatry 188:366–373, 2006

Gourovitch ML, Torrey EF, Gold JM, et al: Neuropsychological performance of monozygotic twins discordant for bipolar disorder. Biol Psychiatry 45:639–646, 1999

Grober E, Buschke H, Crystal H, et al: Screening for dementia by memory testing. Neurology 38:900–903, 1988

Harmer CJ, Clark L, Grayson L, et al: Sustained attention deficit in bipolar disorder is not a working memory impairment in disguise. Neuropsychologia 40:1586–1590, 2002

Jones BP, Duncan CC, Mirsky AF, et al: Neuropsychological profiles in bipolar affective disorder and complex partial seizure disorder. Neuropsychology 8:55–64, 1994

Kessing LV: Cognitive impairment in the euthymic phase of affective disorder. Psychol Med 28:1027–1038, 1998

Kopelman MD, Corn TH: Cholinergic "blockade" as a model for cholinergic depletion: a comparison of the memory deficits with those of Alzheimer-type dementia and the alcoholic Korsakoff syndrome. Brain 111:1079–1110, 1988

Krabbendam L, Honig A, Wiersma J, et al: Cognitive dysfunctions and white matter lesions in patients with bipolar disorder in remission. Acta Psychiatr Scand 101:274–280, 2000

Kwapil TR, Hegley DC, Chapman LJ, et al: Facilitation of word recognition by semantic priming in schizophrenia. J Abnorm Psychol 99:215–221, 1990

Larson ER, Shear PK, Krikorian R, et al: Working memory and inhibitory control among manic and euthymic patients with bipolar disorder. J Int Neuropsychol Soc 11:163–172, 2005

Martinez-Aran A, Vieta E, Colom F, et al: Cognitive dysfunctions in bipolar disorder: evidence of neuropsychological disturbances. Psychother Psychosom 69:2–18, 2000

Martinez-Aran A, Vieta E, Colom F, et al: Cognitive impairment in euthymic bipolar patients: implications for clinical and functional outcome. Bipolar Disord 6:224–232, 2004a

Martinez-Aran A, Vieta E, Reinares M, et al: Cognitive function across manic or hypomanic, depressed, and euthymic states in bipolar disorder. Am J Psychiatry 161:262–270, 2004b

McGrath J, Chapple B, Wright M: Working memory in schizophrenia and mania: correlation with symptoms during the acute and subacute phases. Acta Psychiatr Scand 103:181–188, 2001

Mojtabai R, Bromet EJ, Harvey PD, et al: Neuropsychological differences between first-admission schizophrenia and psychotic affective disorders. Am J Psychiatry 157:1453–1460, 2000

Monks PJ, Thompson JM, Bullmore ET, et al: A functional MRI study of working memory task in euthymic bipolar disorder: evidence for task-specific dysfunction. Bipolar Disord 6:550–564, 2004

Murphy FC, Sahakian BJ, Rubinsztein JS, et al: Emotional bias and inhibitory control processes in mania and depression. Psychol Med 29:1307–1321, 1999

Pirkola T, Tuulio-Henriksson A, Glahn D, et al: Spatial working memory function in twins with schizophrenia and bipolar disorder. Biol Psychiatry 58:930–936, 2005

Quraishi S, Frangou S: Neuropsychology of bipolar disorder: a review. J Affect Disord 72:209–226, 2002

Rey A: L'Examen Clinique en Psychologie. Paris, Presses Universitaires de France, 1964

Rubinsztein JS, Michael A, Paykel ES, et al: Cognitive impairment in remission in bipolar affective disorder. Psychol Med 30:1025–1036, 2000

Sapin LR, Berrettini WH, Nurnberger JI Jr, et al: Mediational factors underlying cognitive changes and laterality in affective illness. Biol Psychiatry 22:979–986, 1987

Seidman LJ, Kremen WS, Koren D, et al: A comparative profile analysis of neuropsychological functioning in patients with schizophrenia and bipolar psychoses. Schizophr Res 53:31–44, 2002

Seidman LJ, Lanca M, Kremen WS, et al: Organizational and visual memory deficits in schizophrenia and bipolar psychoses using the Rey-Osterrieth complex figure: effects of duration of illness. J Clin Exp Neuropsychol 25:949–964, 2003

Smith DJ, Muir WJ, Blackwood DH: Neurocognitive impairment in euthymic young adults with bipolar spectrum disorder and recurrent major depressive disorder. Bipolar Disord 8:40–46, 2006

Sweeney JA, Kmiec JA, Kupfer DJ: Neuropsychologic impairments in bipolar and unipolar mood disorders on the CANTAB neurocognitive battery. Biol Psychiatry 48:674–684, 2000

Tham A, Engelbrektson K, Mathe AA, et al: Impaired neuropsychological performance in euthymic patients with recurring mood disorders. J Clin Psychiatry 58:26–29, 1997

Thompson JM, Gallagher P, Hughes JH, et al: Neurocognitive impairment in euthymic patients with bipolar affective disorder. Br J Psychiatry 186:32–40, 2005

Torrent C, Martinez-Aran A, Daban C, et al: Cognitive impairment in bipolar II disorder. Br J Psychiatry 189:254–259, 2006

van Gorp WG, Altshuler L, Theberge DC, et al: Cognitive impairment in euthymic bipolar patients with and without prior alcohol dependence: a preliminary study. Arch Gen Psychiatry 55:41–46, 1998

van Gorp WG, Altshuler L, Theberge DC, et al: Declarative and procedural memory in bipolar disorder. Biol Psychiatry 46:525–531, 1999

Watson S, Thompson JM, Ritchie JC, et al: Neuropsychological impairment in bipolar disorder: the relationship with glucocorticoid receptor function. Bipolar Disord 8:85–90, 2006

Wechsler D: Wechsler Adult Intelligence Scale, Revised. San Antonio, TX, Psychological Corporation, 1981

Wechsler D: The Wechsler Memory Scale, Revised. New York, Psychological Corporation, 1987

Wolfe J, Granholm E, Butters N, et al: Verbal memory deficits associated with major affective disorders: a comparison of unipolar and bipolar patients. J Affect Disord 13:83–92, 1987

4

The Endophenotype Concept

Examples From Neuropsychological and Neuroimaging Studies of Bipolar Disorder

David C. Glahn, Ph.D.
Katherine E. Burdick, Ph.D.
Carrie E. Bearden, Ph.D.

Although bipolar disorder is strongly influenced by genetic factors, the imprecision of categorical psychiatric diagnoses may be a limiting factor in understanding the genetic basis of the illness. Genetic investigation of endophenotypes—quantitative traits hypothesized to lie intermediately between the gene and the disease syndromes—is a promising alternative or complement to studies of the categorical disease phenotype. In this chapter, we review evidence that neuropsychological and neuroimaging measures represent viable candidate endophenotypes that may be useful in genetic studies of bipolar disorder.

The genetics of bipolar disorder is considered to be complex in the sense that multiple traits and multiple genes are thought to each independently contribute small but important cumulative effects to the overall clinical manifestations of illness (i.e., the phenotype). As such, bipolar disorder does not fall within the realm of classical Mendelian (i.e., autosomal or sex-linked) genetic transmission across generations. Molecular genetic studies have focused on regions of interest to the diagnosis itself (i.e., so-called candidate genes), which are associated with gene products (i.e., proteins or enzymes) involved in the synthesis, catabolism, or function of key neurotransmitter systems, and have focused on small variations of DNA (polymorphisms; often single-nucleotide polymorphisms [SNPs]) that have shown functional significance. Genetic association studies seek to compare (or link) such genetic codings (genotypes) with observable signs of disease (phenotypes). Our interest in the genetics of neurocognitive function pertains to cognition as one potential element of observable disease characteristics that may be familial (i.e., overrepresented within families—such as fluency in a native language, or a predilection for certain occupations, or allegiance to sports teams) and heritable (i.e., directly transmitted via the gene pool).

Family studies have repeatedly shown that bipolar disorder is inherited (Bertelsen et al. 1977). Individuals who are related to persons with bipolar disorder are significantly more likely to have bipolar disorder themselves than those in the general population. Furthermore, the level of risk or liability for bipolar illness increases with the genetic proximity to an affected individual. For example, an individual with a bipolar parent has a 10- to 20-fold increased risk for developing bipolar illness (Merikangas et al. 2002). However, an identical or monozygotic twin of a bipolar patient has approximately a threefold increase in risk for the illness compared with a nontwin sibling (Bertelsen et al. 1977; Kalidindi and McGuffin 2003). Indeed, the concordance rate for identical twins is between 67% and 85% (Bertelsen et al. 1977; Kalidindi and McGuffin 2003), suggesting that bipolar disorder is strongly genetically mediated.

These data suggest two important conclusions regarding the genetic components of bipolar disorder. First, bipolar disorder is not entirely determined by genes. More formally stated, genetic liability alone does not wholly account for affection status; environmental factors must also play a role. This assertion can be deduced from the imperfect concordance rates among identical twins. If risk for bipolar disorder were due entirely to genetic variation, then there would never be genetically identical individuals (monozygotic twins) who differ in illness status. Although at this time researchers do not have a clear view of what environmental events may precipitate the illness, possible risk factors include severe physiological stress (e.g., hypoxia, traumatic brain injury, other major traumas), significant drug or alcohol usage, and noteworthy psychological stressors (e.g., death of a loved one). However, this is a very incomplete and rather imprecise list of potential environmental factors, and the exact stressor for any given patient may never be known. Nonetheless, the notion that bipolar disorder is not entirely genetic is important to keep in mind when considering the causes of the illness.

A second conclusion that can be drawn from family studies of bipolar disorder is that individuals with the genetic predisposition for the illness do not necessarily manifest the illness. One could argue that this second assertion is simply the inverse of the first statement, that both genetic and environmental influences are necessary for bipolar disorder. However, focusing on the notion that individuals who have the genetic predisposition for the illness do not necessarily have the diagnosis suggests several important clues about how to search for genes for bipolar disorder. First, genetic studies that focus exclusively on diagnostic categorization (i.e., the presence or absence of bipolar disorder, based on structured clinical diagnostic interviews) may classify some subjects as not bipolar (because they do not manifest a full bipolar syndrome) when in fact they do carry genetic risk variants (risk alleles) linked with the disorder. Similarly, clinical diagnoses may include subjects whose outward symptoms may resemble those of bipolar disorder (known as phenocopies) but who in fact lack the true bipolar genotype. Such misclassification ultimately results not only in diagnostic confusion and lack of reproducibility across research studies, but also reduced statistical power to discover genes. A number of statistical geneticists have argued that the sample sizes needed for genetic studies of bipolar disorder should be very large in order to combat the problem of reduced power (Risch 1990; Risch and Merikangas 1996).

A second and genetically more sophisticated approach would be to use other traits that correlate with illness status but might be more sensitive than psychiatric illness. These traits are often conceptualized as risk factors for an illness and are termed *allied phenotypes* in the wider human genetics community. In the late 1960s, Gottesman and Shields coined the term *endophenotype* to describe these "hidden" (*endo-*) traits for psychiatric genetic research (Gottesman and Shields 1972; Gottesman et al. 1987).

An endophenotype is conceptualized as an indicator of biological processes mediating between genotype and phenotype (diagnosis). Using endophenotypic markers may be advantageous because they are generally less complex than their associated phenotype and thus may be more readily linked to a specific genetic locus (Gottesman and Gould 2003; Lenox et al. 2002). In addition, endophenotypes for complex human psychiatric disorders could potentially be extended to animal models (Gottesman and Gould 2003), advancing our understanding of the neurobiology of psychiatric disorders and furthering the development of novel medications (Nestler et al. 2002). Furthermore, endophenotypes may be necessary to resolve the status of family members in genetic studies of bipolar disorder. Genetic studies of bipolar disorder could focus on mapping endophenotypes rather than strict phenotypes (i.e., diagnostic information).

Unlike other areas of medicine, psychiatry at present has no biochemical markers or laboratory tests on which to base its diagnoses (Bearden et al. 2004). Instead, subjective assessments form the basis of both clinical and research psychiatric diagnoses (Gottesman and Gould 2003). Twin studies of bipolar disorder have shown dramatically different concordance rates, depending on which diagnostic criteria were utilized, how the samples were ascertained, and how assessments were conducted (Figure 4–1). Differences across studies also reflect changing diagnostic criteria over time. For example, the early twin study by Bertelsen et al. (1977), one of the most highly cited studies demonstrating the high heritability of bipolar disorder, utilized nonstructured clinical interviews and diagnosed affectedness according to principles established by Emil Kraepelin in the early twentieth century. More recent twin studies (e.g., Kieseppä et al. 2005) have relied on semistructured interviews and have utilized modern diagnostic criteria (e.g., the DSM-IV-TR [American Psychiatric Association 2000]), which require a specific number and duration of symptoms in order to pass the threshold for a diagnosis of the disorder. These studies have identified substantially lower concordance rates, for both monozygotic and dizygotic twins, than did Bertelsen et al. (1977).

Because endophenotypic markers are often quantitative, they allow for powerful statistical analysis strategies (e.g., quantitative trait loci) that are not readily available for qualitative phenotypic markers such as diagnostic category (Almasy and Blangero 2001). Furthermore, once identified, endophenotypes could refine diagnostic accuracy and potentially identify individuals at risk for an illness prior to symptom onset. By providing a means to identify more quantitative measures, endophenotypes could allow a window into the genetically influenced biological processes underlying bipolar disorder.

The National Institute of Mental Health convened a work group to develop a strategic plan for genetic mood disorders research (Merikangas et al. 2002). Among the many recommendations, the work group pointed to the need for the widespread use of an endophenotype-based approach to facilitate the identification of susceptibility genes. Given the advantages of endophenotype-based strategies for elucidating the genetic underpinnings of psychiatric disorders, we review the existing evidence for the feasibility of one class of endophenotypic markers—that is, neuropsychological tests—for use in bipolar illness. For a cognitive measure, or any marker for that matter, to be considered an endophenotype, it must be shown to 1) be highly heritable, 2) be associated with the illness, 3) be independent of clinical state, and 4) indicate that the impairment cosegregates with the illness within a family, with nonaffected family members showing impairment relative to the general population (Gershon and Goldin 1986; Glahn et al. 2004; Gottesman and Gould 2003; Leboyer et al. 1998; Lenox et al. 2002).

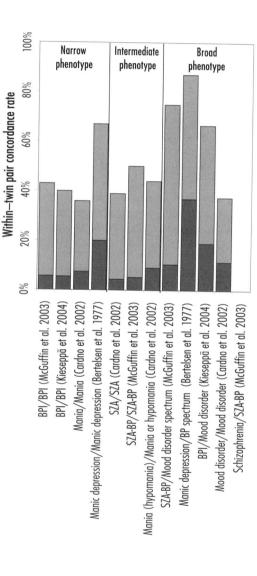

FIGURE 4–1. Differing concordance rates across twin studies of bipolar disorder as a function of varying definitions of the phenotype.

Using the narrowly defined bipolar phenotype, twin-pair concordance rates for monozygotic twins are moderate, ranging from 36% to 43%. However, when the definition of concordance is expanded to include the broader spectrum of mood disorders, concordance rates (and thus heritability estimates) substantially increase. This indicates that categorical diagnoses, as defined by the narrow phenotype, may not adequately capture the full range of phenotypic variation associated with genetic susceptibility to mood disorder. The y-axis displays concordance rates for psychiatric diagnoses in Twin 1 versus Twin 2. BP=bipolar; BPI=bipolar I disorder; SZA=schizoaffective disorder; SZA-BP=schizoaffective disorder, bipolar subtype.

Source. Adapted from Bearden CE, Freimer NB: "Endophenotypes for Psychiatric Disorders: Ready for Primetime?" *Trends in Genetics* 22:306–312, 2006. Used with permission of Elsevier Limited.

In this chapter, we provide an overview of evidence that neuropsychological and neuroimaging measures constitute endophenotypes for genetic studies of bipolar disorder. To that end, we review how well these measures fit the criteria discussed above.

Criterion 1: Heritability

Neurocognitive Traits

Twin, family, and adoption studies have documented that 45%–80% of the individual differences in adult intelligence test performance are due to genetic factors (Bouchard and McGue 1981; Bouchard et al. 1990; Devlin et al. 1997; McClearn et al. 1997). Recently, behavioral geneticists have begun investigating the heritability of specific neurocognitive domains to elucidate the genetic influences of these more basic mental abilities (Luciano et al. 2001). Such studies indicate that genetics strongly influences a wide variety of cognitive tests of processing speed (heritability, $h^2 = 26$–76 [Luciano et al. 2001; Posthuma et al. 2001; Swan and Carmelli 2002]), attention/vigilance ($h^2 = 16$–89 [Fan et al. 2001]), executive control ($h^2 = 33$–68 [Swan and Carmelli 2002]), working memory ($h^2 = 2$–60 [Ando et al. 2001; Jacob et al. 2001; Neubauer et al. 2000]) and declarative memory ($h^2 = 56$–65 [Swan et al. 1999]).

Brain Structure

The size, shape, and complexity of the primate brain vary considerably across individuals, and a significant portion of this variability is influenced by genetic factors. Although very early stages of brain development are predominantly mediated by genetic programs (Rubenstein and Rakic 1999; Rubenstein et al. 1999), later stages of development, organization, and brain maturation result from a complex interaction of genetic and environmental influences (Rakic et al. 1988). Studies in nonhuman primates provided heritability estimates for brain weight ranging between 0.42 and 0.75 (Cheverud et al. 1990; Mahaney et al. 1993; Tuulio-Henriksson et al. 2002). Human imaging studies have expanded on these initial findings, reporting high heritabilities for whole brain volumes (average heritability [range] = 0.78 [0.56–1.00] [Baaré et al. 2001a; Bartley et al. 1997; Geschwind et al. 2002; Hulshoff Pol et al. 2004; Narr et al. 2002; Posthuma et al. 2000; Wright et al. 2002]; gray matter volume = 0.88 [0.82–1.00] [Baaré et al. 2001b; Hulshoff Pol et al. 2004; Posthuma et al. 2000]; white matter volume = 0.85 [0.82–0.87] [Baaré et al. 2001a; Hulshoff Pol et al. 2004; Posthuma et al. 2000]), with somewhat lower heritabilities for lobular volumes (frontal = 0.65 [0.64–0.66] [Geschwind et al. 2002]; temporal = 0.58 [0.56–0.60] [Geschwind et al. 2002]; parietal = 0.52 [0.50–0.53] [Geschwind et al. 2002]; occipital=0.33 [Geschwind et al. 2002]; and cerebellar=0.74 [0.66–0.87] [Posthuma et al. 2000; Wright et al. 2002]). Reduced heritability estimates for lobular structures might be associated with the reliability of delineating lobular regions rather than an intrinsic reduction in the genetic influences of these regions. In contrast, ventricular volume seems to be mediated almost entirely by environmental factors (Baaré et al. 2001a; for contrary evidence, see Styner et al. 2005.) Estimated heritability for sulcal shape or length seems to vary considerably based on the sulcus in question (0.22 [0.10–0.77] [Bartley et al. 1997]), although these measurements traditionally suffer from poor reliability. White matter hyperintense lesions, also known as *subcortical leukoencephalopathy,* are highly heritable in older, but not younger, subjects (0.76 [0.73–0.78] [Atwood et al. 2004; Carmelli et al. 1998]).

Thompson et al. (2001) used an elastic deformation procedure to model the genetic influences on neuroanatomical variation between healthy monozygotic and dizygotic twin pairs at each voxel on the surface of the cortex. This analysis indicated that genetic factors significantly influence cortical structure in subregions of the prefrontal and temporal lobes, particularly Broca's and Wernicke's language areas. However, other areas within these structures were less heritable, suggesting that heritability estimates based on gross lobular regions of interest blur more subtle local differences.

Taken together, these data suggest that both neuropsychological and neuroanatomical measures are strongly influenced by genetics and thus meet the first criterion for endophenotypes.

Criterion 2: Association With Bipolar Disorder

Neuropsychological Impairments

Although it is unclear at this time how common cognitive impairments are among individuals diagnosed with bipolar disorder, a significant portion of patients with bipolar disorder complain of cognitive difficulties (Burdick et al. 2005; Martinez-Aran et al. 2005; see also Chapter 12 in this volume, "Summary and Assessment Recommendations for Practitioners"). Furthermore, formal neuropsychological deficits have also been documented in asymptomatic patients who do not complain of cognitive difficulties (Burdick et al. 2005; Martinez-Aran et al. 2005), indicating that neuropsychological impairments may be more widespread than clinical experience suggests. Indeed, there is now significant evidence that cognitive dysfunction occurs across several domains among patients with bipolar disorder and that these impairments seem to be somewhat independent of mood state and psychotropic medication usage (as reviewed in this volume in Chapter 5, "Impact of Mood, Anxiety, and Psychotic Symptoms on Cognition in Patients With Bipolar Disorder"; Chapter 7, "Adverse Cognitive Effects of Psychotropic Medications"; and Chapter 8, "Pharmacological Strategies to Enhance Neurocognitive Function"). A recent review concluded that the most consistent trait in bipolar disorder appear to be verbal learning and memory, sustained attention, and executive functioning (Quraishi and Frangou 2002). Thus far, measures of these cognitive domains appear to be the most likely candidate neurocognitive endophenotypes for bipolar disorder (Glahn et al. 2004).

Neuroanatomy

In vivo volumetric magnetic resonance imaging (MRI) studies have reported subtle structural brain changes in prefrontal, medial temporal, and limbic regions in individuals with bipolar disorder (Brambilla et al. 2005), suggesting disturbances in neuronal survival or resilience (Duman 2002; Duman et al. 1997; Manji et al. 2000). However, findings are rather inconsistent, with the most solid evidence indicating increased rates of white matter hyperintensities and mild ventricular enlargement (Bearden et al. 2001; McDonald et al. 2004; Strakowski et al. 2005). Inconsistencies in the literature may be due to small sample sizes, clinical heterogeneity, psychotropic medication usage, and cross-sectional designs.

Strakowski et al. (2005) noted that abnormalities in some neuroanatomical regions (e.g., subgenual prefrontal cortex, striatum, amygdala) exist early in the course of illness and may predate illness onset. Other anatomical regions (e.g., cerebellar vermis, lateral ventricles, inferior prefrontal regions) appear to degenerate with repeated affective episodes. These regions may represent the effects of illness progression. Based on these observations and converging data from functional and physiological imaging, Strakowski et al. (see Figure 1–1 in Chapter 1, "Overview and Introduction: Dimensions of Cognition and Measures of Cognitive Function") have proposed a model of bipolar disorder that involves dysfunction within striatal-thalamic-prefrontal networks and the associated limbic modulating regions (amygdala, midline cerebellum), suggesting that diminished prefrontal modulation of subcortical and medial temporal structures within the anterior limbic network (e.g., amygdala, anterior striatum, thalamus) results in the dysregulation of mood found in bipolar disorder.

Criterion 3: Independence of Clinical State

Variation of Clinical State and Cognition

There is clear evidence that individuals with bipolar disorder exhibit widespread neurocognitive dysfunction during acute episodes of mania (Clark et al. 2001) and depression (Borkowska and Rybakowski 2001), and the discovery that these deficits endure in euthymic bipolar patients raises the possibility that cognitive impairment may represent a trait rather than a state variable (Quraishi and Frangou 2002). Euthymic bipolar patients exhibit limitations in several cognitive domains (Kerry et al. 1983; Paradiso et al. 1997; Sapin et al. 1987), including measures of executive function (El-Badri et al. 2001; Goodwin and Jamison 1990; Hawkins et al. 1997; Krabbendam et al. 2000; Rubinsztein et al. 2000), declarative memory (El-Badri et al. 2001; Goodwin and Jamison 1990; Hawkins et al. 1997; Krabbendam et al. 2000; Rubinsztein et al. 2000; van Gorp et al. 1998, 1999; Zubieta et al. 2001), and sustained attention (Clark et al. 2002; Harmer et al. 2002; Wilder-Willis et al. 2001). Yet, even cognitive impairments found in patients with euthymic bipolar disorder may be confounded by clinical variables, such as manifestations of subclinical symptoms or broader epiphenomena of an individual's illness history (e.g., illness duration, number of hospitalizations). Euthymic bipolar patients often present with minor affective symptoms, which may adversely affect performance on cognitive measures (Clark et al. 2002; Ferrier et al. 1999; Frangou et al. 2005a). Patients who have been euthymic for months prior to assessment have marked neuropsychological impairments (Thompson et al. 2005), particularly in the areas of attention, executive functioning, and memory. Indeed, Thompson et al. (2005) reported that about 12% of euthymic bipolar patients are impaired (below the fifth percentile of normative performance); however, the level of deficit varies widely based on the actual tests used.

Although use of psychotropic medications can impact neurocognitive functioning, systematic investigation of the cognitive impact of these agents in patients with bipolar disorder has been limited (see Chapter 7 in this volume). A qualitative review concluded that although lithium had a negative effect on memory and speed of information processing, patients were often unaware of these deficits (Honig et al. 1999). Engelsmann et al. (1988) found that mean memory test scores remained quite stable over a 6-year interval in lithium-treated bipolar patients. Further, after the researchers controlled for age and initial memory scores, there were no significant differences between patients with short-term and those with long-term lithium treatment on any measure, suggesting that long-term lithium usage is unlikely to cause progressive cognitive decline (Engelsmann et al. 1988). Although few studies have examined neurocognitive performance in unmedicated bipolar patients, we previously found comparably impaired verbal memory in patients receiving psychotropic medication ($n = 32$) and those who were drug-free ($n = 17$) (Bearden et al. 2006). Taken together, these findings suggest that cognitive deficits and underlying abnormalities in neuronal activation in patients with bipolar illness are not primarily attributable to the use of psychotropic medications. However, large-scale, longitudinal investigations of bipolar patients on different medication regimens are warranted to fully address this question.

An issue related to independence of mood state involves the longitudinal stability of heritable traits, which, by definition, are non–state dependent. Several studies have demonstrated the persistence of cognitive deficits in subjects with bipolar disorder, not only across varying phases of illness (see Chapter 11 of this volume, "Cognition Across the Life Span: Clinical Implications for Older Adults With Bipolar Disorder") but also within subjects over the span of years. Notably, Balanzá-Martínez et al. (2005) conducted a 3-year prospective follow-up of 30 subjects with bipolar I disorder or schizophrenia and 26 healthy volunteer comparison subjects and found stability across most cognitive domains studied within each diagnostic group. Similarly, Burdick et al. (2006) conducted a 5-year prospective study of 32 bipolar or schizophrenia probands in which those with bipolar disorder showed stability in performance measures of attention, with greater variability in other cognitive domains, whereas those with schizophrenia showed a decline in executive function but stability in other cognitive dimensions. Longer-term studies with larger sample sizes are needed to affirm the persistence of impaired attentional versus other subservient dimensions of cognition in patients with bipolar disorder.

Brain Anatomy and Mood State

There is little evidence that changes in mood state have an impact on brain structure (Brambilla et al. 2005). However, more severe clinical course has been associated with specific neuroanatomical changes (e.g., increased ventricular size [Strakowski et al. 2002]), potentially suggesting that affective episodes might be associated with increased neuronal degeneration. However, to date, no longitudinal neuroanatomical study has been conducted to determine whether increased ventricular size is a risk factor for or the result of a more virulent clinical course. For example, individuals with bipolar disorder who have a history of psychotic symptoms during mood episodes have larger lateral ventricles than bipolar patients without psychotic symptoms (Strasser et al. 2005). Thus, it is possible that enlarged ventricles are associated with a number of pathophysiological changes found in a subgroup of patients with bipolar disorder, although the relationship between ventricular size and illness history is unclear at this time.

Some evidence suggests that psychotropic treatments commonly prescribed for bipolar symptoms may impact brain volume. For example, in a study of patients with bipolar disorder, Moore et al. (2000) observed that lithium significantly increased total gray matter volume by 3% on average after 4 weeks. Sassi et al. (2002) found larger total gray matter volume in lithium-treated bipolar patients than in either untreated patients or healthy controls. In a partially overlapping sample, decreased left anterior cingulate volumes were observed in untreated bipolar patients compared with healthy controls, whereas no differences were found between lithium-treated patients and the control subjects (Sassi et al. 2004). Recent findings by our group also point to lithium-associated volumetric increases in the anterior limbic network (Bearden et al. 2007). Together, these reports suggest that lithium treatment may alter MRI brain volume measures, and that some of the inconsistencies among prior neuroanatomical studies of patients with bipolar disorder may be due to competing processes of disease-related atrophy and/or tissue reduction, pitted against possible neurotrophic or neuroprotective effects of mood-stabilizing medication.

Criterion 4: Impairment Within Families

Neuropsychological Impairment

The study of bipolar patients in isolation from their families cannot determine whether neurocognitive deficits in the euthymic state are the result of an underlying trait of confounding factors, such as the acute or chronic effects of medications, permanent structural changes wrought by prior episodes of acute illness, psychosocial sequelae of previous affective episodes, or subsyndromal symptoms such as alterations in sleep cycle. Further, documenting neuropsychological impairment in patients with bipolar disorder does not, in and of itself, suggest that these impairments are genetically mediated. To show that cognitive (or neuroanatomical) impairments are sensitive to the genetic liability for bipolar disorder, these impairments must be observed in family members who do not have bipolar disorder. Additionally, impairments should be more pronounced in individuals who are genetically closer to the bipolar patients (e.g., first-degree relatives) than in more distant individuals (e.g., third-degree relatives). At this time, no studies have been conducted to investigate the cosegregation of affection status and cognitive impairment in bipolar families. However, there is growing evidence that first-degree relatives (e.g., siblings, parents) have mild executive (Clark et al. 2005; Ferrier et al. 2004; Zalla et al. 2004) and memory (Ferrier et al. 2004; Gourovitch et al. 1999; McIntosh et al. 2005) deficits. Other studies have found little evidence of attention, executive, or memory deficits in unaffected siblings of persons with bipolar disorder (Frangou et al. 2005b; Keri et al. 2001; Kieseppä et al. 2005; McIntosh et al. 2005)

Neuroanatomical Abnormalities

Coffman et al. (1990) conducted one of the earliest studies demonstrating cofnitive impairment across multiple domains in adults with bipolar disorder, and these investigators further correlated observed cognitive deficits with diminished frontal lobe volume by MRI. McDonald et al. (2004) used structural MRI to investigate the relationship between genetic risk for schizophrenia or bipolar disorder and neuroanatomical variation. They reported that whereas genetic risk for schizophrenia was associated with distributed gray matter volume deficits in the bilateral frontostriatothalamic and left lateral temporal regions, liability for bipolar disorder was associated with gray matter deficits only in the right anterior cingulate gyrus and ventral striatum (McDonald et al. 2004). In addition, risk for both disorders was associated with white matter volume reduction in the left frontal and temporoparietal regions, suggesting that these two disorders show both unique and overlapping patterns of brain structural pathology related to variable genetic risk. In a subsequent analysis of these same data, McDonald et al. (2006) did not find evidence for ventricular enlargement in either the patients with bipolar disorder or their unaffected relatives.

Structural MRI studies also have been undertaken to examine white matter tissue abnormalities—identified as so-called hyperintense T_2 signals—which may be subtle but common among individuals with bipolar disorder in periventricular regions, potentially reflecting astrogliosis, demyelination, or other degenerative changes (Altshuler et al. 1995). A comparison of white matter hyperintensities in bipolar subjects and in their healthy siblings or controls found more frequent hyperintensities among patients than in either of the other groups. However, when hyperintensities were evident among siblings or patients, they were more often located in right-sided than in left-sided cerebral regions (Gulseren et al. 2006).

Conclusions

There is growing evidence that neuropsychological measures of executive functioning and declarative memory could be endophenotypes for bipolar disorder (Glahn et al. 2005). These measures are heritable, are relatively independent of clinical state, and are impaired in both patients with bipolar disorder and their unaffected relatives. Although larger-scale family studies need to be completed, a number of groups are actively collecting these data, and initial reports look promising. In contrast, neuroanatomical findings in patients with bipolar disorder are rather inconsistent, and changes found in unaffected relatives have not been separately reported in patients. These inconsistencies are likely due to relatively small sample sizes, extreme differences in image analysis strategies used across samples, and heterogeneity among patients studied, both within and across studies. Nonetheless, several groups are currently collecting large neuroanatomical data sets in the hopes that these data will have the power to detect potential changes. Thus, although current evidence supports the use of neuropsychological tests in the search for genes predisposing to bipolar disorder, the use of specific neuroanatomical measures associated with bipolar disorder would necessarily be exploratory.

We have discussed the utility of endophenotypes for finding genes that increase risk for bipolar disorder. However, specific endophenotypes may also be useful for characterizing subgroups of patients with bipolar disorder. For example, it is possible that those persons with bipolar disorder who have working memory impairments may also have unique symptom profiles or course of illness. Indeed, we recently reported that those patients with bipolar disorder with a history of psychotic symptoms have spatial working memory deficits similar in magnitude to those of patients with schizophrenia (Glahn et al. 2006). In contrast, those patients without a history of psychosis were not impaired on this measure. These data suggest that psychotic symptoms may have etiological implications, and that the biological changes associated with psychosis may be indexed through spatial working memory tests.

Currently, there is a good deal of interest in discovering genes predisposing to psychiatric illness. Methods used for gene discovery vary significantly, and our discussion to this point has focused on linkage methods with analyses of quantitative traits (i.e., neurocognitive and neuroimaging endophenotypes). However, a candidate gene strategy, based on the known function of particular genes important for brain development and neurotransmitter function, is an alternative approach to determining whether specific candidate genes confer risk for mental illness. In context, endophenotypic measures can provide valuable information by helping to characterize the behavioral or biological implications of a specific polymorphism. A relevant example involves the catechol O-methyltransferase (COMT) gene, located on chromosome 22q11, which is involved in the degredation of dopamine and norepinephrine. A large body of evidence suggests that COMT is associated with cognitive performance in patients with schizophrenia and in healthy volunteers, but new evidence also implicates a genetic association involving COMT and cognition in patients with bipolar disorder. Burdick et al. (2007) genotyped 52 bipolar I probands and 102 healthy controls across four SNPs within the COMT gene, assessed the relationship between COMT genotype and diagnosis, and then tested for effects on cognition. They observed a modest but significant association between a specific SNP (rs165599) and bipolar I disorder, with the g allele being overrepresented in patients versus controls. Further, they found a relationship between the risk allele at this SNP and poorer performance on measures of verbal memory, particularly with regard to prefrontal aspects of learning. These data provide molecular genetic evidence of the utility of cognition as an endophenotype in bipolar disorder.

The endophenotype strategy is a highly promising concept that awaits further validation (Hasler et al. 2006). By identifying candidate neurobiological endophenotypes that are associated with genetic risk for bipolar disorder, it is likely that we will also be able to refine phenotypic definitions of the illness. Improving our current nosological system by incorporating intermediate pathophysiological markers is of fundamental importance, as this will likely facilitate gene discovery, ultimately leading to the development of alternative treatments and preventive strategies for this highly disabling mental illness.

Take-Home Points

- Endophenotypes are intermediate or "hidden" traits associated with an illness that may help to refine the genetic elements of a disease. Cognitive dysfunction represents an endophenotype of bipolar disorder because it is heritable, associated with the disease, occurs independently from clinical (affective) state, and aggregates within families.

- Genetic factors may hold particular importance for prefrontal and temporal cortex regions, including centers of language comprehension and expression.

- The most consistent structural neuroimaging findings in bipolar disorder have been observations of white matter hyperintensities and mild ventricular enlargement. Other, more inconsistent findings also implicate abnormal volumes in prefrontal, medial temporal, and limbic regions.

- Lithium appears to increase gray matter volume in patients with bipolar disorder, presumably via its neurotrophic or neuroprotective effects.

- Healthy first-degree relatives of bipolar probands may demonstrate mild executive and memory deficits. Data are less conclusive about whether or not siblings of bipolar probands display problems with attention and what degree of memory and executive function problems is noted in bipolar patients. MRI studies show that white matter hyperintensities (reflecting possible neurodegeneration) are not more common in healthy siblings of bipolar probands, although when such anomalies occur in siblings, they are more often on the right side.

- Although the use of cognition as an endophenotype in the context of molecular genetic studies is in its relative infancy, data from studies investigating genes with known biological functions (e.g., COMT) have begun to emerge in support of this approach.

References

Almasy L, Blangero JC: Endophenotypes as quantitative risk factors for psychiatric disease: rationale and study design. Am J Med Genet 105:42–44, 2001

Altshuler LL, Curran JG, Hauser P, et al: T2 hyperintensities in bipolar disorder: magnetic resonance imaging comparison and literature meta-analysis. Am J Psychiatry 152:1139–1144, 1995

American Psychiatric Association: Diagnostic and Statistical Manual of Mental Disorders, 4th Edition, Text Revision. Washington, DC, American Psychiatric Association, 2000

Ando J, Ono Y, Wright MJ: Genetic structure of spatial and verbal working memory. Behav Genet 31:615–624, 2001

Atwood LD, Wolf PA, Heard-Costa NL, et al: Genetic variation in white matter hyperintensity volume in the Framingham Study. Stroke 35:1609–1613, 2004

Baaré WF, Hulshoff Pol HE, Boomsma DI, et al: Quantitative genetic modeling of variation in human brain morphology. Cereb Cortex 11:816–824, 2001a

Baaré WF, van Oel CJ, Hulshoff Pol HE, et al: Volumes of brain structures in twins discordant for schizophrenia. Arch Gen Psychiatry 58:33–40, 2001b

Balanzá-Martínez V, Tabarés-Seisdedos R, Selva-Vera G, et al: Persistent cognitive dysfunctions in bipolar I disorder and schizophrenic patients: a 3-year follow-up study. Psychother Psychosom 74:113–119, 2005

Bartley A, Jones D, Weinberger D: Genetic variability of human brain size and cortical gyral patterns. Brain 120:257–269, 1997

Bearden CE, Hoffman KM, Cannon TD: The neuropsychology and neuroanatomy of bipolar affective disorder: a critical review. Bipolar Disord 3:106–150; discussion 151–153, 2001

Bearden CE, Reus VI, Freimer NB: Why genetic investigation of psychiatric disorders is so difficult. Curr Opin Genet Dev 14:280–286, 2004

Bearden CE, Glahn DC, Monkul ES, et al: Sources of declarative memory impairment in bipolar disorder: mnemonic processes and clinical features. J Psychiatr Res 40:47–58, 2006

Bearden CE, Thompson PM, Dalwani M, et al: Greater cortical gray matter density in lithium-treated patients with bipolar disorder. Biol Psychiatry 62:7–16, 2007

Bertelsen A, Harvald B, Hauge M: A Danish twin study of manic-depressive disorders. Br J Psychiatry 130:330–351, 1977

Borkowska A, Rybakowski JK: Neuropsychological frontal lobe tests indicate that bipolar depressed patients are more impaired than unipolar. Bipolar Disord 3:88–94, 2001

Bouchard TJ Jr, McGue M: Familial studies of intelligence: a review. Science 212:1055–1059, 1981

Bouchard TJ Jr, Segal NL, Lykken DT: Genetic and environmental influences on special mental abilities in a sample of twins reared apart. Acta Genet Med Gemellol (Roma) 39:193–206, 1990

Brambilla P, Glahn DC, Balestrieri M, et al: Magnetic resonance findings in bipolar disorder. Psychiatr Clin North Am 28:443–467, 2005

Burdick KE, Endick CJ, Goldberg JF: Assessing cognitive deficits in bipolar disorder: are self-reports valid? Psychiatry Res 136:43–50, 2005

Burdick KE, Goldberg JF, Harrow M, et al: Neurocognition as a stable endophenotype in bipolar disorder and schizophrenia. J Nerv Ment Dis 194:255–260, 2006

Burdick KE, Funke B, Goldberg JF, et al: COMT genotype increases risk for bipolar I disorder and influences neurocognitive performance. Bipolar Disord 9:370–376, 2007
Cardno AG, Rijsdijk FV, Sham PC, et al: A twin study of genetic relationships between psychotic symptoms. Am J Psychiatry 159:539–545, 2002
Carmelli D, DeCarli C, Swan GE, et al: Evidence for genetic variance in white matter hyperintensity volume in normal elderly male twins. Stroke 29:1177–1181, 1998
Cheverud JM, Falk D, Hildebolt C, et al: Heritability and association of cortical petalias in rhesus macaques (*Macaca mulatta*). Brain Behav Evol 35:368–372, 1990
Clark L, Iversen SD, Goodwin GM: A neuropsychological investigation of prefrontal cortex involvement in acute mania. Am J Psychiatry 158:1605–1611, 2001
Clark L, Iversen SD, Goodwin GM: Sustained attention deficit in bipolar disorder. Br J Psychiatry 180:313–319, 2002
Clark L, Sarna A, Goodwin GM: Impairment of executive function but not memory in first-degree relatives of patients with bipolar I disorder and in euthymic patients with unipolar depression. Am J Psychiatry 162:1980–1982, 2005
Coffman JA, Bornstein RA, Olson SC, et al: Cognitive impairment and cerebral structure by MRI in bipolar disorder. Biol Psychiatry 27:1188–1196, 1990
Devlin B, Daniels M, Roeder K: The heritability of IQ. Nature 388:468–471, 1997
Duman RS: Synaptic plasticity and mood disorders. Mol Psychiatry 7:29–34, 2002
Duman RS, Heninger GR, Nestler EJ: A molecular and cellular theory of depression. Arch Gen Psychiatry 54:597–606, 1997
El-Badri SM, Ashton CH, Moore PB, et al: Electrophysiological and cognitive function in young euthymic patients with bipolar affective disorder. Bipolar Disord 3:79–87, 2001
Engelsmann F, Katz J, Ghadirian AM, et al: Lithium and memory: a long-term follow-up study. J Clin Psychopharmacol 8:207–212, 1988
Fan J, Wu Y, Fossella JA, et al: Assessing the heritability of attentional networks. BMC Neurosci 2:14, 2001
Ferrier IN, Stanton BR, Kelly TP, et al: Neuropsychological function in euthymic patients with bipolar disorder. Br J Psychiatry 175:246–251, 1999
Ferrier IN, Chowdhury R, Thompson JM, et al: Neurocognitive function in unaffected first-degree relatives of patients with bipolar disorder: a preliminary report. Bipolar Disord 6:319–322, 2004
Frangou S, Donaldson S, Hadjulis M, et al: The Maudsley Bipolar Disorder Project: executive dysfunction in bipolar disorder I and its clinical correlates. Biol Psychiatry 58:859–864, 2005a
Frangou S, Haldane M, Roddy D, et al: Evidence for deficit in tasks of ventral, but not dorsal, prefrontal executive function as an endophenotypic marker for bipolar disorder. Biol Psychiatry 58:838–839, 2005b
Gershon E, Goldin L: Clinical methods in psychiatric genetics, I: robustness of genetic marker investigative strategies. Acta Psychiatr Scandinavica 74:113–118, 1986
Geschwind DH, Miller BL, DeCarli C, et al: Heritability of lobar brain volumes in twins supports genetic models of cerebral laterality and handedness. Proc Natl Acad Sci USA 99:3176–3181, 2002

Glahn DC, Bearden CE, Niendam TA, et al: The feasibility of neuropsychological endophenotypes in the search for genes associated with bipolar affective disorder. Bipolar Disord 5:171–182, 2004

Glahn DC, Bearden CE, Caetano S, et al: Declarative memory impairment in pediatric bipolar disorder. Bipolar Disord 7:546–554, 2005

Glahn DC, Bearden CE, Cakir S, et al: Differential working memory impairment in bipolar disorder and schizophrenia: effects of lifetime history of psychosis. Bipolar Disord 8:117–123, 2006

Goodwin FK, Jamison KR: Manic-Depressive Illness. New York, Oxford University Press, 1990

Gottesman II, Gould TD: The endophenotype concept in psychiatry: etymology and strategic intentions. Am J Psychiatry 160:636–645, 2003

Gottesman II, Shields J: Schizophrenia and Genetics: A Twin Study Vantage Point. New York, Academic Press, 1972

Gottesman II, McGuffin P, Farmer AE: Clinical genetics as clues to the "real" genetics of schizophrenia (a decade of modest gains while playing for time). Schizophr Bull 13:23–47, 1987

Gourovitch ML, Torrey EF, Gold JM, et al: Neuropsychological performance of monozygotic twins discordant for bipolar disorder. Biol Psychiatry 45:639–646, 1999

Gulseren S, Gurcan M, Gulseren L, et al: T2 hyperintensities in bipolar patients and their healthy siblings. Arch Med Res 37:79–85, 2006

Harmer CJ, Clark L, Grayson L, et al: Sustained attention deficit in bipolar disorder is not a working memory impairment in disguise. Neuropsychologia 40:1586–1590, 2002

Hasler G, Drevets WC, Gould TD, et al: Toward constructing an endophenotype strategy for bipolar disorders. Biol Psychiatry 60:93–105, 2006

Hawkins KA, Hoffman RE, Quinlan DM, et al: Cognition, negative symptoms, and diagnosis: a comparison of schizophrenic, bipolar, and control samples. J Neuropsychiatry Clin Neurosci 9:81–89, 1997

Honig A, Arts BM, Ponds RW, et al: Lithium induced cognitive side-effects in bipolar disorder: a qualitative analysis and implications for daily practice. Int Clin Psychopharmacol 14:167–171, 1999

Hulshoff Pol HE, Brans RG, van Haren NE, et al: Gray and white matter volume abnormalities in monozygotic and same-gender dizygotic twins discordant for schizophrenia. Biol Psychiatry 55:126–130, 2004

Jacob N, van Gestel S, Derom C, et al: Heritability estimates of intelligence in twins: effect of chorion type. Behav Genet 31:209–217, 2001

Kalidindi S, McGuffin P: The genetics of affective disorders: present and future, in Behavioral Genetics in the Post-Genomic Era. Edited by Plonim R, DeFries JC, Craig IW, et al. Washington, DC, American Psychological Association, 2003, pp 481–501

Keri S, Kelemen O, Benedek G, et al: Different trait markers for schizophrenia and bipolar disorder: a neurocognitive approach. Psychol Med 31:915–922, 2001

Kerry RJ, McDermott CM, Orme JE: Affective disorders and cognitive performance. A clinical report. J Affect Disord 5:349–352, 1983

Kieseppä T, Partonen T, Haukka J, et al: High concordance of bipolar I disorder in a nationwide sample of twins. Am J Psychiatry 161:1814–1821, 2004

Kieseppä T, Tuulio-Henriksson A, Haukka J, et al: Memory and verbal learning functions in twins with bipolar-I disorder, and the role of information-processing speed. Psychol Med 35:205–215, 2005

Krabbendam L, Honig A, Wiersma J, et al: Cognitive dysfunctions and white matter lesions in patients with bipolar disorder in remission. Acta Psychiatr Scand 101:274–280, 2000

Leboyer M, Bellivier F, Nosten-Bertrand M, et al: Psychiatric genetics: search for phenotypes. Trends Neurosci 21:102–105, 1998

Lenox RH, Gould TD, Manji HK: Endophenotypes in bipolar disorder. Am J Med Genet 114:391–406, 2002

Luciano M, Wright M, Smith GA, et al: Genetic covariance among measures of information processing speed, working memory, and IQ. Behav Genet 31:581–592, 2001

Mahaney MC, Williams-Blangero S, Blangero J, et al: Quantitative genetics of relative organ weight variation in captive baboons. Hum Biol 65:991–1003, 1993

Manji HK, Moore GJ, Chen G: Clinical and preclinical evidence for the neurotrophic effects of mood stabilizers: implications for the pathophysiology and treatment of manic-depressive illness. Biol Psychiatry 48:740–754, 2000

Martinez-Aran A, Vieta E, Colom F, et al: Do cognitive complaints in euthymic bipolar patients reflect objective cognitive impairment? Psychother Psychosom 74:295–302, 2005

McClearn GE, Johansson B, Berg S, et al: Substantial genetic influence on cognitive abilities in twins 80 or more years old. Science 276:1560–1563, 1997

McDonald C, Bullmore ET, Sham PC, et al: Association of genetic risks for schizophrenia and bipolar disorder with specific and generic brain structural endophenotypes. Arch Gen Psychiatry 61:974–984, 2004

McDonald C, Marshall N, Sham PC, et al: Regional brain morphometry in patients with schizophrenia or bipolar disorder and their unaffected relatives. Am J Psychiatry 163:478–487, 2006

McGuffin P, Rijsdijk F, Andrew M, et al: The heritability of bipolar affective disorder and the genetic relationship to unipolar depression. Arch Gen Psychiatry 60:497–502, 2003

McIntosh AM, Harrison LK, Forrester K, et al: Neuropsychological impairments in people with schizophrenia or bipolar disorder and their unaffected relatives. Br J Psychiatry 186:378–385, 2005

Merikangas KR, Chakravarti A, Moldin SO, et al: Future of genetics of mood disorders research. Biol Psychiatry 52:457–477, 2002

Moore GJ, Bebchuk JM, Wilds IB, et al: Lithium-induced increase in human brain grey matter. Lancet 356:1241–1242, 2000

Narr KL, Cannon TD, Woods RP, et al: Genetic contributions to altered callosal morphology in schizophrenia. J Neurosci 22:3720–3729, 2002

Nestler E, Gould E, Manji H, et al: Preclinical models: status of basic research in depression. Biol Psychiatry 52:503–528, 2002

Neubauer A, Spinath F, Riemann R, et al: Genetic and environmental influences on two measures of speed of information processing and their relation to psychometric intelligence: evidence from the German Observational Study of Adult Twins. Intelligence 28:267–289, 2000

Paradiso S, Lamberty GJ, Garvey MJ, et al: Cognitive impairment in the euthymic phase of chronic unipolar depression. J Nerv Ment Dis 185:748–754, 1997

Posthuma D, de Geus EJ, Neale MC, et al: Multivariate genetic analysis of brain structure in an extended twin design. Behav Genet 30:311–319, 2000

Posthuma D, Neale MC, Boomsma DI, et al: Are smarter brains running faster? heritability of alpha peak frequency, IQ, and their interrelation. Behav Genet 31:567–579, 2001

Quraishi S, Frangou S: Neuropsychology of bipolar disorder: a review. J Affect Disord 72:209–226, 2002

Rakic P: Specification of cerebral cortical areas. Science 241:170–176, 1988

Risch N: Linkage strategies for genetically complex traits, I: multilocus models. Am J Hum Genet 46:222–228, 1990

Risch NJ, Merikangas KR: The future of genetic studies of complex human diseases. Science 273:1516–1517, 1996

Rubenstein JL, Rakic P: Genetic control of cortical development. Cereb Cortex 9:521–523, 1999

Rubenstein JL, Anderson S, Shi L, et al: Genetic control of cortical regionalization and connectivity. Cereb Cortex 9:524–532, 1999

Rubinsztein JS, Michael A, Paykel ES, et al: Cognitive impairment in remission in bipolar affective disorder. Psychol Med 30:1025–1036, 2000

Sapin LR, Berrettini WH, Nurnberger JI Jr, et al: Mediational factors underlying cognitive changes and laterality in affective illness. Biol Psychiatry 22:979–986, 1987

Sassi RB, Nicoletti MA, Brambilla P, et al: Increased gray matter volume in lithium-treated bipolar disorder patients. Neurosci Lett 329:243–245, 2002

Sassi RB, Brambilla P, Hatch JP, et al: Reduced left anterior cingulate volumes in untreated bipolar patients. Biol Psychiatry 56:467–475, 2004

Strakowski SM, DelBello MP, Zimmerman ME, et al: Ventricular and periventricular structural volumes in first- versus multiple-episode bipolar disorder. Am J Psychiatry 159:1841–1847, 2002

Strakowski SM, Delbello MP, Adler CM: The functional neuroanatomy of bipolar disorder: a review of neuroimaging findings. Mol Psychiatry 10:105–116, 2005

Strasser HC, Lilyestrom J, Ashby ER, et al: Hippocampal and ventricular volumes in psychotic and nonpsychotic bipolar patients compared with schizophrenia patients and community control subjects: a pilot study. Biol Psychiatry 57:633–639, 2005

Styner M, Lieberman JA, McClure RK, et al: Morphometric analysis of lateral ventricles in schizophrenia and healthy controls regarding genetic and disease-specific factors. Proc Natl Acad Sci USA 102:4872–4877, 2005

Swan GE, Carmelli D: Evidence for genetic mediation of executive control: a study of aging male twins. J Gerontol B Psychol Sci Soc Sci 57:P133–P143, 2002.

Swan GE, Reed T, Jack LM, et al: Differential genetic influence for components of memory in aging adult twins. Arch Neurol 56:1127–1132, 1999

Thompson JM, Gallagher P, Hughes JH, et al: Neurocognitive impairment in euthymic patients with bipolar affective disorder. Br J Psychiatry 186:32–40, 2005

Thompson PM, Cannon TD, Narr KL, et al: Genetic influences on brain structure. Nat Neurosci 4:1253–1258, 2001

Tuulio-Henriksson A, Haukka J, Partonen T, et al: Heritability and number of quantitative trait loci of neurocognitive functions in families with schizophrenia. Am J Med Genet 114:483–490, 2002 van Gorp WG, Altshuler L, Theberge DC, et al: Cognitive impairment in euthymic bipolar patients with and without prior alcohol dependence. A preliminary study. Arch Gen Psychiatry 55:41–46, 1998

van Gorp WG, Altshuler L, Theberge DC, et al: Declarative and procedural memory in bipolar disorder. Biol Psychiatry 46:525–531, 1999

Wilder-Willis KE, Sax KW, Rosenberg HL, et al: Persistent attentional dysfunction in remitted bipolar disorder. Bipolar Disord 3:58–62, 2001

Wright IC, Sham P, Murray RM, et al: Genetic contributions to regional variability in human brain structure: methods and preliminary results. Neuroimage 17:256–271, 2002

Zalla T, Joyce C, Szoke A, et al: Executive dysfunctions as potential markers of familial vulnerability to bipolar disorder and schizophrenia. Psychiatry Res 121:207–217, 2004

Zubieta JK, Huguelet P, O'Neil RL, et al: Cognitive function in euthymic bipolar I disorder. Psychiatry Res 102:9–20, 2001

5

Impact of Mood, Anxiety, and Psychotic Symptoms on Cognition in Patients With Bipolar Disorder

Gin S. Malhi, M.B.Ch.B., B.Sc. (Hons), F.R.C.Psych., F.R.A.N.Z.C.P., M.D.
Catherine M. Cahill, M.Sc., M.Psychol.
Philip Mitchell, M.B., B.S., M.D., F.R.A.N.Z.C.P., F.R.C.Psych.

In recent years, the Kraepelinian concept of bipolar disorder (as manic-depressive psychosis) has been questioned with respect to a number of presumed differences from schizophrenia (dementia praecox), including the diagnostic specificity of cognitive impairment. Emerging evidence suggests that in addition to experiencing state-related cognitive deficits, patients with bipolar disorder have residual cognitive compromise during euthymia. As noted in Chapter 4 of this volume, "The Endophenotype Concept: Examples from Neuropsychogical and Neuroimaging Studies of Bipolar Disorder," cognitive deficits also appear evident in unaffected first-degree relatives of patients with bipolar disorder, providing further indirect support for the possibility of an illness trait vulnerability, one facet of which manifests cognitively. In this chapter, we briefly examine the neuropsychological profile of bipolar disorder, drawing attention to the deficits of clinical salience but at the same time noting the many limitations of the clinical research that has been conducted thus far. A significant confounding factor that affects most studies is that of medication; this issue is discussed more fully in this volume in Chapter 7, "Adverse Cognitive Effects of Psychotropic Medications," and Chapter 8, "Pharmacological Strategies to Enhance Neurocognitive Function." Additional confounds of note include subsyndromal interepisode symptoms and the possibility of neuroanatomical change, which together have prompted investigations of possible endophenotypes of cognitive dysfunction in affected patients and associated high-risk populations (Robinson and Ferrier 2006). We begin, however, by considering the context within which cognitive deficits manifest—namely, the patients.

The Patient Perspective

Before we embark on a discussion of research findings, it is important to consider the experience of patients who have bipolar disorder. This topic is noteworthy because, although we discuss in this chapter the findings from many studies that report changes in neurocognition, patients express their problems in relatively simple terms using direct language, and the nuances of their experience are not easily captured by the standard tools used by professionals. The following brief vignettes highlight some of the cognitive dysfunction experienced by patients with bipolar disorder during their daily routines and working lives. The important aspects to note are the subtlety of the deficits, the difficulty that individuals have in accepting their deficits, and the profound impact these deficits can have on everyday function.

Case Vignette 1

A 42-year-old bank manager with a wife and two children describes himself as successful. He enjoys his job and is financially secure. He has been stable while receiving medication (lithium, intermittently in conjunction with antidepressants) and has reasonable insight into his illness. He was diagnosed with bipolar disorder 3 years after the onset of symptoms and began treatment almost immediately. He now complains of difficulties with attention and memory, which are most notable with clients at work, and finds it hard to retain simple day-to-day facts and figures. He has compensated by writing most things down and looking things up when necessary and usually gets by; however, he occasionally draws attention to himself because of cognitive slips, especially in meetings. He recalls that he had a "brilliant memory" while attending college and could work long hours without making any mistakes. In fact, many of his student colleagues used to copy his lecture notes. He blames the medication in part for his cognitive difficulties but reveals that he believes there is something fundamentally wrong with his thinking.

Case Vignette 2

A 19-year-old recently enrolled university student with a 1-year history of bipolar I disorder complains of feeling anxious and low in mood and notes that this has "disastrous effects" on her studies. She scored top marks in her high school and deferred attending university for a year because of ill health. She has modest insight into her mental illness and is still "coming to terms with the label of bipolar disorder." She states that when well she is "perfectly fine" but that the slightest change in mood resulting in irritability or anxiety renders her "unable to function." Interestingly, when she is moderately high she feels "fine" but acknowledges that her work is of poor quality. Medication is not really a potential contributor to her thinking problems because she has generally refused to take medication long term and remains essentially medication free. She describes her inability to function cognitively as follows: "I'm just not how I used to be. I'm quietly going mad because something is eating away at my brain."

The cognitive impairments alluded to in these two accounts are at first pass relatively mild. However, it is important to recognize the cumulative functional impact of even very subtle cognitive deficits in patients with bipolar disorder, because over a long period of time they can have extremely disabling consequences. It is therefore imperative that we better understand the cognitive profile of bipolar disorder.

The Cognitive Profile of Bipolar Disorder

The Impact of Mood Symptoms

The discovery of deficits that persist during periods of euthymia in patients with bipolar disorder has suggested that a trait pattern could serve as a marker of this illness (Malhi et al. 2004). Although such a potential diagnostic hallmark remains elusive, there is evidence that particular deficits persist during euthymia and across all mood states in bipolar disorder. Individual characteristics of the disorder, such as years of illness, number of episodes, and their associated impact on cognitive function, have not been extensively researched. However, increased episodes and greater numbers of hospitalizations have been associated with poorer cognitive functioning in domains such as visual memory (Rubinsztein et al. 2000) and verbal memory (Martinez-Aran et al. 2004b). Age at onset of illness has not yet been shown to have an impact on the cognitive outcome of bipolar patients, and evidence that duration of illness is inversely related to cognitive outcome is equivocal (Clark et al. 2001; Martinez-Aran et al. 2004a, 2004b). A key limitation of the studies to date is that findings are cross-sectional; that is, few of the studies record a decline from previous levels of functioning, making it difficult to conclude whether deficits existed premorbidly, occur only in the presence of mood symptoms, or reflect general cognitive decline.

There is some evidence to suggest that cognitive impairment persists over time, which supports the hypothesis that cognitive impairment is indeed a trait marker of the illness (Balanzá-Martinez et al. 2005; see also Chapter 4 of this volume). Most studies focus on comparing a group of bipolar patients with a control group of subjects who are healthy, have depression, or have schizophrenia. These studies and the evidence they provide for deficits in each mood phase of bipolar disorder are reviewed below.

Euthymia

Despite substantial evidence of cognitive deficits during acute affective episodes, much of the early research in the cognitive function of bipolar disorder assumed that when patients recovered, they returned to normal functioning in all domains and regained intact cognitive abilities. However, more recent studies have cast doubt on this assumption, suggesting that during euthymia, deficits may persist in sustained attention, verbal memory, verbal fluency, and executive functioning (Martinez-Aran et al. 2004b; van Gorp et al. 1999). In particular, euthymic patients have been shown to make a high number of perseverative errors on the Wisconsin Card Sorting Test (Martinez-Aran et al. 2002a). This finding suggests a processing deficit consistent with an earlier report by Sapin et al. (1987), whose study showed that euthymic bipolar patients rely on specific details rather than general information to generate a response when trying to solve problems. Theories about processing efficiency propose that euthymic bipolar patients are perhaps "slower" because of the added cognitive load required to sustain attention to a stimulus (Fleck et al. 2005). Memory deficits, especially in verbal memory, have also been consistently found in euthymic bipolar patients (Ali et al. 2001; Clark et al. 2002; Malhi et al. 2007a).

Depression

Cognitive deficits associated with depression vary with the patient's age, severity of depression, and comorbidity; however, even mild depression in unmedicated patients is associated with significant impairment (Smith et al. 2006). Older adult patients with mild depression, regardless of past affective polarity, demonstrate impaired letter fluency but not semantic fluency, in contrast to their unimpaired, nondepressed counterparts (Ravdin et al. 2003). Memory and concentration problems are among the core symptoms of depression and are reflected in the cognitive profile of depressive disorders. Deficits have been found in performance on measures of memory and of sustained attention or concentration (Murphy et al. 1999). Concentration difficulties are perhaps even more pronounced in patients with bipolar depression, who appear to have additional deficits in shifting attention and paying attention to specific stimuli (Murphy and Sahakian

2001; Sweeney et al. 2000). In addition, to the extent that executive dysfunction may be a core deficit in bipolar disorder (see Chapter 2 of this volume, "Attentional and Executive Functioning in Bipolar Disorder"), its manifestations relative to depressive symptoms warrant careful evaluation. Consider the following vignette.

Case Vignette 3

Several months after having been treated successfully for a manic episode with olanzapine at 10 mg/day, a 43-year-old medically healthy male professional with bipolar I disorder complained during psychotherapy of depressed mood, low energy, and anxiety about completing usual work obligations. On interview, he denied vegetative signs, low self-esteem, suicidal thoughts, hopelessness, or physical sluggishness. There were no signs of mania or hypomania and no psychosis. He also denied problems with attention, memory, or wandering thoughts, but said that he felt it difficult to initiate tasks, that he would "read the same paragraph over and over again" with poor comprehension, and that he avoided contact with clients for fear he could not follow through with normal work expectations. On exam, he was alert and oriented but had blunted affect with normal speech and normal movements. He had no difficulty reciting months backward, recalling immediate objects, or recalling presidents. His score on the Beck Depression Inventory (Beck et al. 1996) was 13, indicating a mild degree of depressive symptom severity.

In this patient, subsyndromal depressive features were evident—a common occurrence in the months following a manic episode (Frye et al. 2006). The patient's subjective problems with initiating, planning, and executing complex but routine work-related activities were suggestive of executive dysfunction in the context of depression. A decision was made not to initiate traditional antidepressants, based on evidence of their propensity to exacerbate mania symptoms in the recent aftermath of mania (MacQueen et al. 2002) and limited known efficacy for bipolar depression, as found in the National Institute of Mental Health (NIMH) Systematic Treatment Enhancement Program for Bipolar Disorder (STEP-BD; Sachs et al. 2007). Consideration was given to adding lamotrigine to olanzapine based on the former's putative antidepressant effects (Calabrese et al. 1999) and cognitive benefits during treatment for bipolar depression (Khan et al. 2004). However, a decision was made instead to augment the effects of olanzapine with the novel psychostimulant modafinil based on provisional data indicating modafinil's acute antidepressant efficacy and safety in bipolar depression (Frye et al. 2007), potential to counteract the sedating effects of atypical antipsychotics (Sevy et al. 2005), and cognitive benefits (for further discussion, see Chapter 8 of this volume). Improvement was evident within several days at a dosage of 100 mg/day, with no signs of psychomotor activation or hypomania.

Cognitive signs associated with depression may also be useful when considering broader diagnostic concepts related to bipolar disorder. Using a "softer" definition of bipolarity, Smith et al. (2006) identified a population with bipolar spectrum disorder, based on Ghaemi et al.'s (2002) description of these patients as having, for example, 1) recurrent major depressive disorder and a history of bipolar traits, such as antidepressant-induced mania; 2) a first-degree relative with bipolar disorder; and 3) frequent recurrences of depressive episodes. Smith et al. compared a young cohort of patients with bipolar spectrum disorders and a group with major depressive disorder and found evidence to suggest that bipolar spectrum disorders involved more pervasive neuropsychological deficits, particularly in verbal memory and executive functioning. Interestingly, a euthymic major depressive disorder control group was less cognitively impaired than the bipolar spectrum group but more impaired than healthy controls (Smith et al. 2006). In addition, studies have reported more profound psychomotor slowing in bipolar than in unipolar depressed patients, as measured by tests of processing speed (e.g., the Digit Symbol subtest of the Wechsler Adult Intelligence Scale) (Fleck et al. 2005). Compared with patients with unipolar depression or healthy controls, bipolar depressed patients have been shown to perform more poorly on effortful verbal tasks. Deficits in visuospatial and nonverbal learning in both bipolar depressed and major depressive disorder populations have also been identified (Borkowska and Rybakowski 2001).

Cognitive biases affecting depressive thinking, along the lines of those described by Aaron Beck et al. (1979), may explain some of the characteristic performance patterns found in samples of depressed patients (Chamberlain and Sahakian 2004). An example of a cognitive bias in operation may be Murphy et al.'s (1999) discovery of faster response times to sad words by patients during depression in contrast to faster response times to happy words during mania. Further, in comparison to patients with schizophrenia or Parkinson's disease, elderly patients with major depressive disorder who are given feedback about the accuracy of their responses appear more adversely affected by negative feedback, increasing the likelihood of a subsequent incorrect response (Steffens et al. 2001). This is perhaps an indication that cognitive performance can be modulated by affect (for further discussion of how this phenomenon may pertain to psychotherapy, see Chapter 6 of this volume, "Improving Psychotherapy Practice and Technique for Bipolar Disorder: Lessons From Cognitive Neuroscience").

Suicide and Executive Dysfunction

Greater impairment in executive function has been demonstrated in depressed patients with suicidal ideation than in nonsuicidal depressed patients (Marzuk et al. 2005), as well as in depressed patients with high-lethality past suicide attempts than in depressed patients with either low-lethality past suicide attempts or no past suicide attempts (Keilp et al. 2001). Suicidal depressed patients manifest impaired executive function that is more suggestive of deficits in the dorsolateral prefrontal cortex than in the orbitofrontal cortex (see Chapter 1 of this volume, "Overview and Introduction: Dimensions of Cognition and Measures of Cognitive Function"), consistent with regions of probable serotonergic dysfunction (Raust et al. 2007). Intact executive function is needed in order to initiate and plan behaviors as complex as intentional suicide, although impulsive suicidal behaviors are quite often more common than premeditated suicide attempts in patients with mood disorder (Simon et al. 2001). Additionally, deficits in motor sequence learning (Naismith et al. 2006) may impede the capacity of depressed and suicidal patients to consider alternative solutions and responses to life stresses or situations that trigger feelings of hopelessness. Insofar as increased ruminations could mediate the increased risk for suicidal behaviors among anxious patients with bipolar disorder (Simon et al. 2007a), intact executive function may play an important role for inhibiting the progression of ruminative suicidal thoughts to self-destructive acts (Green et al. 2007).

Mania

The investigation of cognition in mania is inherently difficult because of associated psychotic features, distractibility, and impulsivity, which have significantly hindered but not totally prevented research of this phase of bipolar illness. Predictably, manic patients have been found to have difficulty in concentrating or attending (Clark and Goodwin 2004; Sax et al. 1995) and to be more impulsive when making decisions (Clark et al. 2001; see also Chapter 2 of this book). However, mania has also been linked with information processing and executive functioning deficits that include, in particular, difficulties with problem solving, attentional set shifting, and controlling inhibition (Clark et al. 2001; McGrath et al. 1997; Sweeney et al. 2000). Consequently, patients with mania perform poorly on decision-making tasks, and their performance deteriorates as their Young Mania Scale scores increase (Malhi et al. 2004). This suggests that manic symptomatology is closely associated with cognition and that its impact is incremental as symptom severity increases (Rubinsztein et al. 2001).

Studies of mnemonic function in manic patients provide evidence of deficits in working memory and episodic memory (Clark et al. 2001; McGrath et al. 2001), with preliminary evidence suggesting that mixed symptoms further heighten these deficits (Berk et al. 2005; Sax et al. 1995). The cognitive impact of mixed states has received limited empirical study. However, in a study that compared mixed/manic patients with depressed bipolar patients, Sweeney et al. (2000) found that mixed patients demonstrated deficits in episodic and working memory, spatial attention, and problem solving. Similarly, in a study comparing three patient groups—manic, mixed, and bipolar depressed—and healthy controls, Basso et al. (2002) reported comparable cognitive deficits among all three patient groups, which all differed from control subjects on a number of cognitive domains. Interestingly, a number of studies have failed to identify any difference between manic patients and healthy controls on either memory or overall intellectual ability (Green and Walker 1986; Taylor et al. 1981). Further information about hypothesized neuropsychological deficits during mania in bipolar disorder may be gleaned from emerging literature that compares mania with schizophrenia.

The extent to which deficits have been reported in specific cognitive domains across depressed, manic, and euthymic phases of bipolar disorder is summarized in Table 5–1. Greater cognitive impairment has been reported in bipolar than unipolar depression (at least with respect to bipolar I disorder) (Brand and Jolles 1987; Calev et al. 1989; Wolfe et al. 1987); therefore, greater functional impairment may be evident in bipolar than unipolar depression (Mitchell and Malhi 2004). The identified deficits fit well with the theoretical underpinnings of psychological interventions for depression (Chamberlain and Sahakian 2004) that describe altered cognition in depression such that negative stimuli are interpreted as internal, stable, and global entities (e.g., Beck et al. 1979). Additionally, depression and mania confer mood state–dependent cognitive biases that are reflected in response to stimuli (Murphy et al. 1999), such that negative feedback in depression, for instance, appears to have an impact on future performance. Curiously, manic patients may also possess a cognitive predisposition to negative stimuli. Bentall et al. (2005) administered a task involving recall of self-descriptive words in which depressed patients endorsed more negative words as descriptive of themselves and recalled more negative words, whereas manic patients endorsed more positive words in reference to themselves but recalled more negative ones. Relatedly, Goldberg et al. (2008) found that bipolar manic patients more often endorsed negative than positive attitudes and core beliefs, resembling cognitive schemas similar to those seen in depressed patients.

The Impact of Psychotic Symptoms

As noted in Chapter 1 of this volume, affective or anxiety symptoms have been shown to adversely affect cognitive performance more profoundly than does acute psychosis; however, a handful of recent studies, but not all (Selva et al. 2007), have reported that a history of psychotic symptomatology does indeed impact specific cognitive function in patients with bipolar I disorder and, importantly, also influences health-related quality of life and functioning (e.g., Depp et al. 2006). Specifically, during periods of euthymia, bipolar patients with a history of psychotic symptoms demonstrate significant impairment relative to bipolar patients without psychosis on specific aspects of frontal executive function and spatial working memory (Bora et al. 2007; Glahn et al. 2007). In contrast, bipolar patients with or without psychosis performed comparably on measures of attention, fluency, memory, and psychomotor speed (Bora et al. 2007; Glahn et al. 2007; Selva et al. 2007). A history of psychosis also has been associated with impaired verbal fluency in other studies (Rocca et al. 2008). Further, patients with bipolar disorder who have a positive family history of any psychotic disorder in a first-degree relative have been shown to perform significantly worse than patients with no such family history (Tabarés-Seisdedos et al. 2003). Taken together, these data support the notion that a history of psychosis in patients with bipolar disorder, or in their first-degree relatives, worsens the cognitive course of the illness with regard to specific neurocognitive impairments. This notion is compatible with the existence of some common genetic factors along the "psychosis continuum," including psychotic affective disorders and major psychotic illnesses such as schizophrenia.

There is also evidence to suggest that psychosocial outcome in schizophrenia is predicted more robustly by general cognitive functioning than by individual cognitive domains (Green et al. 2000). It is plausible that this also applies to assessments of bipolar disorder, although the extent of cognitive domains impaired in individuals with bipolar disorder appears less global than that seen in schizophrenia (Burdick et al. 2006; Dickerson et al. 2004).

A Comparison of Bipolar Disorder and Schizophrenia

Substantial evidence links psychotic features to poor outcome in psychotic disorders such as schizophrenia. Broadly speaking, in schizophrenia, verbal learning appears to be associated with poor social functioning, whereas in bipolar disorder, social functioning relates more directly to problem solving and poor planning. As a consequence, diminished reasoning in approaching daily difficulties and stressors may significantly contribute to the often debilitating functional impact of bipolar disorder.

Evidence suggests that although remitted patients with bipolar disorder show cognitive deficits, they perform better on tests of cognitive functioning than patients with schizophrenia, and the cognitive profile of bipolar disorder reflects specific, rather than global, deficits (Chamberlain and Sa-

TABLE 5–1. Studies finding cognitive impairments in phases of bipolar disorder

Impairment	Phase of bipolar disorder		
	Depression	Mania	Euthymia
Sustained attention	Malhi et al. 2007a	Addington and Addington 1997 Bora et al. 2006 Clark et al. 2001 McGrath et al. 1997	Bora et al. 2006 Clark et al. 2002 Clark et al. 2005 Ferrier et al. 1999
Selective attention	None	Addington and Addington 1997	None
Visuospatial memory	Goldberg et al. 1993	Badcock et al. 2005 Gourovitch et al. 1999 McGrath et al. 2001	Deckersbach et al. 2004a Glahn et al. 2006 Rubinsztein et al. 2000 Thompson et al. 2006
Verbal fluency	Martinez-Aran et al. 2002b Wolfe et al. 1987	None	Martinez-Aran et al. 2002a Rossell 2006
Inhibitory control	None	Malhi et al. 2007a Murphy et al. 1999	None
Cognitive flexibility	Malhi et al. 2007a Martinez-Aran et al. 2004a Savard et al. 1980	Malhi et al. 2007a Martinez-Aran et al. 2004a McGrath et al. 1997	Ferrier et al. 1999 Goswami et al. 2006 Martinez-Aran et al. 2002a Martinez-Aran et al. 2004a Martinez-Aran et al. 2004b Morice 1990
Problem solving	Goldberg et al. 1993	None	None
Verbal learning	Bearden et al. 2006 Martinez-Aran et al. 2002a	Clark et al. 2001	Deckersbach et al. 2004b Deckersbach et al. 2005

TABLE 5–1.　Studies finding cognitive impairments in phases of bipolar disorder *(continued)*

Impairment	Phase of bipolar disorder		
	Depression	**Mania**	**Euthymia**
Verbal memory	Calev et al. 1989 Martinez-Aran et al. 2004a Strauss et al. 1984	Atre-Vaidya et al. 1998 Martinez-Aran et al. 2004a	Clark et al. 2002 Ferrier et al. 1999 Goswami et al. 2006 Gourovich et al. 1999 Martinez-Aran et al. 2004a Martinez-Aran et al. 2004b van Gorp et al. 1999 Wolfe et al. 1987

hakian 2004; Dickerson et al. 2004; Olley et al. 2005b; Quraishi and Frangou 2002). A review by Krabbendam et al. (2005) indicates that patients with schizophrenia performed worse in 9 of 11 cognitive domains when compared with patients with bipolar disorder, whose deficits were more circumscribed. In this regard, psychopathology symptoms have been proposed as being more important than cognition for determining social functioning (Laes and Sponheim 2006). It appears that the impact of cognitive deficits on social functioning may differ in patients with bipolar disorder and patients with schizophrenia, because even though both groups perform similarly on measures of social functioning, patients with schizophrenia perform worse on measures of social acceptability and effectiveness (Dickerson et al. 2001).

There is also evidence, however, that cognitive deficits may be more associated with symptom type than with diagnosis, which is particularly true of psychotic features in these disorders (Kravariti et al. 2005). In an investigation of executive functioning, bipolar manic patients had greater similarity in cognitive profile to patients with disorganized schizophrenia than to either bipolar depressed patients or patients with schizophrenia demonstrating prominent negative symptoms of bipolar illness (Kravariti et al. 2005). This similarity has been replicated in a task demanding the ability to attend to and manipulate information to generate a correct response (Glahn et al. 2006). These findings therefore corroborate earlier studies that describe similarities between the cognitive profiles of schizophrenia and bipolar disorder, although many studies suggest that these studies are perhaps biased and reflect more severely affected bipolar patient samples.

The Impact of Anxiety Symptoms

Anxiety has long been recognized as a factor known to interfere with normal cognitive functioning. Indeed, before clinicians can reliably diagnose the presence of bona fide cognitive deficits in patients with mood disorder, they must carefully screen for the presence of anxiety symptoms or related features. Consider the following example.

Case Vignette 4

A 49-year-old married man with an approximately 20-year history of bipolar II disorder sought consultation for depression. He had been taking divalproex at 1,500 mg/day, producing a serum trough valproate level of 74 µg/dL, to which lamotrigine was added at 25 mg every other day for the first 2 weeks, followed by 25 mg/day for the following 2 weeks. In the course of treatment, he reported long-standing problems with memory, predating his current pharmacology and particularly involving tasks of emotional importance to him. Examples included difficulty remembering meeting dates or deadlines and trouble recalling the content of meetings with coworkers. "Bedside" assessment revealed that the patient had no errors with encoding information but modest difficulty with short-term recall, intact with cueing. A prior psychiatrist, wondering about a possible diagnosis of attention-deficit/hyperactivity disorder, undertook a trial of mixed amphetamine salts, which produced a "hyperalert" sensation but no effect otherwise. Further inquiry revealed a substantial degree of free-floating anxiety with near-constant fears of making errors at work. The patient described an excessive pattern of worry that was difficult to control, as well as feelings of restlessness.

Several of his depressive symptoms were noted to overlap with features of generalized anxiety disorder, and it was suggested to him that his problems with memory could be artifactually related to untreated comorbid anxiety. His regimen of divalproex and lamotrigine was augmented with quetiapine in order to target ongoing symptoms of bipolar depression (Calabrese et al. 2005; Thase et al. 2006) as well as coincident anxiety symptoms that were consistent with comorbid generalized anxiety disorder (Hirschfeld et al. 2006). Cognitive strategies (including list making and relaxation techniques) also were begun for managing the patient's anxiety and its potential expression through memory gaps in high-fear situations.

Anxiety symptoms or full syndromes are common in patients with bipolar disorder, appearing in half or more of individuals surveyed in community-based samples (Grant et al. 2005). The Epidemiologic Catchment Area survey results indicated that the rates of anxiety disorders comorbid with bipolar disorder were 21% for obsessive-compulsive disorder and 21% for panic disorder (Chen and Dilsaver 1995a, 1995b). This compares with rates of 0.8% and 2.6% for obsessive-compulsive disorder and panic disorder, respectively, in the general population. In another study of patients with bipolar I disorder, 24% were found to have one comorbid anxiety disorder, most often panic disorder (affecting 16% of patients) (Henry et al. 2003). Kessler et al. (1994) reported that lifetime occurrence of anxiety disorders can be as high as 92% for people with bipolar I disorder, compared with 25% in the general population. However, to date, no studies have investigated the cognitive profile of bipolar disorder and comorbid anxiety, even though it is widely acknowledged that anxiety can alter cognitive performance, and hence anxiety is routinely assessed during neuropsychological evaluations.

Anxiety has been shown to be associated with psychopathology in mood spectrum disorders with psychotic features (Cassano et al. 1999). In bipolar disorder, anxiety is related to poor functional outcome (Feske et al. 2000) and suicidality (Simon et al. 2007b). Specifically, generalized and social anxiety disorders appear associated with current suicidal ideation and behaviors in outpatients with bipolar disorder. However, this association becomes no longer significant when age at first episode of mood disorder and current bipolar recovery are factored into analyses, suggesting that the severity of bipolar illness may be mediating the link between anxiety and suicidality. Earlier age at onset of bipolar disorder was also associated with increased comorbidity of generalized social anxiety and panic disorder in the NIMH STEP-BD program (Perlis et al. 2004; Simon et al. 2004) and has also been linked with poor outcome (Otto et al. 2006).

The association of anxiety with bipolar disorder is important both theoretically and clinically. Anxiety is known to impact negatively and significantly on the cognitive interpretation of feared stimuli, and it is likely that this, in combination with the cognitive deficits that commonly occur in bipolar disorder, contributes to the poorer prognosis that patients with comorbid anxiety manifest. Clinicians must also be aware that the use of benzodiazepines as anxiolytic treatments for patients with bipolar disorder may directly impair arousal, attention, and memory (as described more fully in Chapter 7 of this volume), and hence such potential iatrogenic factors require consideration in the evaluation of cognitive problems in anxious patients with bipolar disorder.

Future Directions for Cognitive Profiling of Bipolar Disorder

As discussed in Chapter 4 of this volume, the concept of an endophenotype for both affective and psychotic disorders has become a matter of increasing interest. Impairments in both executive and cognitive domains have been found in patients with schizophrenia and their unaffected first-degree relatives (Rosa et al. 2004; Zalla et al. 2004). In bipolar disorder, the unaffected monozygotic twins of bipolar probands have been shown to have deficits in verbal memory and visuospatial functioning (Gourovitch et al. 1999). However, there has been less thorough investigation of whether these are stable deficits indicative of trait dysfunction in bipolar disorder, as contrasted with longitudinal studies of schizophrenia that reveal persistent dysfunction across multiple domains, including working memory and executive function (Bartok et al. 1996; Basso et al. 1998; Burdick et al. 2006). Recent longitudinal studies and neuroimaging investigations in bipolar disorder indicate a trait deficit (Malhi et al. 2007a, 2007b).

Importantly, it must be noted that longitudinal and association studies are predicated on the assumption that neurocognition represents a stable trait (Gottesman and Gould 2003). In schizophrenia, impaired facial recognition has been put forward as a putative neurocognitive trait (Addington and Addington 1998) and, similarly, nonverbal memory (Purdon et al. 2000) and verbal fluency (Cuesta et al. 2001) deficits appear to change little over time or with treatment. Burdick et al. (2006) suggested that neurocognitive performance in bipolar disorder is more related to attentional processes than other functions, such as memory or executive processes, which may be more subject to variability. Indeed, improvement in cognitive performance has been demonstrated in bipolar mania (Liu et al. 2002). The stability of attentional performance contrasts with suggestions by Drs. Glahn, Burdick, and Bearden in Chapter 4 of this volume that executive functioning or working memory and verbal learning or explicit memory may represent the most viable endophenotype for neurocognition in bipolar disorder.

In a recent review, Robinson and Ferrier (2006) identified a consistent relationship between mania and impaired verbal explicit memory and executive functioning. They highlighted that euthymic bipolar patients have greater difficulty with encoding, whereas manic patients appear to have more difficulty with retention. In comparison, depressed bipolar patients experience consistently reduced performance on visual memory, spatial working memory, verbal learning, and executive tasks.

Further evidence that neurocognitive impairment may be a trait marker has begun to emerge from research into childhood and adolescent presentations of bipolar disorder (Cahill et al. 2007). Difficulties with attentional set shifting, visuospatial memory, verbal learning, and memory have been demonstrated in this population (Dickstein et al. 2004; McClure et al. 2005a), and many of the deficits mirror those that have been demonstrated in adult populations. Also, McClure et al. (2005b) found that adolescents with bipolar disorder display deficits in emotion recognition and response flexibility, and Ernst et al. (2004) found that this population has greater sensitivity to negative feedback on a gambling task than controls, despite comparable performance overall.

Conclusions

In this chapter, we have focused on mood, anxiety, and psychotic symptoms and how they relate to cognition in bipolar disorder. Other comorbidities, such as substance abuse, personality disorders, and history of trauma, are likely to impact negatively on cognition in bipolar disorder and, in addition to the comorbidities we reviewed, are worthy of further investigation to improve understanding of the mechanisms underlying their cognitive impact. Cognitive profiling of bipolar disorder is beginning to yield preliminary insights into the disorder and to contribute to the construction of an as yet incomplete illustration characterized by specific deficits in attention and verbal explicit memory (Malhi et al. 2006) (see Figure 5–1). These findings require replication in different subsets of bipolar populations but in the meantime suggest that future research should focus on better characterization of bipolar disorder in order to improve diagnosis

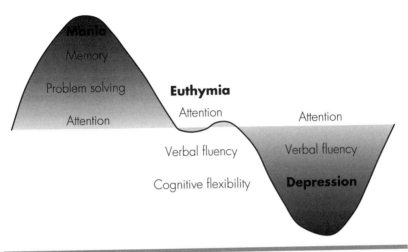

FIGURE 5–1.   Clinical picture of key neuropsychological deficits across phases of bipolar disorder.

and treatment options. It is crucial to develop more sensitive and perhaps more socially appropriate tests, such as those tapping into theory of mind (Olley et al. 2005a; see also Chapter 6 of this volume).

In practice, the message is simple: Bipolar disorder is profoundly disabling not only when patients are visibly unwell but also when they are seemingly recovered. It is important to inquire about patients' cognitive compromise with questions concerning attention and memory and to inform patients that these difficulties are not necessarily a consequence of medication. Greater awareness and monitoring are likely to be of assistance, as are acknowledgment of these impairments and neuropsychological assessment.

Take-Home Points

- Bipolar depression is associated with more severe and extensive cognitive impairment than seen in unipolar depression, particularly with respect to problems with memory and concentration, including deficits in verbal memory, sustained attention, shifting attention, and executive dysfunction.

- Executive dysfunction and orbitofrontal deficits may contribute to the probability of impulsive (rather than premeditated and planned) suicide attempts in bipolar depressed patients.

- Manic symptoms exacerbate underlying bipolar vulnerabilities toward disinhibition, poor decision making, impaired problem solving and attentional set shifting, deficits in working memory and episodic memory, and executive dysfunction. However, deficits in these domains persist, albeit to a lesser degree, during periods of euthymia.

• Bipolar manic patients tend to recall self-descriptive words and display core belief patterns that closely resemble those seen in depressed patients. These patterns of affective bias may contribute to cognitive impairment in other domains (e.g., difficulty in set shifting).

• A personal or family history of psychosis may be associated with more extensive cognitive impairment in patients with bipolar disorder.

• Anxiety symptoms or comorbid syndromes can directly impair cognitive function and must be considered when assessing reasons for cognitive deficits. Treatment of comorbid anxiety features may also help to improve apparent cognitive problems that might otherwise be misattributed to other aspects of psychopathology in bipolar disorder, such as affective symptoms or psychosis.

References

Addington J, Addington D: Attentional vulnerability indicators in schizophrenia and bipolar disorder. Schizophr Res 23:197–204, 1997

Addington J, Addington D: Facial affect recognition and information processing in schizophrenia and bipolar disorder. Schizophr Res 17:171–181, 1998

Ali SO, Denicoff KD, Altshuler LL, et al: Relationship between prior course of illness and neuroanatomic structures in bipolar disorder: a preliminary study. Neuropsychiatry Neuropsychol Behav Neurol 14:227–232, 2001

Atre-Vaidya N, Taylor MA, Seidenberg MA, et al: Cognitive deficits, psychopathology, and psychosocial functioning in bipolar mood disorder. Neuropsychiatry Neuropsychol Behav Neurol 11:120–126, 1998

Badcock J, Michiel PT, Rock D: Spatial working memory and planning ability: contrasts between schizophrenia and bipolar I disorder. Cortex 41:753–763, 2005

Balanzá-Martínez V, Tabarés-Seisdedos R, Selva-Vera G, et al: Persistent cognitive dysfunctions in bipolar I disorder and schizophrenic patients: a 3-year follow-up study. Psychother Psychosom 74:113–119, 2005

Bartok J, Sands J, Harrow M, et al: Executive functioning deficits in schizophrenia patients 15 years after initial hospitalization. J Int Neuropsychol Soc 2:22, 1996

Basso M, Nasrallah HA, Olson SC, et al: Neuropsychological correlates of negative, disorganized and psychotic symptoms in schizophrenia. Schizophr Res 31:99–111, 1998

Basso MR, Lowery N, Neel J, et al: Neuropsychological impairment among manic, depressed, and mixed episode inpatients with bipolar disorder. Neuropsychology 16:84–91, 2002

Bearden C, Glahn DC, Monkul ES, et al: Patterns of memory impairment in bipolar disorder and unipolar major depression. Psychiatry Res 142:139–150, 2006

Beck AT, Rush AJ, Shaw BF, et al: Cognitive Therapy of Depression. New York, Guilford, 1979

Beck AT, Steer RA, Brown GK: Beck Depression Inventory, 2nd Edition. San Antonio, TX, Psychological Corporation, 1996

Bentall R, Kinderman P, Manson K: Self-discrepancies in bipolar disorder: comparison of manic, depressed, remitted and normal participants. Br J Clin Psychol 44:457–473, 2005

Berk M, Dodd S, Malhi GS: 'Bipolar missed states': the diagnosis and clinical salience of bipolar mixed states. Aust N Z J Psychiatry 39:215–221, 2005

Bora E, Vahip S, Akdeniz F: Sustained attention deficits in manic and euthymic patients with bipolar disorder. Prog Neuropsychopharmacol Biol Psychiatry 30:1097–1102, 2006

Bora E, Vahip S, Akdeniz F, et al: The effect of previous psychotic mood episodes on cognitive impairment in euthymic bipolar patients. Bipolar Disord 9:468–477, 2007

Borkowska A, Rybakowski JK: Neuropsychological frontal lobe tests indicate that bipolar depressed patients are more impaired than unipolar. Bipolar Disord 3:88–94, 2001

Brand N, Jolles J: Information processing in depression and anxiety. Psychol Med 17:145–153, 1987

Burdick K, Goldberg JF, Harrow M, et al: Neurocognition as a stable endophenotype in bipolar disorder and schizophrenia. J Nerv Ment Dis 194:255–260, 2006

Cahill CM, Green MJ, Jairam R, et al: Do cognitive deficits in juvenile bipolar disorder persist into adulthood? J Nerv Ment Dis 195:891–896, 2007

Calabrese JR, Bowden CL, Sachs GS, et al; for Lamictal 602 Study Group: A double-blind placebo-controlled study of lamotrigine monotherapy in outpatients with bipolar I depression. J Clin Psychiatry 60:79–88, 1999

Calabrese JR, Keck PE Jr, Macfadden W, et al: A randomized, double-blind, placebo-controlled trial of quetiapine in the treatment of bipolar I or II depression. Am J Psychiatry 162:1351–1360, 2005

Calev A, Nigal D, Chazan S: Retrieval from semantic memory using meaningful and meaningless constructs by depressed, stable bipolar and manic patients. Br J Clin Psychol 28:67–73, 1989

Cassano G, Pini S, Saettoni M, et al: Multiple anxiety disorder comorbidity in patients with mood spectrum disorders with psychotic features. Am J Psychiatry 156:474–476, 1999

Chamberlain S, Sahakian BJ: Cognition in mania and depression: psychological models and clinical implications. Curr Psychiatry Rep 6:451–458, 2004

Chen Y, Dilsaver SC: Comorbidity for obsessive-compulsive disorder in bipolar and unipolar disorders. Psychiatry Res 59:57–64, 1995a

Chen Y, Dilsaver SC: Comorbidity of panic disorder in bipolar illness: evidence from the Epidemiologic Catchment Area Survey. Am J Psychiatry 152:280–282, 1995b

Clark L, Goodwin G: State- and trait-related deficits in sustained attention in bipolar disorder. Eur Arch Psychiatry Clin Neurosci 254:61–68, 2004

Clark L, Iversen SD, Goodwin GM: A neuropsychological investigation of prefrontal cortex involvement in acute mania. Am J Psychiatry 158:1605–1611, 2001

Clark L, Iversen SD, Goodwin GM: Sustained attention deficit in bipolar disorder. Br J Psychiatry 180:313–319, 2002

Clark L, Kempton MJ, Scarnà A, et al: Sustained attention-deficit confirmed in euthymic bipolar disorder but not in first-degree relatives of bipolar patients or euthymic unipolar depression. Biol Psychiatry 57:183–187, 2005

Cuesta M, Peralta V, Zarzuela A: Effects of olanzapine and other antipsychotics on cognitive function in chronic schizophrenia: a longitudinal study. Schizophr Res 48:17–28, 2001

Deckersbach T, McMurrich S, Oqutha J, et al: Characteristics of non-verbal memory impairment in bipolar disorder: the role of encoding strategies. Psychol Med 34:823–832, 2004a

Deckersbach T, Savage CR, Reilly-Harrington N, et al: Episodic memory impairment in bipolar disorder and obsessive-compulsive disorder: the role of memory strategies. Bipolar Disord 6:233–244, 2004b

Deckersbach T, Savage CR, Dougherty DD, et al: Spontaneous and directed application of verbal learning strategies in bipolar disorder and obsessive-compulsive disorder. Bipolar Disord 7:166–175, 2005

Depp CA, Davis CE, Mittal D, et al: Health-related quality of life and functioning of middle-aged and elderly adults with bipolar disorder. J Clin Psychiatry 67:215–221, 2006

Dickerson F, Sommerville J, Origoni AE, et al: Outpatients with schizophrenia and bipolar I disorder: do they differ in their cognitive and social functioning? Psychiatry Res 102:21–27, 2001

Dickerson F, Boronow JJ, Stallings CC, et al: Cognitive functioning in schizophrenia and bipolar disorder: comparison of performance on the Repeatable Battery for the Assessment of Neuropsychological Status. Psychiatry Res 129:45–53, 2004

Dickstein DP, Treland JE, Snow J, et al: Neuropsychological performance in pediatric bipolar disorder. Biol Psychiatry 55:32–39, 2004

Ernst M, Dickstein DP, Munson S, et al: Reward-related processes in pediatric bipolar disorder: a pilot study. J Affect Disord 82 (suppl 1):S89–S101, 2004

Ferrier IN, Stanton BR, Kelly TP, et al: Neuropsychological function in euthymic patients with bipolar disorder. Br J Psychiatry 175:246–251, 1999

Feske U, Frank E, Mallinger AG, et al: Anxiety as a correlate of response to the acute treatment of bipolar I disorder. Am J Psychiatry 157:956–962, 2000

Fleck D, Shear PK, Strakowski SM: Processing efficiency and sustained attention in bipolar disorder. J Int Neuropsychol Soc 11:49–57, 2005

Frye MA, Yatham LN, Calabrese JR, et al: Incidence and time course of subsyndromal symptoms in patients with bipolar I disorder: an evaluation of 2 placebo-controlled maintenance trials. J Clin Psychiatry 67:1721–1728, 2006

Frye MA, Grunze H, Suppes T, et al: A placebo-controlled evaluation of adjunctive modafinil in the treatment of bipolar depression. Am J Psychiatry 164:1242–1249, 2007

Ghaemi SN, Ko JY, Goodwin FK: "Cade's disease" and beyond: misdiagnosis, antidepressant use, and a proposed definition for bipolar spectrum disorder. Can J Psychiatry 47:125–134, 2002

Glahn D, Bearden CE, Cakir S, et al: Differential working memory impairment in bipolar disorder and schizophrenia: effects of lifetime history of psychosis. Bipolar Disord 8:117–123, 2006

Glahn DC, Bearden CE, Barguil M, et al: The neurocognitive signature of psychotic bipolar disorder. Biol Psychiatry 62:910–916, 2007

Goldberg JF, Gerstein RK, Wenze SJ, et al: Dysfunctional attitudes and cognitive schemas in bipolar manic and unipolar depressed outpatients: implications for cognitively based psychotherapies. J Nerv Ment Dis 196:207–210, 2008

Goldberg TE, Gold JM, Greenberg J, et al: Contrasts between patients with affective disorders and patients with schizophrenia on a neuropsychological test battery. Am J Psychiatry 150:1355–1362, 1993

Goswami U, Sharma A, Khastigir U, et al: Neuropsychological dysfunction, soft neurological signs and social disability in euthymic patients with bipolar disorder. Br J Psychiatry 188:366–373, 2006

Gottesman I, Gould TD: The endophenotype concept in psychiatry: etymology and strategic intentions. Am J Psychiatry 160:636–645, 2003

Gourovitch ML, Torrey EF, Gold JM, et al: Neuropsychological performance of monozygotic twins discordant for bipolar disorder. Biol Psychiatry 45:639–646, 1999

Grant BF, Stinson FS, Hasin DS, et al: Prevalence, correlates, and comorbidity of bipolar I disorder and Axis I and II disorders: results from the National Epidemiologic Survey on Alcohol and Related Conditions. J Clin Psychiatry 66:1205–1215, 2005

Green M, Walker E: Attentional performance in positive- and negative-symptom schizophrenia. J Nerv Ment Dis 174:208–213, 1986

Green M, Kern RS, Braff DL, et al: Neurocognitive deficits and functional outcome in schizophrenia: are we measuring the "right stuff"? Schizophr Bull 26:119–136, 2000

Green MJ, Cahill CM, Malhi GS: The cognitive and neurophysiological basis of emotion dysregulation in bipolar disorder. J Affect Disord 103:29–42, 2007

Henry C, van den Bulke D, Bellivier F, et al: Anxiety disorders in 318 bipolar patients: prevalence and impact on illness severity and response to mood stabilizer. J Clin Psychiatry 64:331–335, 2003

Hirschfeld RM, Weisler RH, Raines SR, et al: Quetiapine in the treatment of anxiety in patients with bipolar I or II depression: a secondary analysis from a randomized, double-blind, placebo-controlled study. J Clin Psychiatry 67:355–362, 2006

Keilp JG, Sackheim HA, Brodsky BS, et al: Neuropsychological dysfunction in depressed suicide attempters. Am J Psychiatry 158:735–741, 2001

Kessler R, McGonagle KA, Zhao S, et al: Lifetime and 12-month prevalence of DSM-III-R psychiatric disorders in the United States: results from the National Comorbidity Survey. Arch Gen Psychiatry 51:8–19, 1994

Khan DA, Ginsberg LD, Asnis GM, et al: Effect of lamotrigine on cognitive complaints in patients with bipolar I disorder. J Clin Psychiatry 65:1483–1490, 2004

Krabbendam L, Arts B, van Os J, et al: Cognitive functioning in patients with schizophrenia and bipolar disorder: a quantitative review. Schizophr Res 80:137–149, 2005

Kravariti E, Dixon T, Frith C, et al: Association of symptoms and executive function in schizophrenia and bipolar disorder. Schizophr Res 74:22–31, 2005

Laes J, Sponheim SR: Does cognition predict community function only in schizophrenia? a study of schizophrenia patients, bipolar affective disorder patients, and community control subjects. Schizophr Res 84:121–131, 2006

Liu S, Chiu CH, Chang CJ, et al: Deficits in sustained attention in schizophrenia and affective disorders: stable versus state-dependent markers. Am J Psychiatry 159:975–982, 2002

MacQueen GM, Young LT, Marriott M, et al: Previous mood state predicts response and switch rates in patients with bipolar depression. Acta Psychiatr Scand 105:414–418, 2002

Malhi GS, Ivanovski B, Szekeres V, et al: Bipolar disorder: it's all in your mind? The neuropsychological profile of a biological disorder. Can J Psychiatry 49:813–819, 2004

Malhi GS, Cahill C, Ivanovski B, et al: A neuropsychological "image" of bipolar disorder. Clinical Approaches in Bipolar Disorders 5:2–13, 2006

Malhi GS, Ivanovski B, Hazdi-Pavlovic D, et al: Neuropsychological deficits and functional impairment in bipolar depression, hypomania and euthymia. Bipolar Disord 9:114–125, 2007a

Malhi GS, Lagopoulos J, Sachdev P, et al: Is a lack of disgust something to fear? An fMRI facial emotion recognition study in euthymic bipolar disorder patients. Bipolar Disord 9:345–357, 2007b

Martinez-Aran A, Penadés R, Vieta E, et al: Executive function in patients with remitted bipolar disorder and schizophrenia and its relationship with functional outcome. Psychother Psychosom 71:39–46, 2002a

Martinez-Aran A, Vieta E, Colom F, et al: Neuropsychological performance in depressed and euthymic bipolar patients. Neuropsychobiology 46 (suppl 1):16–21, 2002b

Martinez-Aran A, Vieta E, Colom F, et al: Cognitive impairment in euthymic bipolar patients: implications for clinical and functional outcome. Bipolar Disord 6:224–232, 2004a

Martinez-Aran A, Vieta E, Reinares M, et al: Cognitive function across manic or hypomanic, depressed, and euthymic states in bipolar disorder. Am J Psychiatry 161:262–270, 2004b

Marzuk PM, Hartwell N, Leon AC, et al: Executive functioning in depressed patients with suicidal ideation. Acta Psychiatr Scand 112:294–301, 2005

McClure EB, Treland JE, Snow J, et al: Deficits in social cognition and response flexibility in pediatric bipolar disorder. Am J Psychiatry 162:1644–1651, 2005a

McClure EB, Treland JE, Snow J, et al: Memory and learning in pediatric bipolar disorder. J Am Acad Child Adolesc Psychiatry 44:461–469, 2005b

McGrath J, Scheldt S, Welham J, et al: Performance on tests sensitive to impaired executive ability in schizophrenia, mania and well controls: acute and subacute phases. Schizophr Res 26:127–137, 1997

McGrath J, Chapple B, Wright M: Working memory in schizophrenia and mania: correlation with symptoms during the acute and subacute phases. Acta Psychiatr Scand 103:181–188, 2001

Mitchell PB, Malhi GS: Bipolar depression: phenomenological overview and clinical characteristics. Bipolar Disord 6:530–539, 2004

Morice R: Cognitive inflexibility and pre-frontal dysfunction in schizophrenia and mania. Br J Psychiatry 157:50–54, 1990

Murphy FC, Sahakian BJ: Neuropsychology of bipolar disorder. Br J Psychiatry 41(suppl):120–127, 2001

Murphy FC, Sahakian BJ, Rubinsztein JS, et al: Emotional bias and inhibitory control processes in mania and depression. Psychol Med 29:1307–1321, 1999

Naismith SL, Hickie IB, Ward PB, et al: Impaired implicit sequence learning in depression: probe for frontostriatal dysfunction? Psychol Med 36:313–323, 2006

Olley AL, Malhi GS, Bachelor J, et al: Executive functioning and theory of mind in euthymic bipolar disorder. Bipolar Disord 7 (suppl 5):43–52, 2005a

Olley AL, Malhi GS, Mitchell PB, et al: When euthymia is just not good enough: the neuropsychology of bipolar disorder. J Nerv Ment Dis 193:323–330, 2005b

Otto MW, Simon NW, Wisniewski SR, et al: Prospective 12-month course of bipolar disorder in out-patients with and without comorbid anxiety disorders. Br J Psychiatry 189:20–25, 2006

Perlis RH, Miyahara S, Marangell LB, et al: Long-term implications of early onset in bipolar disorder: data from the first 1000 participants in the Systematic Treatment Enhancement Program for Bipolar Disorder (STEP-BD). Biol Psychiatry 55:875–881, 2004

Purdon S, Jones BD, Stip E, et al; for The Canadian Collaborative Group for research in schizophrenia: Neuropsychological change in early phase schizophrenia during 12 months of treatment with olanzapine, risperidone, or haloperidol. Arch Gen Psychiatry 57:249–258, 2000

Quraishi S, Frangou S: Neuropsychology of bipolar disorder: a review. J Affect Disord 72:209–226, 2002

Raust A, Slama F, Mathieu F, et al: Prefrontal cortex dysfunction in patients with suicidal behavior. Psychol Med 37:411–419, 2007

Ravdin LD, Katzen HL, Agrawal P, et al: Letter and semantic fluency in older adults: effects of mild depressive symptoms and age-stratified normative data. Clin Neuropsychol 17:195–202, 2003

Robinson L, Ferrier IN: Evolution of cognitive impairment in bipolar disorder: a systematic review of cross-sectional evidence. Bipolar Disord 8:103–116, 2006

Rocca CC, Macedo-Soares MB, Gorenstein C, et al: Verbal fluency dysfunction in euthymic bipolar patients: a controlled study. J Affect Disord 107:187–192, 2008

Rosa A, Peralta V, Cuesta MJ, et al: New evidence of association between COMT gene and prefrontal neurocognitive function in healthy individuals from sibling pairs discordant for psychosis. Am J Psychiatry 161:1110–1112, 2004

Rossell SL: Category fluency performance in patients with schizophrenia and bipolar disorder: the influence of affective categories. Schizophr Res 82:135–138, 2006

Rubinsztein JS, Michael A, Paykel ES, et al: Cognitive impairment in remission in bipolar affective disorder. Psychol Med 30:1025–1036, 2000

Rubinsztein J, Fletcher PC, Rogers RD, et al: Decision-making in mania: a PET study. Brain 124:2550–2563, 2001

Sachs GS, Nierenberg AA, Calabrese JR, et al: Effectiveness of adjunctive antidepressant treatment for bipolar depression. N Engl J Med 356:1711–1722, 2007

Sapin LR, Berrettini WH, Nurnberger JI Jr, et al: Mediational factors underlying cognitive changes and laterality in affective illness. Biol Psychiatry 22:979–986, 1987

Savard RJ, Rey AC, Post RM: Halstead-Reitan Category Test in bipolar and unipolar affective disorders: relationship to age and phase of illness. J Nerv Ment Dis 168:297–304, 1980

Sax KW, Strakowski SM, McElroy SL, et al: Attention and formal thought disorder in mixed and pure mania. Biol Psychiatry 37:420–423, 1995

Selva G, Salazar J, Balanzá-Martinez V, et al: Bipolar I patients with and without a history of psychotic symptoms: do they differ in cognitive functioning? J Psychiatr Res 41:265–272, 2007

Sevy S, Rosenthal MH, Alvir J, et al: Double-blind, placebo-controlled study of modafinil for fatigue and cognition in schizophrenia patients treated with psychotropic medications. J Clin Psychiatry 66:839–843, 2005

Simon NM, Otto MW, Wisniewski SR, et al: Anxiety disorder comorbidity in bipolar disorder patients: data from the first 500 participants in the Systematic Treatment Enhancement Program for Bipolar Disorder (STEP-BD). Am J Psychiatry 161:1–8, 2004

Simon NM, Pollack MH, Ostacher MJ, et al: Understanding the link between anxiety symptoms and suicidal ideation and behaviors in outpatients with bipolar disorder. J Affect Disord 97:91–99, 2007a

Simon NM, Zalta AK, Otto MW, et al: The association of comorbid anxiety disorders with suicide attempts and suicidal ideation in outpatients with bipolar disorder. J Psychiatr Res 41:255–264, 2007b

Simon OR, Swann AC, Powell KE, et al: Characteristics of impulsive suicide attempts and attempters. Suicide Life Threat Behav 32 (suppl 1):49–59, 2001

Smith D, Muir WJ, Blackwood DH: Neurocognitive impairment in euthymic young adults with bipolar spectrum disorder and recurrent major depressive disorder. Biol Psychiatry 8:40–46, 2006

Steffens D, Wagner HR, Levy RM, et al: Performance feedback deficit in geriatric depression. Biol Psychiatry 50:358–363, 2001

Strauss ME, Bohannon WE, Stephens JH, et al: Perceptual span in schizophrenia and affective disorders. J Nerv Ment Dis 172:431–435, 1984

Sweeney JA, Kmiec JA, Kupfer DJ: Neuropsychologic impairments in bipolar and unipolar mood disorders on the CANTAB neurocognitive battery. Biol Psychiatry 48:674–684, 2000

Tabarés-Seisdedos R, Balanzá-Martínez V, Salazar-Fraile J, et al: Specific executive/attentional deficits in patients with schizophrenia or bipolar disorder who have a positive family history of psychosis. J Psychiatr Res 37:479–486, 2003

Taylor MA, Redfield J, Abrams R: Neuropsychological dysfunction in schizophrenia and affective disease. Biol Psychiatry 16:467–478, 1981

Thase ME, Macfadden W, Weisler RH, et al: Efficacy of quetiapine monotherapy in bipolar I and II depression: a double-blind, placebo-controlled study (the BOLDER II study). J Clin Psychopharmacol 26:600–609, 2006

Thompson JM, Hamilton CJ, Gray JM, et al: Executive and visuospatial sketchpad resources in euthymic bipolar disorder: implications for visuospatial working memory architecture. Memory 14:437–451, 2006

van Gorp WG, Altshuler L, Theberge DC, et al: Declarative and procedural memory in bipolar disorder. Biol Psychiatry 46:525–531, 1999

Wolfe J, Granholm E, Butters N, et al: Verbal memory deficits associated with major affective disorders: a comparison of unipolar and bipolar patients. J Affect Disord 13:83–92, 1987

Zalla T, Joyce C, Szöke A, et al: Executive dysfunctions as potential markers of familial vulnerability to bipolar disorder and schizophrenia. Psychiatry Res 121:207–217, 2004

6

Improving Psychotherapy Practice and Technique for Bipolar Disorder

Lessons From Cognitive Neuroscience

Joseph F. Goldberg, M.D.

Cory F. Newman, Ph.D.

Gin S. Malhi, M.B.Ch.B., B.Sc. (Hons), F.R.C.Psych., F.R.A.N.Z.C.P., M.D.

David J. Miklowitz, Ph.D.

In recent years, several forms of psychotherapy specific to bipolar disorder have been developed that demonstrate efficacy in reducing affective symptoms, fostering relapse prevention, and improving quality of life when integrated with appropriate pharmacotherapy. Structured psychotherapies draw on knowledge about cognitive and interpersonal deficits associated with bipolar disorder and employ largely remedial techniques to counter maladaptive behaviors, attitudes, and emotional experiences. Psychotherapy in this sense represents an active learning paradigm—for example, acquiring new skills to better anticipate and negotiate the effects of stress, or replacing negative attitudes and assumptions with new and more fair and balanced perspectives and insights about oneself and one's capabilities. Undertaking such activities in most psychotherapies presupposes the patient's capacity to sustain attention, manipulate abstract concepts, shift sets, iden-

tify environmental cues, test hypotheses, and appreciate the emotional valence of memories (as in the case of traumatic experiences or repetitive
maladaptive behaviors). In group-based psychoeducational therapies or
family-focused therapies, each individual must also have the capacity to recognize the effects that his or her behaviors have on others, consider alternative viewpoints, and identify thoughts, feelings, and motivations held by
others as being separate from his or her own.

Formal training in the practice of psychotherapy—whether psychody-
namic, supportive, cognitive-behavioral, interpersonal, group based, or
family based—seldom incorporates education about those very deficits in
executive function and related operations in which patients must engage to
participate meaningfully in the work of psychotherapy. A broadened awareness of such neurocognitive processes may help practitioners understand
the mechanics of psychotherapy from a new vantage point, and help shape
and modify technique by taking into account cognitive limitations and
points of leverage for more successful psychotherapy outcomes.

General Points of Consideration for Psychotherapists

Problems with attention, verbal memory, and executive function are common in patients with bipolar disorder across all phases of illness but may be
especially pronounced during acute phases of affective episodes. Gross impairment in attention and selective attention, as seen during mania, limits
the extent to which bipolar patients can bring to bear the information processing skills central to most psychotherapies. By contrast, severe depressive phases do not seem to impair patients' capacity to derive functional
benefits from intensive psychotherapy, despite the presumed adverse effects of depression on cognitive efficiency (Miklowitz et al. 2006).

Neurocognitively important phenomena often emerge during the
course of psychotherapy, such as the inability to acknowledge and appreciate alternative points of view about oneself and about the world. Cognitive-behavioral, interpersonal, or family-focused psychotherapies for
depression typically reframe patients' negative attitudes or emotional experiences as reflecting the effects of a biologically based illness, thereby falling
within a disease model, and guide patients toward alternative outlooks and
perspectives about themselves vis-à-vis the environment. Analogously,
dynamically oriented psychotherapies tend to conceptualize maladaptive
patterns of thinking or behavior as reflecting factors such as poor insight
(e.g., denying, or failing to recognize and appreciate, one's own role in a
dispute) or intrapsychic conflict (e.g., repetitive patterns of self-sabotaging
behavior that result in undesirable outcomes). Most structured as well as

contemporary dynamic psychotherapies encourage practitioners to consider whether symptoms such as social isolation, apathy, or low motivation may be explainable as signs of untreated affective illness within the disease model, before speculating about psychological (e.g., conflict-based) etiologies for such phenomena. In a similar way—but one that may be more challenging to recognize—the neurocognitive deficits of bipolar disorder may also contribute to patients' problems with relationships, decision making, or role functioning. Consider, for example, a euthymic patient with bipolar disorder whose spouse complains that the patient lacks empathy and ignores others' concerns and feelings. Worthy of dynamic exploration are the patient's thoughts and feelings about such complaints, his or her perceptions about their validity, and whether similar problems arise globally across settings or are circumscribed in nature. At the same time, frank cognitive deficits involving social inattentiveness may exist that appear tantamount to poor empathy or outright indifference, insofar as judgments about oneself relative to others depend on activation of specific neural networks, as described further in the subsection of this chapter titled "Social Cognition and Impaired Capacity for Understanding Others' Intentions (Theory of Mind)."

One task of psychotherapy involves gauging a patient's capacity for empathy, alongside other neurocognitive domains, as part of the process for generating hypotheses about potential reasons for deficits. Knowledge of neurocognitive corollaries to communication problems that may arise during psychotherapy can give psychotherapists a broadened perspective in making such determinations.

In the following sections, we discuss a number of representative common themes addressed in psychotherapy that hold particular relevance to neurocognitive processes: rigidity of thinking and cognitive flexibility; social cognition and impaired capacity for understanding others' intentions; difficulty incorporating feedback; impaired judgment; and perseveration, impulsivity, and disinhibition.

Rigidity of Thinking and Cognitive Flexibility

Psychotherapists often seek to guide patients toward greater insight about decisions or behaviors they engage in that seem maladaptive, or motivations that appear counterproductive to their own interests, when such realizations are not readily apparent. Patients' refusals to acknowledge such maladaptations and their possible motives are sometimes assumed by psychotherapists to reflect denial or to be resistance to confronting behaviors or psychological experiences that may be emotionally unpleasant. However, it may sometimes be appropriate to consider whether there also exist frank neurocognitive obstacles for incorporating new perspectives.

Cognitive flexibility involves the capacity to process unexpected conditions within the environment and redirect one's attention to recognize novel aspects of a problem and its possible solutions (Canas et al. 2003). Inflexible patterns of thinking may be mediated by emotional or intrapsychic factors (e.g., either a deliberate or unwitting refusal to consider alternative perspectives that may be emotionally difficult or narcissistically intolerable); however, psychotherapists must be equally alert to the potential among individuals with bipolar disorder for difficulty in shifting cognitive sets, a type of executive dysfunction mediated largely by prefrontal cortical dysfunction. Clinicians also must be alert to the potential for cognitive inflexibility to reflect a psychotic process, as may occur when patients demonstrate such severe rigidity of thought, with an inability to consider alternative points of view because of an unwavering level of belief conviction, that it constitutes delusional thinking. Anxious ruminations and obsessive thoughts differ from delusional thought by virtue of the preserved capacity for reality testing and the ability to shift attention to entertain alternative perspectives.

Social Cognition and Impaired Capacity for Understanding Others' Intentions (Theory of Mind)

Theory of mind (ToM) is the cognitive ability to infer mental states to others and oneself with respect to emotion, thought, and intention. ToM dysfunction has been linked to symptoms of schizophrenia—in particular, negative symptoms and symptoms of disorganization (Mazza et al. 2001; Sarfati et al. 1997). Patients with impaired ToM may show difficulty with interpersonal intuition and may even appear to lack empathy, as when recognizing the emotional effect their words or actions may have on others.

Often in psychotherapy, patients struggle to understand reasons for emotional responses and reactions they receive from people in their lives. One element in such instances may involve the ability to "read" the emotions of others based on facial expression, body language, verbal tone, and an awareness of the effect one's own behavior has on others, and to recognize the beliefs, desires, and intentions of other people as separable from one's own concerns. Consider, for example, an ebullient, boisterous, hypomanic passenger on a long airplane flight who intrusively attempts to engage the passenger next to him in a conversation laden with excessive disclosure of personal information, then becomes irritated and frustrated when his overtures are rebuffed. The capacity to gauge others' reactions to interpersonal exchanges and respond appropriately involves a complex convergence of skills related to empathy, social judgment, and the ability to incorporate feedback, any or all of which may be compromised in individuals with bipolar illness. This type of interpersonal awareness is central to the interpersonal and social rhythm therapy approach (Frank et al. 2000, 2005).

ToM deficits have been well characterized across illness phases in bipolar disorder. Early studies included small, heterogeneous samples of individuals with bipolar disorder (Fletcher et al. 1995; Mazza et al. 2001) who were often subsumed within groups identified as having "psychosis" or groups that served as controls for comparison groups with schizophrenia (Drury et al. 1998; Sarfati et al. 1999). More recent studies that have examined bipolar patients across mood states (Kerr et al. 2003) as well as when the individuals are euthymic (Inoue et al. 2004) have noted ToM deficits that persist during remission and may predispose the patients to poorer social functioning (Inoue et al. 2006).

ToM deficits compromise social interactions that may be essential for healthy social adjustment (Inoue et al. 2006). This ToM deficit in bipolar euthymia appears to be associated with executive dysfunction (Olley et al. 2005). ToM deficits in people with bipolar disorder are most likely part of a more global cognitive impairment that includes problems with sustained attention and executive function (Bora et al. 2005; Clark et al. 2002). The neurobiology of empathy further bears on ToM, insofar as the process of making judgments about oneself appears to depend on activation of subregions of the medial prefrontal cortex and left temporal cortex, whereas judgments about others involves activation of the left lateral prefrontal cortex and medial occipital cortex (Ochsner et al. 2004; Schulte-Rüther et al. 2007).

One means of studying brain function during ToM tasks involves the use of functional magnetic resonance imaging (fMRI) while subjects are asked to interpret the social meaning conveyed within cartoons of human interactions. As illustrated in Figure 6–1, subjects with bipolar disorder differ from healthy control subjects in regions of cerebral blood flow during such tasks—notably, patients appear to show diminished blood flow in the middle frontal gyrus, which clinically may translate to diminished understanding of the social context of stimuli. Limited prefrontal elaboration of emotional meaning in euthymic bipolar patients has been recently demonstrated in two fMRI studies (Malhi et al. 2007a, 2007b), suggesting that this may be a trait deficit or at least a dysfunction that necessitates longer-term treatment for remediation.

Further related to ToM, successful social behavior entails the ability to differentiate various expressed facial emotions. Generalized impairment in the perception of emotions has been demonstrated in depressed subjects (Persad and Polivy 1993), as well as in patients with bipolar mania (Lembke and Ketter 2002) and during euthymic phases of bipolar disorder (Harmer et al. 2002). In further investigation of this phenomenon, Venn et al.

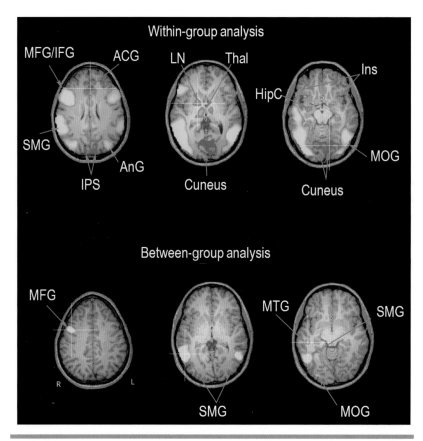

FIGURE 6-1.   Differences between subjects with bipolar disorder and healthy controls during interpretation of theory of mind cartoons.

Activation foci depicting within- and between-group blood oxygen level–dependent changes for control subjects (lentiform nucleus [LN], thalamus [Thal], insula [Ins], hippocampus [HipC], middle temporal gyrus [MTG], supramarginal gyrus [SMG], middle occipital gyrus [MOG]) versus bipolar patients (anterior cingulate gyrus [ACG], intraparietal sulcus [IPS], cuneus). All activations depicted represent the contrast between theory of mind task and random motion (blue denotes bipolar patients and yellow-orange denotes healthy subjects). The between-group analysis differences favored the healthy subjects. The within-group data were Bonferroni corrected to z scores greater than 4.0, corresponding to corrected whole brain P-value < 0.05. The random effects (between-group) results indicate regions of significantly increased activity for the control subjects compared with bipolar patients. All images are radiologically oriented. AnG=angular gyrus; L=left; MFG/IFG=middle/inferior frontal gyrus; R=right.

(2004) examined whether differences in facial emotional recognition are dependent on mood state or whether this impairment is an underlying trait in bipolar disorder. Compared with healthy matched control individuals, the remitted bipolar group showed no difference in sensitivity to any specific emotion (happiness, surprise, sadness, fear, anger, or disgust). Although a statistical trend was evident in the bipolar subjects' ability to recognize fear, this was not significantly greater than that of the other emotions. This study does not lend support for misinterpretation of facial emotions as an underlying trait in the development of bipolar illness, but it does suggest that errors in distinguishing facial expressions among depressed and manic patients may be mood-congruent influences. The discrepancy found between the results of Venn et al. (2004) and those of other investigators may be due to methodological differences, sample sizes, medication effects, and collapsing of the bipolar subgroups.

Difficulty Incorporating Feedback

The capacity to appreciate and utilize feedback (as measured during performance task paradigms) generally appears intact among depressed patients; however, compared with matched controls, depressed patients make more performance errors when negative feedback is accompanied by inaccurate or misleading information (Murphy et al. 2003) and by negative affect (Elliott et al. 1997). Cognitive models of depression point out that depressed patients magnify the significance of failures and overestimate the importance and generalizability of failures, and may have greater difficulty making use of negative feedback when it is linked with a strong "affective" element as opposed to a strong "informational" element (Murphy et al. 2003). In the setting of psychotherapy, patients who struggle with negative feedback may benefit from having therapists guide them to identify and filter negative affective bias from feedback that might otherwise be constructive and informative.

Impaired Judgment

Faulty decision making is sometimes considered to be willful volitional behavior. It is often difficult for clinicians to discern whether socially or professionally inappropriate behaviors reflect a deliberate attempt to deceive or harm others (e.g., in the case of embezzlement) or, rather, a lapse in judgment that more accurately reflects the failure to consider the adverse consequences of certain risky acts. ToM research suggests that poor social cognition may partly arise from a diminished ability to recognize normal fear—that is, individuals who fail to detect and meaningfully appreciate fearful responses in others may themselves be more prone to behave in ways that appear socially incognizant (Corden et al. 2006).

Rich et al. (2006) found that adolescents with bipolar disorder perceived greater hostility in neutral faces and reported more fear when viewing them than age- and sex-matched control subjects. In an fMRI paradigm, the bipolar patients were distinguished from the controls by their greater activation in the left amygdala, nucleus accumbens, putamen, and ventral prefrontal cortex when rating facial hostility. They also showed greater activation in the left amygdala and bilateral nucleus accumbens when rating their fear of faces.

Perseveration, Impulsivity, and Disinhibition

Lesions to the frontal lobe (specifically, the orbitofrontal cortex) classically are associated with impulsive and socially inappropriate behaviors. Similarly, decreased activation of the rostral and orbitofrontal cortex as seen in bipolar mania may contribute to impaired planning, judgment, and insight, as well as more primitive or inappropriate responses to internal drives (Blumberg et al. 1999). Impulsivity and loss of inhibition in themselves appear to be trait phenomena in patients with bipolar disorder seen across manic, depressed, and euthymic mood states (Peluso et al. 2007), and as such may reflect a type of fundamental impairment in executive function (Mur et al. 2007).

A therapeutically important neurocognitive corollary to managing impulsivity bears on the concept of mindfulness as described originally by Marsha Linehan and colleagues in the treatment of suicidality and distress intolerance in patients with borderline personality disorder (e.g., see Linehan et al. 2006). Turning one's attention toward (rather than away from) unpleasant affects represents an example of manipulating the attention network (e.g., redirection or reorienting, focusing attention, and sustaining attention on a chosen target). The use of mindfulness as a form of meditation applicable to psychotherapy also represents an example of deliberately engaging the attention network (Ivanovski and Malhi 2007; Teasdale et al. 1995). A study by Williams et al. (2008) found that mindfulness-based cognitive-behavioral therapy (CBT) effectively treated anxiety symptoms in patients with bipolar disorder.

Learning and Emotional Memory

A further neurocognitive dimension pertinent to psychotherapy involves the concept of emotional learning and fear extinction. LeDoux (1992) first proposed a model in which memories of learned events (e.g., classical conditioning or associative learning) are more indelible and less prone to disruption when learning occurs during states of high emotional arousal. The so-called fear circuit is thought to bypass neocortical structures and instead route through limbic structures such as the central nucleus of the amygdala

(LeDoux 1998; Willensky et al. 2006). Perhaps the most compelling examples of fear-based learning in humans involve trauma and phobic avoidance.

Trauma

Histories of abuse or trauma—often a focus of psychotherapeutic attention
among patients with mood disorder—may be evident in nearly half of
adults with bipolar disorder (Garno et al. 2005). Childhood trauma poses
a risk factor for the development of comorbid posttraumatic stress disorder
in adults with bipolar disorder (Goldberg and Garno 2005) and may
worsen the course of bipolar illness (Post and Leverich 2006). Fear-based
memories (i.e., traumatic memories) may be especially difficult to alter
through traditional learning paradigms in psychotherapy, partly by virtue
of the limbic basis for their original acquisition and consolidation. Similarly, the emotional reexperiencing of a trauma (e.g., flashbacks) may also
act to solidify such memories (i.e., through rehearsal).

So-called corrective emotional experiences compellingly pair learning
with emotional engagement. Psychotherapeutic interventions may therefore have the greatest impact when conducted in a nonaversive environment that fosters the acquisition, consolidation, and retention of new
information. Moreover, effective cognitive-behavioral strategies generally
require multiple iterations (i.e., active rehearsal) of relaxation techniques,
or systematic desensitization, paired with the conditioned stimulus and its
maladaptive response, in order to reverse fear- or limbic-based learning that
has occurred in the context of trauma.

The therapeutic alliance itself may serve, among other functions, as a
means to engage limbic circuitry within the learning paradigm of psychotherapy, both by suppressing fear (i.e., instilling basic trust) and by linking
a learning paradigm with an emotionally powerful experience.

Fear, Anxiety, and Emotional Perseveration

The medial prefrontal cortex is thought to modify behavior in response to
fearful or aversive stimuli by inhibiting amygdala output (Sotres-Bayon et
al. 2006). Intact functioning of the ventromedial prefrontal cortex is
thought to inhibit fear responses, a concept described as *emotional perseveration* (Morgan et al. 2003). Studies that involve task-switching and inhibitory control paradigms show that increasing working memory load
interferes with executive control over attention (Hester and Garavan
2005), meaning that in the midst of excessive worry, it becomes especially
difficult to selectively redirect one's focus of attention, and emotional distress may dominate over the capacity to utilize effective coping skills for
solving problems and managing perceived crises. Such observations bear
on neuropsychological dimensions of anxiety states and syndromes, which

may be present as comorbid phenomena in more than half of individuals with bipolar disorder (Grant et al. 2005).

In the case of anxiety and anxious ruminations, it may be difficult to suppress the processing of information that is evoked by active rehearsal, causing material (e.g., negative thoughts) to remain in working memory with little capacity for executive suppression. Consequently, effective behavioral strategies to counter such phenomena may require not only learning new ideas and ways of thinking, but also—particularly in the context of executive impairment—pairing maladaptive patterns with new, competing ideas or experiences that carry an emotional valence (again, the concept of corrective emotional experiences). Traditional behavioral techniques to treat simple phobias aim to extinguish fear responses by engaging limbic processing through the use of exposure and desensitization. A broadened application of such ideas may be useful as a means to counteract faulty emotion processing—presumably, also by engaging limbic structures through emotional involvement during learning. From a mechanical standpoint, a goal of psychotherapy involves training patients to engage executive processes more efficiently in order to better regulate emotional distress, and at the same time acquire new ways of thinking about old problems in an emotionally engaged context.

Formal cognitive therapy draws, sometimes implicitly, on the manipulation of executive processes by teaching patients to redirect attention, shift sets, and link emotional states with the process of challenging the logic behind faulty assumptions. Specific applications of cognitive therapy, in the context of neurocognitive deficits associated with bipolar disorder, are described in the following section.

Applications Within Cognitive-Behavioral Therapy

As developed by Aaron Beck and colleagues (1979) for understanding and treating major depression, and subsequently adapted for individuals with bipolar disorder, CBT draws on identifying and modifying or restructuring biased beliefs and thought patterns distorted by negative attitudes and faulty assumptions about oneself vis-à-vis the world. Such thought patterns become identified, challenged, and redirected in the context of therapy sessions through a process of critical evaluation and decision making. When undertaken with adjunctive pharmacotherapy, cognitive therapy—similar to interpersonal and social rhythm therapy (IPSRT) or family-focused therapy (FFT)—has been shown to hasten the time until remission from acute bipolar depression (Miklowitz et al. 2007b) and improve social functioning and life satisfaction (Miklowitz et al. 2007a).

Two studies have examined CBT in relapse prevention within randomized controlled trials. Lam et al. (2005) found that CBT was more effective than treatment as usual (TAU) in delaying relapses over 12 months, although the effects were weakened over 30 months. Nonetheless, patients in CBT spent fewer days ill and had better functioning than patients in TAU. Observed increases in relapse rates over an ensuing 18 months may favor ongoing or "booster" sessions after completion of an acute initial treatment module (Lam et al. 2005).

Scott et al. (2006), in a five-site United Kingdom study, found that patients in CBT fared no better than those in TAU in terms of relapse prevention. Notably, CBT appeared to delay relapses among patients with fewer than 12 episodes, whereas TAU delayed relapses relative to CBT in patients with 12 or more episodes. Thus, Lam et al.'s (2005) results were only replicated for Scott et al.'s subgroup of less recurrent (or younger) patients.

Neurocognitive Mechanics of Cognitive Therapy

Cognitive distortions develop and become reinforced over time in daily life through selective attention and reiteration, such as by repeatedly discounting or dismissing positive experiences and by overattending to and overgeneralizing from negative experiences. Much of the work that occurs during cognitive therapy hinges on a person's ability to consider novel and alternative points of view in response to familiar but stressful stimuli (e.g., perceived losses, disappointments, or misappraisals of social or professional opportunities). At its most fundamental level, cognitive therapy involves the "unlearning" of negative attitudes and biases about oneself relative to the world, and replacement or restructuring of faulty beliefs with alternative ones that are free from bias. Such a skill is akin to learning a new language or becoming facile with driving a car on the opposite side of the road from usual. In essence, patients identify new patterns of thinking and then practice replacing old patterns with the new ones until the process becomes automatic—that is, explicit memory processes eventually become implicit. Performing such operations requires the capacity to manipulate information and draw alternative inferences from events and experiences, operations that are influenced by factors such as selective attention, emotional learning, working memory, and cognitive flexibility or set shifting. These abilities may be more intact among patients who have been less neurologically compromised by repeated episodes of the disorder, and, indeed, Scott et al. (2006) found that CBT was less effective than TAU among patients with 12 or more prior episodes.

One component of change in cognitive therapy involves learning new patterns of thinking in response to specific stimuli, a process that initially may be likened to learning a new language or mechanical skill, one that typically begins as an effortful conscious repetition of facts (relying on recitation and *explicit* memory) before achieving fluency through practice and reiteration (i.e., fostering a process that uses *implicit* memory, occurring without conscious effort). Practice effects result from repetitive exercises aimed to replace dysfunctional thought patterns (e.g., "I will never succeed") with more neutral attitudes and assumptions (e.g., "I can improve my skills and make myself more competitive"). A major goal of cognitive therapy, from a neurocognitive standpoint, involves not only replacing one set of thoughts and beliefs with another through a learning paradigm but also improving a patient's aptitude to remove affective bias and suspend perseveration about those beliefs.

Incorporating specific cognitive therapy techniques may be useful to address common neurocognitive problems in individuals with bipolar disorder. By the same token, it may become important to modify standard cognitive therapy techniques to take into account the types of neurocognitive deficits that might otherwise impede the work of psychotherapy. Following are specific examples of such instances.

Impaired Sustained Attention/Vigilance

Distractibility often arises (or worsens from baseline) during phases of mania or hypomania. In session, this phenomenon may manifest itself in the patients' difficulties in staying on topic and/or answering therapists' direct questions. In such instances, therapists should concentrate on bringing patients back on task in a caring yet assertive way. Therapists and patients facilitate the patients' attentional focus by using and referring back to an agenda they formulated together at the start of the session. Therapists also should make ample use of summary statements (e.g., "Here is what we have been trying to discuss and deal with so far today"), followed by asking the patients if they can provide their own overviews of the main points covered in the session. Cognitive therapists give their patients a clear message that therapy is an educational process and not just a supportive conversation. Further, they tell their bipolar patients explicitly that an important goal of cognitive therapy is to learn to think in a more structured and organized fashion.

At home, patients will need to utilize and practice methods for staying on task, such as when they must take care of chores and other responsibilities. To prepare for this, cognitive therapists teach their bipolar patients the engineering principle of redundant systems, so that if one method fails there are others that serve as safeguarding backups. This is a fancy way of saying that bipolar patients need multiple sources of reminders to keep them focused on short-term tasks and goals. These redundant reminders may take the form of flash cards, e-mails to oneself, memos on a personal digital assistant, or any visual reminder that will serve to alert the patient to a task that needs attention. The involvement of family members in treatment may also facilitate recall and follow-through.

Impaired Memory

Clinicians often notice that patients who are in an active symptom episode have difficulty remembering what it was like to be euthymic. The patients may have presented as being hopeful and well reasoned when between depressive and/or manic episodes, but later become convinced that their depressive and/or manic state of mind represents the sole "truth" of their situation. If they are depressed, they may insist that their situation is hopeless, as they dismiss or overlook past examples of their own well functioning. If they are hypomanic or manic, they may ignore the painful consequences of previous decisions made in these states. The implications are significant, in that the constructive lessons that patients have learned when working productively in therapy seem to become moot when their moods become extreme.

To compensate for this problem, therapists assist their patients in creating durable records of both their work in session and their assignments between sessions. Documentation is essential. Toward this end, it is valuable for therapists to have patients make use of notebooks, in which they are directed to write and compile their most constructive observations. Maintaining folders, including copies of exercises such as dysfunctional thought records (see Newman et al. 2001), may also help to remind patients of changes in their thought content related to mood episodes. Patients refer back to these written records of their work in treatment when their recollections of how to enact coping skills otherwise fail them. Similarly, it can be extremely useful to make audio recordings of sessions so that patients can listen to their cognitive therapy sessions multiple times. Not only does this help with memory consolidation, but patients have reported (anecdotally) that it is enlightening to hear themselves when in a different state of mind than when the tape was recorded. Patients come to realize that moods are fleeting and that the more extreme conclusions they draw while in these emotional states need to be tested and reevaluated, rather than accepted as absolute and permanent facts.

Additionally, a hypomanic patient who hears a recording of himself when he was depressed and lamenting his mistakes suddenly may remember why it is important to exercise more prudent behavior. Similarly, a depressed patient who hears his own levelheaded commentary from a past session in which he was euthymic may then feel more hopeful about being able to function well again and may be less apt to make blanket negative statements about himself.

Disinhibition and Impulse-Control Problems

In simple cognitive-behavioral terms, *disinhibition* refers to a person's problems in delaying gratification, in ascertaining potential negative consequences for his or her actions, and in thinking carefully about behavioral options at times of high arousal. At such times, a key skill for patients to develop is the ability to "delay and distract" while he or she buys time to engage in cognitive reflection, to consult with trusted others (including the therapist), and perhaps to receive psychiatric clearance to adjust medications as needed. Neurocognitively, delay-and-distract efforts become attempts to exercise greater executive control over limbically driven behaviors (e.g., learning self-monitoring techniques, prior to the heat of the moment, in order to counter impulsive flares such as road rage).

A useful "preemptive" homework assignment might be to instruct patients to generate a comprehensive list of low-risk alternative activities in which they may engage that will serve to increase their staying power in averting acting on a potentially deleterious impulse. These activities include simple (i.e., not excessively hedonistic or habit-forming) pleasures, such as listening to music, watching a movie, reading a book or periodical, taking a leisurely walk or warm bath, and writing a friendly e-mail message, among others. The hope is that by engaging in such activities, the bipolar patient will forgo doing the more risky activity, such as going on a shopping spree, angrily confronting or being inappropriately seductive toward someone, or using alcohol or other drugs. Linking such alternative activities with emotional or limbic engagement may further serve to consolidate memories of self-soothing for future continuity.

Therapists ask their patients to adopt and implement the principle of "create more, consume less." When individuals are disinhibited (e.g., when chemically impaired, or in a manic state), they will often be tempted to engage in excessively consumptive behaviors, such as eating, drinking, using illicit drugs, spending, or seeking sex. As a result, they risk incurring serious consequences, including reductions in self-esteem in the aftermath. On the other hand, creative behaviors require more effort and thought but are less risky and lead to improved feelings about oneself. Examples include spending time on a project for school or work, writing in a journal or to important others, playing and/or singing music, working on a craft or in a garden, and designing a more pleasant or functional space at home or in the office. Bipolar patients are often quite resistant to these kinds of behavioral recommendations when they are introduced during a manic or hypomanic state. Instead, rehearsing these alternative behaviors when the patient is euthymic can increase the likelihood of their implementation during illness states.

Standard relaxation and breathing control exercises can also help bipolar patients to reduce physiological arousal just enough to be able to say "no" to their own urges to do something overstimulating and potentially risky. Cognitive therapists try to motivate their bipolar patients to choose the more conservative courses of action by appealing to their need to feel strong and effective, such as by saying, "Be the master of your impulses, rather than have your impulses be the master of you."

Hypomanic and manic patients are prone to engage in emotional reasoning, whereby they feel justified in acting and compelled to act on their strongest (but perhaps most problematic) emotions. Unfortunately, such strong emotions may be unfounded and may lead to decisions that cause further loss and shame. In response to this issue, cognitive therapists teach their bipolar patients to notice and study the difference between the *intensity* of their feelings and the *longevity* of their feelings. The patients chart the intensity of their moods (e.g., anger, sexual arousal), on a 0–100 scale over the course of days and weeks. The patients' task is to determine how some of their most seemingly compelling emotions actually hold up over the test of time. Often, patients discover that their moods are variable and that they are better off for having *not* acted rashly on those feelings. Patients should document examples of benefiting from resisting the urge to act on high-amplitude but fleeting moods. Longer-term moods (e.g., resentment about missed opportunities, love and commitment toward family members) then become more of the focus in treatment, as they tie into more enduring states of mind, and more consistent aspects of a patient's real-life situation that need attention.

Executive Dysfunction: Poor Planning

The phenomenon of poor autobiographical recall has been implicated in the problem-solving deficits seen in patients with mood disorders (Williams et al. 2006). Such patients have difficulties in reflecting on their past experiences in anything other than a vague, general, nondescript way. Such a cognitive style reduces their ability to learn specific, constructive lessons from past errors and similarly hinders their capacity for accessing a sense of self-satisfaction based on previous successes. As a result, patients with extreme problems in mood management wind up being prone to act impulsively on the basis of their emotions, which are typically based on old, dysfunctional beliefs. Consequently, these individuals underutilize the methods of rational planning, careful weighing of pros and cons, revising tactics based on past mistakes, anticipating consequences, and cognitive rehearsal (imaginally "walking through" a planned course of action). Thus, cognitive therapists must assist these patients in identifying and practicing the following skills.

- *Instituting a period of "reflective delay" before acting on an emotional impulse.* This may take the form of an informal rule to "get a good, full night's sleep" before acting on an urge (e.g., to buy a car), or waiting at least 48 hours as an experiment to see if one's impulses (and related ideas) subside.
- *Running a "pilot study" rather than the "full experiment."* For example, if a hypomanic patient insists that she wants to quit her job and become a full-time novelist, the therapist may ask her to utilize the period of reflective delay mentioned above, followed by implementing a scaled-back version of the goal, or pilot study (e.g., writing a short story and attempting to get it published in a periodical). This technique serves as a reality check for patients, while allowing them to save face. The patients will not feel unduly controlled by their therapists, thus preserving the positive status of the therapeutic relationship.
- *Writing down a concrete plan of action.* Rather than simply acting, patients learn to write about their goals, including their intended actions to reach those goals, as well as anticipated outcomes (including "unintended consequences"). For example, a patient may say that he wishes to move out of his parents' house to live independently, but he often spends his money unwisely, thus interfering with his goal. In cognitive therapy, this patient might be given the homework assignment of designing a comprehensive personal financial plan, along with a timetable, and specific guidelines for making various expenditures. Further, the assignment may involve writing about potential obstacles or drawbacks to the plan, along with suggested remedies for such problems. When a patient is able to do this assignment, it represents a significant learning experience and serves as a valuable written reminder. If the patient has significant difficulties with this task, it lays bare the patient's deficits in planning and provides concrete evidence against self-aggrandizing beliefs that otherwise resist intervention. Notably, patients may be less receptive to this type of assignment when hypomanic, and, when euthymic, may benefit from becoming accustomed to carrying out such an exercise as an anticipatory intervention.

Impaired Capacity for Empathy

Bipolar patients who become overexuberant often evince a diminished capacity to understand the impact of their behavior on others. For example, a hypomanic patient in a classroom may fail to see how his constant questions are disturbing the progress of a lecture. Similarly, a manic person at a social event may not realize that she is crossing boundaries and causing others distress by boisterously giving personal advice in a bawdy, indiscreet, unsolicited manner. Or a man with bipolar disorder may steadfastly maintain that his multiple extramarital affairs "have nothing to do with" his wife, whose resultant suffering he can neither understand nor tolerate. In such instances, cognitive therapists are greatly challenged to find a way to help such patients to take the perspective of others whom they are adversely affecting. Patients who are lacking in empathy rarely appreciate being told that they need to change their behavior so as to be more thoughtful toward others. However, they may be more likely to examine the perspectives of other people if they see the exercise as a challenge to their intellect and imagination.

For example, therapists can engage their patients in a reverse role-play, where the therapist plays the role of the patient (taking great care not to present an unflattering caricature), while the patient is challenged to adopt the role of the person who presumably is not receiving understanding and consideration from the patient. Many patients at first balk at enacting such role-plays, but some are moved by entreaties to accept the challenge of a technique that "many have tried, but few have mastered."

Impaired Insight

Hypomania and frank mania are associated with (among other problematic symptoms) deficiencies in reality testing. For example, a hypomanic person with no serious athletic training may believe that she is capable of running in an upcoming local half-marathon. When therapists or other well-meaning persons who have the bipolar patient's best interest at heart try to intervene with cautionary feedback, the patient may respond with indignation, believing that she is being treated with an egregious lack of respect and trust. Thus, it is best if the patient's own insights (revealed at times of interepisode euthymia and peak functioning) are documented for later use during times when the patient's judgment is impaired. Toward this end, the following therapeutic principle may be implemented: whenever a patient makes an in-session comment that the therapist finds particularly wise, prudent, or otherwise consistent with the goals of treatment and well functioning, the therapist should "flag" this comment and ask the patient to write it down in a therapy notebook for later use. When the patient begins to slide into a symptom episode and exhibits a reduction in insight, the therapist can recommend that the patient refer back to his or her own notebook for further instruction. This method greatly reduces the risk of a power struggle between therapist and patient, as the "battle" is between the patient's own perceptions, then (when they were more rational) and now (when they are not). The resulting therapeutic dialogue about cognitive restructuring (e.g., on a dysfunctional thought record [DTR]) can proceed in a more respectful, thoughtful, and calm manner.

Although it has more impact when patients themselves arrive at insightful conclusions, there are times when it is necessary to make use of the well-meaning influences of others in the patients' lives. Toward this end, cognitive therapists encourage their bipolar patients to consult with at least two trusted individuals before making any big decisions. One of these chosen people may be the therapist, and it is ideal if another is a patient's spouse or guardian (if applicable). If the patients believe that they would be losing control over their own decision making by asking others for advice in this manner, the therapist is to remind them that the most successful people generally have a team of personal advisers and consultants. Thus, there is no shame in asking one's "inner circle" for crucially important feedback. This technique helps a patient benefit from the insights of others, while also keeping the others (e.g., a spouse) apprised of the patient's plans that may affect them.

In the same way that cognitive therapists use DTRs to address depressive thinking, they may use them to identify and modify hyperpositive thinking (Newman et al. 2001). Thus, instead of using DTRs to reduce pessimism and improve hopefulness, therapists teach bipolar patients to use DTRs to reduce magical thinking (e.g., "I haven't had a problem yet, so I'll just keep doing whatever I want") and to improve forethought (e.g., "I am looking for trouble, when it would be much better if I found a less risky way to have fun").

Applications Within Interpersonal and Family-Focused Treatments

A second theoretical foundation for psychotherapies specific to bipolar disorder, in addition to CBT, stems from identifying and modifying deficits in patients' awareness of social or interpersonal cues, as well as chronobiological factors that may disrupt the regularity of daily activities. Two separate but related psychotherapy modalities drawing on these phenomena include IPSRT (Frank et al. 2000, 2005) and FFT (Miklowitz et al. 2003). From a neurocognitive standpoint, both IPSRT and FFT require that patients identify and learn to cope with life stressors that elicit emotional dysregulation. IPSRT maintains that the most stressful events will be those that are tied to dysregulations of the sleep-wake cycle or to unpredictability in daily routine activities (e.g., overseas flights, birth of a baby, loss of a relationship). For example, a college student in IPSRT might learn that her mood and her sleep-wake cycles change when the school year starts. She might be encouraged to regulate her daily routines as a means of regulating her sleep and wake time. Accomplishing these objectives may require resolving important interpersonal problems that contribute to instability and mood dysregulation (e.g., conflict with a boyfriend, lack of structure formerly imposed by parents).

FFT places more emphasis on a patient's family relationships. The finding that patients are more prone to relapses in high–expressed emotion (highly critical, hostile, or emotionally overinvolved) home environments (Miklowitz et al. 1988; Yan et al. 2004) carries the implication that enhancing the emotional tone and effectiveness of a patient's communication with relatives—and the relatives' communication with the patient—will reduce family tension and contribute to an environment that promotes mood stability. Moreover, educating the patient and relatives about the nature, course, causes, and treatment of bipolar disorder will increase the relatives' empathy for the patient and the limitations imposed by the patient's cognitive functioning. This education may lead to the realization that the patient is not behaving in a willful, oppositional, or purposefully negative manner but rather suffers from a neurochemically based illness.

Cognitive Remediation

A final psychotherapeutic consideration regarding neurocognitive deficits involves the concept of cognitive remediation (CR). Originally described for the treatment of patients with traumatic brain injury and later adapted for the management of deficit states in patients with schizophrenia, CR therapy focuses on the targeted improvement of problems with attention, memory, and executive function. Therapy focuses on the repeated practice of cognitive tasks or the application of training strategies for counteracting cognitive deficits (Pfammatter et al. 2006). In patients with schizophrenia, clinical trials have demonstrated improvement in verbal and nonverbal memory and executive function, in contrast to strictly CBT approaches, which improve overall psychopathology but achieve only modest benefits in neurocognitive domains such as working memory (Penades et al. 2006).

Wykes et al. (2002) examined whether concomitant brain activation changes occur following CR therapy in male patients with schizophrenia compared with a control therapy group and a healthy control group. Patients with schizophrenia were maintained on their antipsychotic medications throughout the study and were randomly assigned to the CR therapy group or control therapy group. Both therapies were 12 weeks long with 40 individual sessions consisting of occupational therapy activities (control therapy) or paper-and-pencil tasks involving practicing information processing strategies in cognitive flexibility, working memory, and planning (CR therapy). At baseline and following the last therapy session, fMRI and tests of executive functioning were completed. At completion of therapy, both groups demonstrated improvements in neuropsychological performance, but there was a definite advantage for those receiving CR in the memory domain. The fMRI data showed that both patient groups had increased brain activation, but particularly the CR group, especially in the frontocortical areas associated with working memory. There were no differences between the patient groups in symptoms or medications. Thus, it seems likely that the brain changes were associated with the psychological rather than the pharmacological treatment.

CR has not been examined in relation to bipolar disorder. Improvements in vocational functioning following depressive episodes were not found for any of the intensive psychotherapies examined in the Systematic Treatment Enhancement Program for Bipolar Disorder (Miklowitz et al. 2007a). More targeted CR approaches that address the unique cognitive deficits of patients with bipolar disorder may be essential to observing vocational improvements.

Conclusions

Knowledge about the types of neurocognitive deficits that are common among individuals with bipolar disorder may help to inform the delivery of more effective and tailored forms of psychotherapy. Identifying potential impairments in attention, executive function, and ToM may help psychotherapists to recognize potential nonobvious contributors to problems in relationships, work functioning, or the management of difficult emotions. Incorporating therapeutic techniques that compensate for possible neurocognitive deficits may allow for more successful outcomes during the course of adjunctive psychotherapy for bipolar disorder.

Take-Home Points

- Severity of depression in bipolar disorder does not limit patients' ability to make effective use of intensive psychotherapy, despite cognitive deficits such as impaired attention or executive dysfunction associated with bipolar depression.

- Cognitive deficits may impinge on psychotherapy efforts in the form of cognitive inflexibility, perseveration, an impaired capacity to shift sets, poor insight, and deficits in social cognition or theory of mind that may hinder an individual's capacity to appreciate the needs and alternative points of view held by other people.

- Cognitive and cognitive-behavioral therapies involve the engagement of attention, the redirection of selective attention (away from negatively biased attitudes), and the use of explicit declarative memory techniques in order to substitute new thought patterns for old ones, eventually creating new implicit memory procedures (akin to acquiring fluency in a new language).

- Effective psychotherapy strategies for patients with bipolar disorder may incorporate recognition of neurocognitive deficits, foster compensatory strategies, and utilize techniques that link emotional learning with new perspectives and ideas that challenge existing, maladaptive patterns of thinking or emotional processing.

References

Beck AT, Rush AJ, Shaw F, et al: Cognitive Therapy of Depression. New York, Guilford, 1979

Blumberg HP, Stern E, Ricketts S, et al: Rostral and orbital prefrontal cortex dysfunction in the manic state of bipolar disorder. Am J Psychiatry 156:1986–1988, 1999

Bora E, Vahip S, Gonul AS, et al: Evidence for theory of mind deficits in euthymic patients with bipolar disorder. Acta Psychiatr Scand 112:110–116, 2005

Canas JJ, Quesada JF, Antolí A, et al: Cognitive flexibility and adaptability to environmental changes in dynamic complex problem-solving tasks. Ergonomics 46:482–501, 2003

Clark L, Iversen SD, Goodwin GM: Sustained attention deficit in bipolar disorder. Br J Psychiatry 180:313–319, 2002

Corden B, Critchley HD, Skuse D, et al: Fear recognition ability predicts differences in social cognitive and neural functioning in men. J Cogn Neurosci 18:889–897, 2006

Drury VM, Robinson EJ, Birchwood M, et al: "Theory of mind" skills during an acute episode of psychosis and following recovery. Psychol Med 28:1101–1112, 1998

Elliott R, Sahakian BJ, Herrod JJ, et al: Abnormal response to negative feedback in unipolar depression: evidence for a diagnosis specific impairment. J Neurol Neurosurg Psychiatry 63:74–82, 1997

Fletcher PC, Happé F, Frith U, et al: Other minds in the brain: a functional imaging study of "theory of mind" in story comprehension. Cognition 57:109–128, 1995

Frank E, Swartz HA, Kupfer DJ: Interpersonal and social rhythm therapy: managing the chaos of bipolar disorder. Biol Psychiatry 48:593–604, 2000

Frank E, Kupfer DJ, Thase ME, et al: Two-year outcomes for interpersonal and social rhythm therapy in individuals with bipolar I disorder. Arch Gen Psychiatry 62:996–1004, 2005

Garno JL, Goldberg JF, Ramirez PM, et al: Impact of childhood abuse on the clinical course of bipolar disorder. Br J Psychiatry 186:121–125, 2005

Goldberg JF, Garno JL: Development of posttraumatic stress disorder in adult bipolar patients with histories of severe childhood abuse. J Psychiatr Res 39:595–601, 2005

Grant BF, Stinson FS, Hasin DS, et al: Prevalence, correlates, and comorbidity of bipolar I disorder and Axis I and II disorders: results from the National Epidemiologic Survey on Alcohol and Related Conditions. J Clin Psychiatry 60:1205–1215, 2005

Harmer CJ, Grayson L, Goodwin GM: Enhanced recognition of disgust in bipolar illness. Biol Psychiatry 51:298–304, 2002

Hester R, Garavan H: Working memory and executive function: the influence of content and load on the control of attention. Mem Cognit 33:221–233, 2005

Inoue Y, Tonooka Y, Yamada K, et al: Deficiency of theory of mind in patients with remitted mood disorder. J Affect Disord 82:403–409, 2004

Inoue Y, Yamada K, Kanba S: Deficit in theory of mind is a risk for relapse of major depression. J Affect Disord 95:125–127, 2006

Ivanovski B, Malhi GH: The psychological and neurophysiological concomitants of mindfulness forms of meditation. Acta Neuropsychiatrica 19:86–91, 2007

Kerr N, Dunbar RI, Bentall RP: Theory of mind deficits in bipolar affective disorder. J Affect Disord 73:253–259, 2003

Lam DH, Hayward P, Watkins ER, et al: Relapse prevention in patients with bipolar disorder: cognitive therapy outcome after 2 years. Am J Psychiatry 162:324–329, 2005

LeDoux JE: Brain mechanisms of emotion and emotional learning. Curr Opin Neurobiol 2:191–197, 1992

LeDoux J: Fear and the brain: where have we been, and where are we going? Biol Psychiatry 44:1229–1238, 1998

Lembke A, Ketter TA: Impaired recognition of facial emotion in mania. Am J Psychiatry 159:302–304, 2002

Linehan MM, Comtois KA, Murray AM, et al: Two-year randomized controlled trial and follow-up of dialectical behavior therapy vs therapy by experts for suicidal behaviors and borderline personality disorder. Arch Gen Psychiatry 63:757–766, 2006

Malhi GS, Lagopoulos J, Owen A, et al: Reduced activation to implicit affect induction in euthymic bipolar patients: an fMRI study. J Affect Disord 97: 109–122, 2007a

Malhi GS, Lagopoulos J, Sachdev P, et al: Is a lack of disgust something to fear? an fMRI facial emotion recognition study in euthymic bipolar disorder patients. Bipolar Disord 9:345–357, 2007b

Mazza M, De Risio A, Surian L, et al: Selective impairments of theory of mind in people with schizophrenia. Schizophr Res 47:299–308, 2001

Miklowitz DJ, Goldstein MJ, Nuechterlein KJ, et al: Family factors and the course of bipolar affective disorder. Arch Gen Psychiatry 45:225–231, 1988

Miklowitz DJ, George EL, Richards JA, et al: A randomized study of family-focused psychoeducation and pharmacotherapy in the outpatient management of bipolar disorder. Arch Gen Psychiatry 60:904–912, 2003

Miklowitz DJ, Otto MW, Wisniewski SR, et al: Psychotherapy, symptom outcomes, and role functioning over one year among patients with bipolar disorder. Psychiatr Serv 57:959–965, 2006

Miklowitz DJ, Otto MW, Frank E, et al: Intensive psychosocial intervention enhances cognitive functioning in patients with bipolar depression: results from a 9-month randomized controlled trial. Am J Psychiatry 164:1340–1347, 2007a

Miklowitz DJ, Otto MW, Frank E, et al: Psychosocial treatments for bipolar depression: a 1-year randomized trial from the Systematic Treatment Enhancement Program. Arch Gen Psychiatry 64:419–426, 2007b

Morgan MA, Schulkin J, DeDoux JE: Ventral medial prefrontal cortex and emotional perseveration: the memory for prior extinction training. Behav Brain Res 146:121–130, 2003

Mur M, Portella MJ, Martinez-Aran A, et al: Persistent neuropsychological deficit in euthymic bipolar patients: executive function as a core deficit. J Clin Psychiatry 68:1078–1086, 2007

Murphy FC, Michael A, Robbins TW, et al: Neuropsychological impairment in patients with major depressive disorder: the effects of feedback on task performance. Psychol Med 33:455–467, 2003

Newman CN, Leahy RL, Beck AT, et al: Bipolar Disorder: A Cognitive Therapy Approach. Washington, DC, American Psychological Association, 2001

Ochsner KN, Knierim K, Ludlow DH, et al: Reflecting upon feelings: an fMRI study of neural systems supporting the attribution of emotion to self and other. J Cogn Neurosci 16:1746–1772, 2004

Olley AL, Malhi GS, Bachelor J, et al: Executive functioning and theory of mind in euthymic bipolar disorder. Bipolar Disord 7 (suppl 5):43–52, 2005

Peluso MA, Hatch JP, Glahn DC, et al: Trait impulsivity in patients with mood disorders. J Affect Disord 100:227–231, 2007

Penades R, Catalan R, Salamero M, et al: Cognitive remediation therapy for outpatients with chronic schizophrenia: a controlled and randomized study. Schizophr Res 87:323–331, 2006

Persad SM, Polivy J: Differences between depressed and nondepressed individuals in the recognition of and response to facial emotional cues. J Abnorm Psychol 102:358–368, 1993

Pfammatter M, Junghan UM, Brenner HD: Efficacy of psychological therapy in schizophrenia: conclusions from meta-analyses. Schizophr Bull 32 (suppl 1):S64–S80, 2006

Post RM, Leverich GS: The role of psychosocial stress in the onset and progression of bipolar disorder and its comorbidities: the need for earlier and alternative modes of therapeutic intervention. Dev Psychopathol 18:1181–1211, 2006

Rich BA, Vinton DT, Roberson-Nay R, et al: Limbic hyperactivation during processing of neutral facial expressions in children with bipolar disorder. Proc Natl Acad Sci USA 103:8900–8905, 2006

Sarfati Y, Hardy-Baylé MC, Besche C, et al: Attribution of intentions to others in people with schizophrenia: a non-verbal exploration with comic strips. Schizophr Res 25:199–209, 1997

Sarfati Y, Hardy-Baylé MC, Brunet E, et al: Investigating theory of mind in schizophrenia: influence of verbalization in disorganized and non-disorganized patients. Schizophr Res 37:183–190, 1999

Schulte-Rüther M, Markowitsch HJ, Fink GR, et al: Mirror neuron and theory of mind mechanisms involved in face-to-face interactions: a functional magnetic resonance imaging approach to empathy. J Cogn Neurosci 19:1354–1372, 2007

Scott J, Paykel E, Morriss R, et al: Cognitive-behavioural therapy for severe and recurrent bipolar disorders: randomised controlled trial. Br J Psychiatry 188:313–320, 2006

Sotres-Bayon F, Cain CK, LeDoux JE: Brain mechanisms of fear extinction: historical perspectives on the contribution of prefrontal cortex. Biol Psychiatry 15:329–336, 2006

Teasdale JD, Segal Z, Williams JM: How does cognitive therapy prevent depressive relapse and why should attentional control (mindfulness) training help? Behav Res Ther 33:25–39, 1995

Venn HR, Gray JM, Montagne B, et al: Perception of facial expressions of emotion in bipolar disorder. Bipolar Disord 6:286–293, 2004

Willensky AE, Schafe GE, Kristensen MP, et al: Rethinking the fear circuit: the central nucleus of the amygdala is required for the acquisition, consolidation, and expression of Pavlovian fear conditioning. J Neurosci 26:12387–12396, 2006

Williams JMG, Barnhofer T, Crane C, et al: The role of overgeneral memory in suicidality, in Cognition and Suicide: Theory, Research, and Therapy. Edited by Ellis TE. Washington, DC, American Psychological Association, 2006, pp 173–192

Williams JM, Alatiq Y, Crane C, et al: Mindfulness-based cognitive therapy (MBCT) in bipolar disorder: preliminary evaluation of immediate effects on between-episode functioning. J Affect Disord 107:275–279, 2008

Wykes T, Brammer M, Mellers J, et al: Effects on the brain of a psychological treatment: cognitive remediation therapy: functional magnetic resonance imaging in schizophrenia. Br J Psychiatry 181:144–152, 2002

Yan LJ, Hammen C, Cohen AN, et al: Expressed emotion versus relationship quality variables in the prediction of recurrence in bipolar patients. J Affect Disord 83: 199–206, 2004

7

Adverse Cognitive Effects of Psychotropic Medications

Joseph F. Goldberg, M.D.

Previous chapters have dealt with the extent to which neurocognitive deficits represent either state-dependent or trait features inherent to bipolar disorder itself. However, most clinical studies have paid only limited attention to the impact of psychotropic medications on neurocognitive function. For both practical and ethical reasons, the study of unmedicated patients with bipolar disorder poses substantial difficulty. As pharmacotherapy options expand across all phases of bipolar disorder, concerns persist about the potential neurocognitive effects—whether adverse, neutral, or beneficial—of major psychotropic agents. In this chapter, I focus on the existing knowledge base from clinical trials regarding adverse neurocognitive effects of lithium, anticonvulsant mood stabilizers, antidepressants, atypical antipsychotics, anticholinergic drugs, and benzodiazepines. Chapter 8 of this volume, "Pharmacological Strategies to Enhance Neurocognitive Function," addresses potential beneficial neurocognitive effects of mood-stabilizing and other psychotropic agents.

Existing studies that report iatrogenic neurocognitive effects of psychotropic agents are in themselves limited by variations in assessment measures and drug doses, frequent combination drug regimens, nonrandomized treatment assignments, and varying populations of healthy controls or diverse clinical groups with disorders other than bipolar disorder (e.g., patients with epilepsy, migraine, neuropathic pain). In addition, inferences about the neurocognitive effects of a psychotropic agent in psychiatric disorders other than bipolar illness (e.g., schizophrenia) further complicate interpretation about disease- versus drug-specific effects.

Measurement of so-called neurocognitive deficits in existing studies also varies widely, from subjective self-reports to formal assessment batteries. Prospective longitudinal studies that covary for changes in cognitive performance relative to changes in mood state represent one strategy for identifying trait neurocognitive features, but data from such studies are rare. Repeated neurocognitive assessments in some instances incur confounds related to practice effects (see Chapter 1 of this volume, "Overview and Introduction: Dimensions of Cognition and Measures of Cognitive Function"), and often such considerations are not addressed (unless, e.g., a placebo comparison group controls for this). Furthermore, clinical parameters such as chronicity or the number of recurrent affective episodes may impinge on neurocognitive dimensions such as verbal fluency and early information processing (Lebowitz et al. 2001; see also Chapter 11 of this volume, "Cognition Across the Life Span: Clinical Implications for Older Adults With Bipolar Disorder"), yet such factors often are not considered in multifactorial analyses. Indeed, it is often difficult to discern the extent to which possible observed neurocognitive deficits reflect underlying illness state, the artifact of chronicity, or pharmacological effects. Amid these considerations, clinicians are left with the practical challenges of ascribing causal effects to psychotropic agents and managing neurocognitive complaints.

Lithium

Clinicians often regard lithium as likely to cause at least some degree of cognitive impairment, although the existing literature reveals that frank deficits due to lithium are relatively modest and circumscribed in nature. Although lithium has not been linked with impaired executive function per se (Frangou et al. 2005), anecdotal observations have suggested that lithium may diminish creativity, and indeed lithium use has been associated with poorer associative productivity and associative idiosyncrasy in euthymic bipolar patients, reversible upon lithium cessation (Kocsis et al. 1993; Shaw et al. 1986). Other studies in healthy controls suggest no decrement in semantic creativity or "aesthetic judgment" after 2 weeks of lithium, despite motor slowing (Judd et al. 1977). A 3-week trial of lithium (mean dosage of 1,569 mg/day) in 15 healthy adults revealed no adverse effects on attention, implicit recall, or explicit memory, but it did reveal mild effects on learning (i.e., practice effects on repetitive testing became less evident) (Stip et al. 2000).

In addition to decrements in associative fluency, other objective neurocognitive deficits seen during lithium treatment include impaired verbal memory, including decreased retrieval of long-term memories (Reus et al. 1979) and short-term memories (Kocsis et al. 1993), and slowed motor performance (e.g., finger-tapping speed) (Christodoulou et al. 1981; Hatcher et al. 1990; Squire et al. 1980). Euthymic bipolar patients treated with lithium monotherapy demonstrate working memory deficits that functional magnetic resonance imaging data suggest may involve failure to engage fronto-executive structures (Monks et al. 2004).

Memory and motor deficits identified during maintenance lithium treatment in patients with bipolar disorder have been shown to improve after lithium cessation (Kocsis et al. 1993). Anecdotal experience suggests that adverse effects such as these also may diminish at least partly with dosage reductions, when feasible. Tremont and Stern (1997) also described the use of adjunctive triiodothyronine (T_3) as a viable strategy to help reduce cognitive complaints associated with lithium. There is no evidence of cumulative neurocognitive impairment associated with long-term lithium exposure (Pachet and Wisniewski 2003). It is worth noting that after acute lithium intoxication (as in the case of overdoses), diffuse neurocognitive deficits that may resemble subcortical dementia can persist for months or even years after cessation of lithium ingestion (Brumm et al. 1998). Lithium neurotoxicity, short of acute intoxication from an overdose, may present with diffuse neurological signs (e.g., tremor, motor slowing, ataxia) as well as gross cognitive disorganization suggestive of acute delirium.

Other studies, however, report no discernible effects of lithium on cognition (Anath et al. 1981; Friedman et al. 1977; Joffe et al. 1988; Marusarz et al. 1981; Telford and Worrall 1978; Young et al. 1977). Notably, subjective reports of memory impairment during lithium therapy have been associated with severity of depression (Engelsmann et al. 1988) and treatment nonadherence (Gitlin et al. 1989), although objective memory deficits have also been reported among euthymic lithium-treated bipolar patients (Senturk et al. 2007). Hatcher et al. (1990) reported reductions in reaction time on a driving simulator task in 16 lithium-treated bipolar patients in remission compared with 22 healthy volunteers. In their review of lithium-associated cognitive deficits, Pachet and Wisniewski (2003) noted that lithium has not been shown to exert an adverse influence on visuospatial/constructional abilities, or on attention and concentration.

A number of neuropsychological studies in euthymic bipolar patients have also performed post hoc analyses to examine potential confounding effects of lithium treatment (Altshuler et al. 2004; Clark et al. 2002). These studies have generally found that patients receiving lithium performed similarly to those not receiving lithium.

Anticonvulsants

Since the mid-1990s, enthusiasm has grown for using certain anticonvulsant drugs over lithium, based partly on clinical impressions that newer agents such as divalproex exert at least comparable antimanic efficacy to lithium but with potentially fewer side effects. Regarding neurocognitive phenomena such as attention and memory, limited anecdotal evidence supports a possible benefit when patients with bipolar disorder are switched from lithium to divalproex (Stoll et al. 1996). However, just as anticonvulsants as a broad class have varied greatly in therapeutic outcomes from controlled trials in individuals with mania or depression, so too have heterogeneous findings been noted in neurocognitive profiles across specific anticonvulsant agents.

Typical clinical challenges of evaluating cognitive complaints in patients with bipolar disorder who are taking anticonvulsants are illustrated in the following vignette.

Case Vignette 1

A 25-year-old female graduate student with bipolar II disorder and binge-eating disorder was referred for evaluation of depression and subjective memory deficits. She had taken a medical leave from school and was living at home with her parents, in anticipation of a protracted course of treatment and recovery, as occurred previously following a hospitalized depressive episode that involved a serious suicide attempt during her freshman year of college. On interview, she was a pleasant, well-related young woman who made good eye contact and had normal speech and motor function. Her mood was depressed and affect was subdued. She complained of poor concentration, lethargy, and feelings of apathy but manifested no suicidal features, hopelessness, or changes in sleep or appetite. Brief assessment of her higher integrative functioning revealed intact attention and psychomotor function but impaired verbal fluency, poor short-term memory, and an increased latency of response to most questions. Her pharmacotherapy regimen consisted of lamotrigine at 50 mg/day (unchanged since an initial antidepressant response about 1 year earlier) and 100 mg of topiramate twice daily (begun 3 months earlier as an "adjunct" mood stabilizer and potential aid for binge eating).

Further history revealed that the onset of her depressed mood and concentration complaints arose in the several weeks following initiation of topiramate. She denied binge-eating or purging behaviors in the preceding 6 months. A suggestion was made to discontinue the topiramate and then reassess her mental status. Two weeks following the cessation of topiramate, she reported euthymic mood, improved energy, and apparent resolution of her cognitive complaints.

Topiramate

The thymoleptic properties of topiramate remain a subject of debate, based on limited favorable open trial data countered by four negative placebo-controlled trials in patients with bipolar mania (Kushner et al. 2006). However, the psychotropic value of topiramate has been reported for comorbid conditions such as binge-eating disorder (McElroy et al. 2006), as described in Case Vignette 1. The potential benefits of topiramate as a viable off-label strategy for problems such as binge eating must be considered alongside risks for adverse cognitive effects. Notably, topiramate has been suggested to have a greater liability for adverse neurocognitive effects than most other newer-generation anticonvulsants (Goldberg and Burdick 2001). In clinical trials for epilepsy or migraine, common adverse effects at dosages up to 400 mg/day included psychomotor slowing, memory impairment (12% of patients), speech and language problems (e.g., word-finding difficulties) (13% of patients), and somnolence or fatigue (29% of patients) (*Physicians' Desk Reference* 2008).

In healthy adult volunteers, topiramate dosed at a mean of 333 mg/day for up to 12 weeks has been associated with a decrement of two standard deviations in performance across a number of neurocognitive measures, representing a clinically significant degree of cognitive impairment (Salinsky et al. 2005). In epilepsy patients, the introduction of topiramate to existing antiepileptic drug regimens has been associated with substantial worsening of verbal and nonverbal fluency, attention and concentration, processing speed, language skills, working memory, and perception (Lee et al. 2003). Among epilepsy patients taking polydrug anticonvulsant regimens, more extensive cognitive problems (e.g., impaired verbal fluency, memory span, and working memory) have been reported when topiramate was included as a component of polytherapy (Kockelmann et al. 2004). Withdrawal of topiramate from epilepsy patients' drug regimens has been associated with significant improvements in attention, verbal fluency, verbal working memory, and spatial short-term memory (Kockelmann et al. 2003).

Evidence suggests that gradual topiramate dosage escalations can help to minimize adverse neurocognitive effects (Aldenkamp et al. 2000; Biton et al. 2001), although cognitive problems (e.g., impaired verbal fluency, working memory, and processing speed) have been reported even at low starting dosages in some patients (e.g., 50 or 100 mg/day) (Lee et al. 2006; Salinsky et al. 2005). Gomer et al. (2007) found no association among epilepsy patients between dosage of topiramate and extent of neurocognitive deficits. Martin et al. (1999) noted in healthy volunteers that despite an approximately threefold decline from baseline in attention, some improvement occurred after several weeks of continued treatment with topiramate. According to some studies (Meador et al. 2003) but not others (Huppertz et al. 2001), the severity of cognitive impairment resulting from topiramate usage diminishes once steady dosages are reached and maintained.

Cessation of topiramate generally leads to reversal of its associated cognitive problems (Burton and Harden 1997; Huppertz et al. 2001; Kockelmann et al. 2003). The exact mechanism by which topiramate may induce diverse neurocognitive deficits is not well understood. Adverse cognitive effects with topiramate are in some respects particularly curious given its potential neuroprotective properties, governed by its ability to enhance brain γ-aminobutyric acid (GABA)–mediated inhibition and also block non–N-methyl-D-aspartate receptor–mediated excitotoxicity (as discussed further in Chapter 8 of this volume).

Although one preliminary report suggests the potential value of topiramate for acute bipolar depression (McIntyre et al. 2002), other reports suggest its potential for inducing or exacerbating depression in patients with epilepsy (Klufas and Thompson 2001) or bipolar disorder (McElroy et al. 2007). In Case Vignette 1, cessation of topiramate was associated with an amelioration of clinical features involving simultaneous depression and disturbances of attention and short-term memory.

Despite its relative lack of efficacy in acute mania, topiramate has garnered interest for its potential benefit in promoting weight loss (McElroy et al. 2007) and for reducing symptoms related to alcoholism. The latter, in theory, is a function of topiramate's indirect modulation of dopamine in the reward pathway, which influences drinking behavior as well as craving (Johnson et al. 2003, 2007). Notably, adverse cognitive effects were observed in only 18.7% ("memory or cognitive impairment") to 26.7% ("psychomotor slowing") of alcohol-dependent subjects in the initial randomized trial conducted by Johnson et al. (2003). One study identified a subjective preference for topiramate over lamotrigine in only 16% of healthy volunteers, which occurred independently of objective neurocognitive performance or body mass index but appeared related to subjective mood benefits (Werz et al. 2006).

Findings from studies of specific neurocognitive domains in healthy adult subjects and patients with epilepsy or bipolar disorder influenced by topiramate are summarized in Tables 7–1 and 7–2, respectively.

Lamotrigine

Clinical trial data of lamotrigine use in patients with bipolar disorder are among the most favorable, and extensive, data regarding use of anticonvulsants with known psychotropic properties. In adult epilepsy trials, "concentration disturbance" was noted as an adverse effect in 2% of patients taking lamotrigine (vs. 1% of patients taking placebo), and confusion was reported in at least 1% of patients with bipolar disorder receiving lamotrigine for relapse prevention for up to 18 months (*Physicians' Desk Reference* 2008). In general, problems involving cognitive function with lamotrigine appear relatively rare, and are typically transient if and when they occur.

Among the few studies of neurocognitive function with lamotrigine use specifically in patients with bipolar disorder, evidence suggests a lack of impairment (and, in fact, even a possible benefit) with respect to verbal fluency and immediate recall (Daban et al. 2006; see Table 7–2). Following 8–16 weeks of open-label treatment with lamotrigine after an acute index manic or bipolar depressive episode, Khan et al. (2004) noted improvement from baseline in a four-item global measure of cognitive function that tapped memory, attention, judgment, and reasoning, while controlling for changes in mood and index episode polarity. Notably, however, the latter study measured cognitive function by self-report rather than objective neurocognitive assessment.

Divalproex

Divalproex is one of the most extensively studied anticonvulsants for the treatment of bipolar disorder. Its extended-release formulation (Depakote ER) was approved for the acute treatment of mania or mixed states in 2006, and efficacy appears linearly associated with serum valproate levels (Allen et al. 2006); however, adverse effects appear to be more common with dosages exceeding about 100 μg/dL. From the standpoint of neurocognitive effects, divalproex has been associated with subtle dosage-related attentional and mild memory deficits, exacerbated by combination therapies (Gallassi et al. 1990; Goldberg and Burdick 2001), impaired verbal memory (Senturk et al. 2007), and slightly delayed decision time, as seen in a 2-week randomized crossover trial of up to 1,000 mg/day in psychiatrically healthy controls (Thompson and Trimble 1981). Cognitive effects of divalproex appear reversible after drug cessation (Gallassi et al. 1990). Divalproex use has not been associated with visuospatial processing deficits (see review by Goldberg and Burdick 2001).

Carbamazepine

In studies based primarily on patients with epilepsy, carbamazepine use has been linked with subtle learning effects (i.e., lack of practice effects on repeated neurocognitive testing), and prolonged stimulus evaluation time (i.e., delayed visuospatial processing) has been shown in studies with healthy adults (see review by Goldberg and Burdick 2001). Carbamazepine also has been reported to induce mild changes in visual memory during evoked potential studies, but has not been shown to impact motor speed (Goldberg and Burdick 2001).

Oxcarbazepine

Oxcarbazepine (the keto analogue of carbamazepine, used occasionally in off-label fashion in some patients with bipolar disorder) does not appear to adversely affect long-term memory in healthy volunteers. In fact, a 2-week study of 300 or 600 mg/day of oxcarbazepine in 12 healthy volunteers was associated with improvement from baseline in attention and motor speed,

TABLE 7–1. Comparative studies of anticonvulsants: healthy adult subjects

Study	Comparison	Design	Findings
Aldenkamp et al. 2002	LTG (n=10; 50 mg/day) vs. DVPX (n=10; 900 mg/day) vs. placebo	N=30, double-blind randomized comparison over 12 days	Better performance on three of four reaction time measures with LTG than placebo. Subjects taking LTG had significantly better auditory reaction times as well as fewer subjective drug complaints than subjects taking DVPX.
Martin et al. 1999	GPN (n=6; 35 mg/kg/day) vs. LTG (n=5; 7.1 mg/kg/day) vs. TPM (n=6; 5.7 mg/kg/day)	N=17, single-blind parallel design over 4 weeks	Poorer performance for TPM than GPN or LTG on letter and category word fluency, visual attention, verbal memory, and psychomotor speed.
Meador et al. 2001	CBZ (mean dosage 696 mg/day) vs. LTG (150 mg/day)	N=25, randomized crossover; two 10-week periods	Better performance for LTG than CBZ on 19 of 40 measures, including cognitive speed, memory, and graphomotor coding; 0 of 40 better for CBZ than LTG.
Meador et al. 2005	LTG (300 mg/day) vs. TPM (300 mg/day)	N=47, randomized crossover; two 12-week periods	Better performance for LTG than TPM on 33 of 41 measures; 0 of 41 better for TPM than LTG.
Salinsky et al. 2005	GPN (all dosed at 3,600 mg/day) vs. TPM (mean dosage 330 mg/day) vs. placebo	N=40, double-blind randomized 12-week comparison	Better performance for GPN than TPM on 12 of 24 measures. TPM associated with poorer digit symbol, study recall, selective reminding, and COWAT.
Smith et al. 2006	LTG (300 mg/day) vs. TPM (300 mg/day)	N=29, double-blind randomized crossover; two 8-week dosage escalation periods followed by 4 weeks of drug continuation	Decreased accuracy and slowed reaction time with TPM vs. LTG on n-back spatial working memory task. No correlation between blood levels and performance.

TABLE 7–1. Comparative studies of anticonvulsants: healthy adult subjects *(continued)*

Study	Comparison	Design	Findings
Werz et al. 2006	LTG (300 mg/day) *vs.* TPM (300 mg/day)	*N*=27, double-blind randomized crossover; two 12-week treatment periods; 23 objective neurocognitive assessments at 4 time points	Greater subjective preference for LTG (70%) than TPM (16%). Preference for LTG associated with better objective performance on 19 of 23 measures.

Note. CBZ=carbamazepine; COWAT=Continuous Word Association Test; DPH=diphenylhydantoin; DVPX=divalproex; GPN=gabapentin; LEV=levetiracetam; LTG=lamotrigine; TPM=topiramate.

TABLE 7–2. Comparative studies of anticonvulsants: patients with epilepsy or bipolar disorder

Study	Comparison	Design	Findings
Aikia et al. 2006	TGB (n=52) vs. CBZ (n=52) vs. no-drug epilepsy patients (n=19)	6-week titration in epilepsy patients of TGB (20–30 mg/day) or CBZ (400–800 mg/day), then 52-week randomized comparison.	Poorer verbal fluency with CBZ than controls. No significant worsening from baseline with either active treatment.
Blum et al. 2006	LTG+CBZ or DPH (n=96) vs. TPM+CBZ or DPH (n=96)	Multicenter randomized double-blind epilepsy study; 8 weeks' titration followed by 8 weeks' continuation therapy. Mean LTG dosage=500 mg/day; mean TPM dosage=300 mg/day.	Better performance on Stroop Color-Word Interference task, COWAT, and Digit Symbol Modalities Test with LTG than TPM. More premature withdrawals due to cognitive adverse effects with TPM (6%) than LTG (0%).
Daban et al. 2006	LTG (n=15) vs. CBZ or DVPX (n=18)	Euthymic bipolar I or II patients treated naturalistically for ≥6 months. Cotherapy with preexisting psychotropics held constant. Dosages not reported.	Better phonemic (but not categorical) verbal fluency with LTG than CBZ or DVPX; better verbal memory/immediate recall (by CVLT) with LTG than CBZ or DVPX.
Fritz et al. 2005	TGB (n=15) vs. TPM (n=15)	Open randomized comparison in epilepsy patients; 7-week TGB titration (mean dosage=32 mg/day), 13-week TPM titration (mean dosage=335 mg/day); neurocognitive battery at baseline and 3 and 6 months.	With TPM, deterioration from baseline in verbal fluency, language comprehension, working memory, and visual block tapping. With TGB, deterioration in verbal memory (delayed free recall).

TABLE 7–2. Comparative studies of anticonvulsants: patients with epilepsy or bipolar disorder (*continued*)

Study	Comparison	Design	Findings
Gomer et al. 2007	LEV (*n*=30) vs. TPM (*n*=21)	Open-label mono- or add-on therapy in epilepsy patients; TPM titrated from 25 mg/day by 25-mg increments every 4 days to 201-mg mean daily dose. LEV begun at 500 mg/day, increased by 250 mg every 3 days to 1,908-mg mean daily dose; neurocognitive battery at baseline and after about 120 days.	Worse cognitive speed, verbal fluency, and short-term memory with TPM than LEV. No diminished neurocognitive performance on any measures with LEV; LEV associated with *improved* attention from baseline.
Kockelmann et al. 2004	Anticonvulsant polypharmacy+TPM (*n*=42) vs. anticonvulsant polypharmacy+LTG (*n*=42)	Retrospective comparison in 84 hospitalized epilepsy patients. Mean TPM dosage=319 mg/day, mean LTG dosage=375 mg/day.	Poorer phonemic verbal fluency, memory spans, and nonverbal working memory with TPM than LTG, independent of drug serum levels. No adverse effects on language or memory function.
Meador et al. 2003	DVPX+CBZ (*n*=29) vs. TPM+CBZ (*n*=34) vs. placebo+CBZ (*n*=13)	63 epilepsy subjects; 8-week titration followed by 12-week continued treatment. DVPX dosed at 2,250 mg/day, TPM dosed at 400 mg/day.	Worse performance on digit symbol and COWAT for TPM+CBZ than for DVPX+CBZ.
Prevey et al. 1996	DVPX (*n*=39) vs. CBZ (*n*=26) vs. normal control subjects (*n*=72)	55 epilepsy patients; randomized double-blind comparison with assessments at 6 and 12 months. Mean 6-month [CBZ]=6.6 μg/mL, mean [valproate]=73.6 μg/mL.	Subtle learning deficits and lack of improvement in practice effects with DVPX. No other differences between agents; no significant declines from baseline.

Note. CBZ=carbamazepine; COWAT=Continuous Word Association Test; CVLT=California Verbal Learning Test; DPH=diphenylhydantoin; DVPX=divalproex; LEV=levetiracetam; LTG=lamotrigine; TGB=tiagabine; TPM=topiramate.

as well as subjective increases in alertness and "clear-headedness and quick-wittedness" (Curran and Java 1993). Elsewhere, a higher dosage (1,200 mg/day) in 10 healthy volunteers over 8 days demonstrated a decline from baseline in motor speed, which was less pronounced than seen with carbamazepine (Mecarelli et al. 2004).

Levetiracetam

Open-label studies of levetiracetam for mood symptoms in patients with bipolar disorder have generally been negative (e.g., Post et al. 2005), although such clinical trials have mainly been conducted in treatment-refractory patients. Preclinical studies suggest that levetiracetam produces no adverse effect on attention (Shannon and Love 2005), whereas studies in epilepsy indicate a relatively benign neurocognitive profile as compared with topiramate (Gomer et al. 2007). Levetiracetam may even lead to improvements in attention, based on studies of approximately 4 months' duration in epilepsy patients (Gomer et al. 2007). In animal models of status epilepticus, levetiracetam demonstrated neuroprotection but did not offset visuospatial deficits related to status epilepticus (Zhou et al. 2007).

Antidepressants

The neurocognitive effects of traditional antidepressants for bipolar depression have received little formal study as separate from global aspects of treatment for depression. Serotonergic antidepressants (e.g., selective serotonin reuptake inhibitors [SSRIs]) or mixed agonists (e.g., serotonin-norepinephrine reuptake inhibitors) are thought to have minimal adverse neurocognitive effects on depressed patients in general (Amado-Boccara et al. 1995; Fudge et al. 1990; Hindmarch 1995). There also exists evidence that at least some SSRIs (notably, citalopram) improve working memory in patients with depression (Zobel et al. 2004), potentially in relation to preclinical evidence that citalopram can increase cholinergic tone in the frontal cortex and dorsal hippocampus (Consolo et al. 1994; Yamaguchi et al. 1997). However, studies of cognitive function during SSRI treatment for anxious or depressed patients (regardless of affective polarity) include at least some suggestion of an adverse effect on episodic (but not semantic or working) memory, while controlling for depressive and anxiety symptoms (Wadsworth et al. 2005).

Tricyclic antidepressants are widely known to exert negative effects on verbal learning and memory in some patients, primarily by virtue of their anticholinergic effects (Richardson et al. 1994), although some studies have concluded that they may improve general cognitive function in unipolar depressed patients despite their adverse effects on mnemonic functions (Gold et al. 1991). Tricyclic antidepressants are seldom used for bipolar depression, given their higher risk for mood destabilization than SSRIs (Peet 1994) and an apparent lack of superior antidepressant efficacy relative to optimized mood stabilizers alone (Ghaemi et al. 2001; Nemeroff et al. 2001).

Deptula and Pomara (1990) pointed out the many limitations of existing studies addressing neurocognitive effects of antidepressants for depressed patients in general (much less for bipolar depression in particular). Limitations included small samples; vague, mixed, or multiple diagnoses among the depression group; and inadequate neuropsychological batteries.

Antipsychotics

There has been growing interest in the potential of atypical antipsychotics to produce neurocognitive benefits, at least among individuals with schizophrenia or schizoaffective disorder who have baseline deficits. Data examining such effects are reviewed in Chapter 8 of this volume. Less empirical information exists about adverse neurocognitive effects of atypical antipsychotics, although several considerations bear on this issue.

First, two studies of remitted patients with bipolar disorder have reported cognitive deficits associated with antipsychotic use. Frangou et al. (2005) assessed 44 remitted bipolar I disorder subjects from the Maudsley Bipolar Disorder Project and found significant associations between antipsychotic use (whether conventional or atypical) and executive dysfunction (in particular, set shifting), potentially due to antipsychotic-induced slowing of processing speed, arising independently of psychosis. Another study by Altshuler et al. (2004) compared neurocognitive function in 40 male patients with euthymic bipolar I disorder, 20 stable male patients with schizophrenia, and 22 healthy male controls. Bipolar subjects had poorer performance than healthy control subjects on measures of executive function and verbal memory, with significantly poorer performance by those bipolar subjects taking antipsychotics. It is uncertain to what extent prior illness severity and course, including a history of psychosis, may have impacted neurocognitive performance in that study.

Second, a study of olanzapine (dosed at 10 mg/day) in healthy control subjects found significant short-term declines in psychomotor speed, verbal fluency, sensorimotor accuracy, visuospatial monitoring, and information processing speed, all independent of sedative effects (Morrens et al. 2007). Interestingly, such findings stand in contrast to most published studies in clinical populations with psychotic disorders, where worsening of neurocognitive function from baseline has not been reported (for further discussion of the potential for cognitive enhancement with atypical antipsychotics in schizophrenia, see Chapter 8 of this volume).

Third, preclinical data also suggest that those atypical antipsychotics with higher binding affinities at the serotonin type 2A (5-HT$_{2A}$) receptor (e.g., olanzapine, clozapine, risperidone) may be more prone to cause decrements in visual recognition memory and planning ability than those agents with lower 5-HT_{2A} binding affinity (e.g., quetiapine, amisulpride) (Tyson et al. 2004). Finally, the practice of combining multiple antipsychotics has received little empirical study with respect to either efficacy or safety, although such prescribing habits appear to be common for patients with serious psychiatric disorders such as schizophrenia (Sernyak and Rosenheck 2004). Notably, in the literature on schizophrenia, patients treated with clozapine demonstrated improvements from baseline in attention, verbal working memory, and verbal learning and memory, although these effects were less robust during coadministration with risperidone (Akdede et al. 2006), suggesting a potential attenuation of cognitive benefits when using multiple atypical antipsychotics.

Anticholinergic Agents

Anticholinergic drugs (e.g., benztropine, diphenhydramine) have long been recognized for their propensity to induce cognitive dulling and gross impairment in attention and multiple subservient neurocognitive functions. In fact, in the National Institute of Mental Health Clinical Antipsychotic Trials of Intervention Effectiveness, improvements from baseline that were initially observed in global neurocognitive function of subjects with schizophrenia were eliminated when anticholinergic drugs were introduced during the first 2 months of the study period (Keefe et al. 2007). Among schizophrenia patients, anticholinergic load has been suggested to account for a substantial proportion of variance associated with performance on tasks related to attention and memory (Minzenberg et al. 2004). Less is known about whether individuals with bipolar disorder differ from schizophrenia patients in their degree of vulnerability to the adverse cognitive effects of anticholinergic medications. Of note, in women taking estrogen, the potential for anticholinergic drugs to impair attention and motor speed may be somewhat attenuated (Dumas et al. 2006).

Benzodiazepines

Benzodiazepines have long been recognized to produce adverse effects on arousal, attention, and memory (for review, see Buffett-Jerrott and Stewart 2002), potentially even causing persistent impairment in verbal and nonverbal memory after withdrawal following long-term use (Barker et al. 2005; Tata et al. 1994). Adverse cognitive effects of benzodiazepines appear to involve memory and psychomotor speed rather than higher-level executive functions such as attention (Curran 1991). In addition, disinhibitory effects of benzodiazepines have been demonstrated not only in individuals with known frontal lobe damage, but also in healthy controls during performance tasks involving reaction time (Deakin et al. 2004). Benzodiazepines are commonly used not only as adjunct pharmacotherapies in acute mania, but also during nonacute or long-term phases of treatment in 25% of patients with bipolar disorder, as observed in the National Institute of Mental Health Systematic Treatment Enhancement Program for Bipolar Disorder (Ghaemi et al. 2006). Accordingly, practitioners should consider the potential short- or long-term as well as historical contribution of benzodiazepines to the development of memory problems and related cognitive complaints. When assessing neurocognitive function, clinicians and researchers alike should undertake testing no sooner than 6 hours after the last dose of any benzodiazepine.

Diagnostic-Pharmacological Mismatches

Clinicians and researchers must bear in mind the potential for certain psychotropic agents to produce adverse cognitive effects, mainly within the context of their use (or misuse) in particular patient groups (e.g., anticholinergic agents in the elderly) or when diagnostic formulations may be wrong, as illustrated by the following example.

Case Vignette 2

A 22-year-old male had been diagnosed with bipolar II depression and comorbid obsessive-compulsive disorder that partially responded to lamotrigine. Prior SSRI trials in conjunction with divalproex produced agitation and sleeplessness without improving the patient's preoccupation with word spellings and numbers, patterns of repetitive counting, or ritualistic perfectionism when reading or writing. His psychiatrist wondered if his obsessive thinking patterns could be an "attention-deficit disorder spectrum equivalent" and added mixed amphetamine salts to lamotrigine. Sleeplessness recurred without other frank mania symptoms, alongside an intensification of the patient's preoccupation about, and time spent with, his obsessions.

This patient presented with no visible evidence of attention-deficit disorder, and indeed his hypervigilance attested not to problems with sustained attention, but rather to issues with executive dysfunction, cognitive inflexibility, and poor capacity to shift attention. Although the potential for stimulants to precipitate mania remains a matter of debate, it is likely that for this patient, dopamine agonism from a mixed amphetamine salt exacerbated his hyperattention to stimuli that he could not efficiently filter and organize, rather than remedied a supposed problem attending to stimuli, which was not in fact present.

Conclusions

With several specific exceptions, most psychotropic agents cause only relatively mild cognitive problems in patients with bipolar disorder. Most notably, these include 1) diminished associative fluency, verbal memory, and motor performance associated with lithium; 2) subtle deficits related to learning, memory, and reaction time associated with divalproex or carbamazepine; 3) motor slowing, memory impairment, and word-finding difficulties with topiramate; 4) overall cognitive dulling with anticholinergic agents; and 5) disinhibition as well as impaired attention and memory with benzodiazepines. Cognitive complaints that may be related to medications are often transient or dose dependent, and monitoring for several weeks may be advisable to determine whether they subside, before assuming the need to discontinue a treatment.

In some studies, use of atypical antipsychotics in individuals with bipolar disorders has been associated with slowed processing speed, verbal memory problems, and executive dysfunction (particularly set shifting); however, studies in schizophrenia suggest the potential for mild but significant improvement in global cognitive functioning. Further investigation is needed to determine whether the fact that atypical antipsychotics produce modest cognitive benefits more clearly in schizophrenia than in bipolar disorder reflects 1) generally more severe global cognitive impairment in schizophrenia than in bipolar disorder, and therefore more opportunity for improvement; 2) differences in study methodologies; 3) a fundamental difference in neurocognitive responses to atypical antipsychotics between schizophrenia and bipolar disorder; 4) the potential for neurocognitively unique effects across different atypical antipsychotics; or 5) other fundamental differences between bipolar disorder and schizophrenia that have not yet been fully identified.

Take-Home Points

- Lithium may reversibly impair associative fluency, verbal memory, short- and long-term memory, and motor speed—deficits that may lessen via dosage reductions. There is no clear evidence of long-term neurocognitive sequelae to chronic lithium use.

- Most anticonvulsants are associated with modest adverse cognitive effects, if any, with the notable exception of topiramate, which may impair language (word-finding difficulties), verbal and nonverbal fluency, attention, concentration, processing speed, working memory, and perception. Deficits in areas such as these may occur in a substantial minority of individuals; they can be minimized in some instances by slow dosage escalations, and they appear reversible with drug cessation. In patients taking other anticonvulsants who develop significant or persistent cognitive complaints, consideration should be given to other possible etiologies, such as additional medications, depressive symptoms, alcohol or substance abuse, or medical/neurological comorbidities.

- Anticholinergic medications and benzodiazepines are among the most likely psychotropic drugs to cause cognitive difficulties, primarily involving diminished arousal and attention, slowed processing speed, and potential impairments in subsidiary cognitive functions such as memory.

- Nontricyclic antidepressants (e.g., SSRIs) have generally been shown to improve, rather than impair, cognitive domains such as attention and working memory, although at least some studies in unipolar depression suggest their potential to impair episodic memory. Whether or not antidepressants may produce different neurocognitive profiles for individuals with bipolar disorder (rather than unipolar depression or other types of disorders) is relatively unstudied and largely unknown.

- In contrast to more globally beneficial cognitive effects seen with atypical antipsychotics in schizophrenia, use of these agents in patients with bipolar disorder has been associated in some studies with executive dysfunction, slowed processing speed, and verbal memory deficits. However, few studies have measured changes in cognitive performance during atypical antipsychotic treatment in patients with bipolar disorder. In addition, because cognitive deficits in schizophrenia are typically more global and pervasive than in bipolar disorder, it is further possible that a lower "floor effect" of baseline dysfunction in schizophrenia may contribute to their observed greater magnitude of improvement in cognitive function from baseline during atypical antipsychotic therapy.

References

Aikia M, Justila L, Salmenpera T, et al: Comparison of the cognitive effects of tiagabine and carbamazepine as monotherapy in newly diagnosed adult patients with partial epilepsy: pooled analysis of two long-term, randomized, follow-up studies. Epilepsia 47:1121–1127, 2006

Akdede BB, Anil Yagcioglu AE, Alptekin K, et al: A double-blind study of combination of clozapine with risperidone in patients with schizophrenia: effects on cognition. J Clin Psychiatry 67:1912–1919, 2006

Aldenkamp AP, Baker G, Mulder OG, et al: A multicenter, randomized clinical study to evaluate the effect on cognitive function of topiramate compared with valproate as add-on therapy to carbamazepine in patients with partial onset seizures. Epilepsia 41:1167–1178, 2000

Aldenkamp AP, Arends J, Bootsma HP, et al: Randomized double-blind parallel-group study comparing cognitive effects of a low-dose lamotrigine with valproate and placebo in healthy volunteers. Epilepsia 43:19–26, 2002

Allen MH, Hirschfeld RM, Wozniak PJ, et al: Linear relationship of valproate serum concentration to response and optimum serum levels for acute mania. Am J Psychiatry 163:272–275, 2006

Altshuler LL, Ventura J, van Gorp WG, et al: Neurocognitive function in clinically stable men with bipolar I disorder or schizophrenia and normal control subjects. Biol Psychiatry 56:560–569, 2004

Amado-Boccara I, Gougoulis N, Poirier Littré MF, et al: Effects of antidepressants on cognitive functions: a review. Neurosci Biobehav Rev 19:479–493, 1995

Anath J, Gold J, Ghadirian AM, et al: Long-term effects of lithium carbonate on cognitive functions. J Psychiatr Treat Eval 3:551–555, 1981

Barker MJ, Greenwood KM, Jackson M, et al: An evaluation of persisting cognitive effects after withdrawal from long-term benzodiazepine use. J Int Neuropsychol Soc 11:281–289, 2005

Biton V, Edwards KR, Montouris GD, et al; for the Topiramate TPS-TR Study Group: Topiramate titration and tolerability. Ann Pharmacother 35:173–179, 2001

Blum D, Meador K, Biton V, et al: Cognitive effects of lamotrigine compared with topiramate in patients with epilepsy. Neurology 67:378–379, 2006

Brumm VL, van Gorp WG, Wirshing W: Chronic neuropsychological sequelae in a case of severe lithium intoxication. Neuropsychiatry Neuropsychol Behav Neurol 11:245–249, 1998

Buffett-Jerrott SE, Stewart SH: Cognitive and sedative effects of benzodiazepine use. Curr Pharm Des 8:45–58, 2002

Burton LA, Harden C: Effect of topiramate on attention. Epilepsy Res 27:29–32, 1997

Christodoulou GN, Kokkevi A, Lykouras EP, et al: Effects of lithium on memory. Am J Psychiatry 138:847–848, 1981

Clark L, Iversen SD, Goodwin GM: Sustained attention deficit in bipolar disorder. Br J Psychiatry 180:313–319, 2002

Consolo S, Bertorelli R, Russi G, et al: Serotonergic facilitation of acetylcholine release in vivo from rat dorsal hippocampus via serotonin 5-HT$_3$ receptors. J Neurochem 62:2254–2261, 1994

Curran HV: Benzodiazepines, memory and mood: a review. Psychopharmacology (Berl) 105:1–8, 1991

Curran HV, Java R: Memory and psychomotor effects of oxcarbazepine in healthy human volunteers. Eur J Clin Pharmacol 44:529–533, 1993

Daban C, Martinez-Aran A, Torrent C, et al: Cognitive functioning in bipolar patients receiving lamotrigine: preliminary studies. J Clin Psychopharmacol 26:178–181, 2006

Deakin JB, Aitken MR, Dowson JH, et al: Diazepam produces disinhibitory cognitive effects in male volunteers. Psychopharmacology (Berl) 173:88–97, 2004

Deptula D, Pomara N: Effects of antidepressants on human performance: a review. J Clin Psychopharmacol 10:105–111, 1990

Dumas J, Hancur-Bucci C, Naylor M, et al: Estrogen treatment effects on anticholinergic-induced cognitive dysfunction in normal postmenopausal women. Neuropsychopharmacology 31:2065–2078, 2006

Engelsmann F, Katz J, Ghadirian AM, et al: Lithium and memory assessment: a long-term follow-up study. J Clin Psychopharmacol 8:207–212, 1988

Frangou S, Donaldson S, Hadjulis M, et al: The Maudsley Bipolar Disorder Project: executive dysfunction in bipolar disorder I and its clinical correlates. Biol Psychiatry 58:859–864, 2005

Friedman MJ, Culver CM, Ferrell RB: On the safety of long-term treatment with lithium. Am J Psychiatry 134:1123–1126, 1977

Fritz N, Glogau S, Hoffmann J, et al: Efficacy and cognitive side effects of tiagabine and topiramate in patients with epilepsy. Epilepsy Behav 6:373–381, 2005

Fudge JL, Perry PJ, Garvey MJ, et al: A comparison of the effect of fluoxetine and trazodone on the cognitive functioning of depressed outpatients. J Affect Disord 18:275–280, 1990

Gallassi R, Morreale A, Lorusso S, et al: Cognitive effects of valproate. Epilepsy Res 5:160–164, 1990

Ghaemi SN, Lenox MS, Baldessarini RJ: Effectiveness and safety of long-term antidepressant treatment in bipolar depression. J Clin Psychiatry 62:565–569, 2001

Ghaemi SN, Hsu DJ, Thase ME, et al: Pharmacologic treatment patterns at study entry for the first 500 STEP-BD participants. Psychol Serv 57:660–665, 2006

Gitlin MJ, Cochran SD, Jamison KR: Maintenance lithium treatment: side effects and compliance. J Clin Psychiatry 50:127–131, 1989

Gold JM, Goldberg TE, Kleinman JE, et al: The impact of symptomatic state and pharmacological treatment on cognitive functioning of patients with schizophrenic and mood disorders, in Handbook of Clinical Trials. Edited by Mohr E, Brouwers T. Amsterdam, Swers, 1991, pp 185–214

Goldberg JF, Burdick KE: Cognitive side effects of anticonvulsants. J Clin Psychiatry 62 (suppl 14):27–33, 2001

Gomer B, Wagner K, Frings L, et al: The influence of antiepileptic drugs on cognition: a comparison of levetiracetam with topiramate. Epilepsy Behav 10:486–494, 2007

Hatcher S, Sims R, Thompson D: The effects of chronic lithium treatment on psychomotor performance related to driving. Br J Psychiatry 157:275–278, 1990

Hindmarch I: The behavioural toxicity of the selective serotonin reuptake inhibitors. Int Clin Psychopharmacol 9 (suppl 4):S13–S17, 1995

Huppertz HJ, Quiske A, Schulze-Bonhagen A: Kognitive Beeinträchtigungen unter Add-on Therapie mit Topiramat. Nervenartz 72:275–280, 2001

Joffe RT, MacDonald C, Kutcher SP: Lack of differential cognitive effects of lithium and carbamazepine in bipolar affective disorder. J Clin Psychopharmacol 8:425–426, 1988

Johnson BA, Ait-Daoud N, Bowden CL, et al: Oral topiramate for treatment of alcohol dependence: a randomised controlled trial. Lancet 361:1677–1685, 2003

Johnson BA, Rosenthal N, Capece JA, et al: Topiramate for treating alcohol dependence: a randomized controlled trial. JAMA 298:1641–1651, 2007

Judd LL, Hubbard B, Janowsky DS, et al: The effect of lithium carbonate on the cognitive functions of normal subjects. Arch Gen Psychiatry 34:355–357, 1977

Keefe RS, Bilder RM, Davis SM, et al: Neurocognitive effects of antipsychotic medications in patients with chronic schizophrenia in the CATIE trials. Arch Gen Psychiatry 64:633–647, 2007

Khan DA, Ginsberg LD, Asnis GM, et al: Effect of lamotrigine on cognitive complaints in patients with bipolar I disorder. J Clin Psychiatry 65:1483–1490, 2004

Klufas A, Thompson D: Topiramate-induced depression (letter). Am J Psychiatry 158:1736, 2001

Kockelmann E, Elger CE, Helmstaedter C: Significant improvement in frontal lobe associated neuropsychological functions after withdrawal of topiramate in epilepsy patients. Epilepsy Res 54:171–178, 2003

Kockelmann E, Elger CE, Helmstaedter C: Cognitive profile of topiramate as compared with lamotrigine in epilepsy patients on antiepileptic drug polytherapy: relationships to blood serum levels and comedication. Epilepsy Behav 5:716–721, 2004

Kocsis JH, Shaw ED, Stokes PE, et al: Neuropsychologic effects of lithium discontinuation. J Clin Psychopharmacol 13:268–275, 1993

Kushner SF, Khan A, Lane R, et al: Topiramate monotherapy in the management of acute mania: results of four double-blind placebo-controlled trials. Bipolar Disord 8:15–27, 2006

Lebowitz BK, Shear PK, Steed MA, et al: Verbal fluency in mania: relationship to number of manic episodes. Neuropsychiatry Neuropsychol Behav Neurol 14:177–182, 2001

Lee HW, Jung DK, Suh CK, et al: Cognitive effects of low-dose topiramate monotherapy in epilepsy patients: a 1-year follow-up. Epilepsy Behav 8:736–741, 2006

Lee S, Sziklas V, Andermann F, et al: The effects of adjunctive topiramate on cognitive function in patients with epilepsy. Epilepsia 44:339–347, 2003

Martin R, Kuzniecky R, Ho S, et al: Cognitive effects of topiramate, gabapentin and lamotrigine in healthy young adults. Neurology 15:321–327, 1999

Marusarz TZ, Wolpert EA, Koh SD: Memory processing with lithium carbonate. J Clin Psychiatry 42:190–192, 1981

McElroy SL, Kotwal R, Keck PE Jr: Comorbidity of eating disorders with bipolar disorder and treatment implications. Bipolar Disord 8:686–695, 2006

McElroy SL, Frye MA, Altshuler LL, et al: A 24-week, randomized, controlled trial of adjunctive sibutramine versus topiramate in the treatment of weight gain in overweight or obese patients with bipolar disorders. Bipolar Disord 9:426–434, 2007

McIntyre RS, Mancini DA, McCann S, et al: Topiramate versus bupropion SR when added to mood stabilizer therapy for the depressive phase of bipolar disorder: a preliminary single-blind study. Bipolar Disord 4:207–213, 2002

Meador KJ, Loring DW, Ray PG, et al: Differential cognitive and behavioral effects of carbamazepine and lamotrigine. Neurology 56:1177–1182, 2001

Meador KJ, Loring DW, Hulihan JF: Differential cognitive and behavioral effects of topiramate and valproate. Neurology 60:1483–1488, 2003

Meador KJ, Loring DW, Vahle VJ, et al: Cognitive and behavioral effects of lamotrigine and topiramate in healthy volunteers. Neurology 64:2108–2114, 2005

Mecarelli O, Vicenzinni E, Pulitano P, et al: Clinical, cognitive, and neurophysiologic correlates of short-term treatment with carbamazepine, oxcarbazepine, and levetiracetam in healthy volunteers. Ann Pharmacother 38:1816–1822, 2004

Minzenberg MJ, Poole JH, Benton C, et al: Association of anticholinergic load with impairment of complex attention and memory in schizophrenia. Am J Psychiatry 161:116–124, 2004

Monks PJ, Thompson JM, Bullmore ET, et al: A functional MRI study of working memory task in euthymic bipolar disorder: evidence for task-specific dysfunction. Bipolar Disord 6:550–564, 2004

Morrens M, Wezenberg E, Verkes RJ, et al: Psychomotor and memory effects of haloperidol, olanzapine, and paroxetine in healthy subjects after short term administration. J Clin Psychopharmacol 27:15–21, 2007

Nemeroff CB, Evans DL, Gyulai L, et al: Double-blind, placebo-controlled comparison of imipramine and paroxetine in the treatment of bipolar depression. Am J Psychiatry 158:906–912, 2001

Pachet AK, Wisniewski AM: The effects of lithium on cognition: an updated review. Psychopharmacology (Berl) 170:225–234, 2003

Peet M: Induction of mania with selective serotonin re-uptake inhibitors and tricyclic antidepressants. Br J Psychiatry 164:549–550, 1994

Physicians' Desk Reference, 61st Edition. Montvale, NJ, Thompson, 2007

Post RM, Altshuler LL, Frye MA, et al: Preliminary observations on the effectiveness of levetiracetam in the open adjunctive treatment of refractory bipolar disorder. J Clin Psychiatry 66:370–374, 2005

Prevey ML, Delaney RC, Cramer JA, et al: Effect of valproate on cognitive functioning: comparison with carbamazepine. Arch Neurol 53:1008–1016, 1996

Reus VI, Targum SD, Weingartner H, et al: The effect of lithium carbonate in memory processes of bipolar affectively ill patients. Psychopharmacology (Berl) 63:39–42, 1979

Richardson JS, Keegan DL, Bowen RC, et al: Verbal learning by major depressive disorder patients during treatment with fluoxetine or amitriptyline. Int Clin Psychopharmacol 9:35–40, 1994

Salinsky MC, Storzbach D, Spencer DC, et al: Effects of topiramate and gabapentin on cognitive abilities in healthy volunteers. Neurology 64:792–798, 2005

Senturk V, Goker C, Bilgic A, et al: Impaired verbal memory and otherwise spared cognition in remitted bipolar patients on monotherapy with lithium or valproate. Bipolar Disord 9 (suppl 1):136–144, 2007

Sernyak MJ, Rosenheck R: Clinicians' reasons for antipsychotic coprescribing. J Clin Psychiatry 65:1597–1600, 2004

Shannon HE, Love PL: Effects of antiepileptic drugs on attention as assessed by a five-choice serial reaction time task in rats. Epilepsy Behav 7:620–628, 2005

Shaw ED, Mann JJ, Stokes PE, et al: Effects of lithium carbonate on associative productivity and idiosyncrasy in bipolar outpatients. Am J Psychiatry 143:1166–1169, 1986

Smith ME, Gevins A, McEvoy LK, et al: Distinct cognitive neurophysiologic profiles for lamotrigine and topiramate. Epilepsia 47:695–703, 2006

Squire LR, Judd LL, Janowsky DS, et al: Effects of lithium carbonate on memory and other cognitive functions. Am J Psychiatry 137:1042–1046, 1980

Stip E, Dufresne J, Lussier I, et al: A double-blind, placebo-controlled study of the effects of lithium on cognition in healthy subjects: mild and selective effects on learning. J Affect Disord 60:147–157, 2000

Stoll AL, Locke CA, Vuckovic A, et al: Lithium-associated cognitive and functional deficits reduced by a switch to divalproex: a case series. J Clin Psychiatry 57:356–359, 1996

Tata PR, Rollings J, Collins M, et al: Lack of cognitive recovery following withdrawal from long-term benzodiazepine use. Psychol Med 24:203–213, 1994

Telford R, Worrall EP: Cognitive functions in manic-depressives: effects of lithium and physostigmine. Br J Psychiatry 133:424–428, 1978

Thompson PJ, Trimble MR: Sodium valproate and cognitive functioning in normal volunteers. Br J Clin Pharmacol 12:819–824, 1981

Tremont G, Stern RA: Use of thyroid hormone to diminish the cognitive side effects of psychiatric treatment. Psychopharmacol Bull 33:273–280, 1997

Tyson PJ, Roberts KH, Mortimer AM: Are the cognitive effects of atypical antipsychotics influenced by their affinity to 5HT-2A receptors? Int J Neurosci 114:593–611, 2004

Wadsworth EJ, Moss SC, Simpson SA, et al: SSRIs and cognitive performance in a working sample. Hum Psychopharmacol 20:561–572, 2005

Werz MA, Schoenberg MR, Meador KJ, et al: Subjective preference for lamotrigine or topiramate in healthy volunteers: relationship to cognitive and behavioral functioning. Epilepsy Behav 8:181–191, 2006

Yamaguchi T, Suzuki M, Yamamoto M: Facilitation of acetylcholine release in rat frontal cortex by indeloxazine hydrochloride: involvement of endogenous serotonin and 5-HT$_4$ receptors. Naunyn Schmiedebergs Arch Pharmacol 356:712–720, 1997

Young LD, Taylor I, Holmstrom V: Lithium treatment of patients with affective illness associated with organic brain symptoms. Am J Psychiatry 134:1405–1407, 1977

Zhou JL, Zhao Q, Holmes GL: Effect of levetiracetam on visual-spatial memory following status epilepticus. Epilepsy Res 73:65–74, 2007

Zobel AW, Schulze-Rauschenbach S, von Widdern OC, et al: Improvement of working but not declarative memory is correlated with HPA normalization during antidepressant treatment. J Psychiatr Res 38:377–383, 2004

8

Pharmacological Strategies to Enhance Neurocognitive Function

Joseph F. Goldberg, M.D.
L. Trevor Young, M.D., Ph.D.

In contrast to Chapter 7 of this volume, "Adverse Cognitive Effects of Psychotropic Medications," the focus in this chapter is on the potential cognitive benefits associated with some anticonvulsants, atypical antipsychotics, antidepressants, and other psychotropic agents. At present, no pharmacological compounds have been approved by the U.S. Food and Drug Administration (FDA) to treat cognitive problems in patients with bipolar disorder (or schizophrenia), and no sufficiently dramatic data are available to compel their routine off-label use as antidotes for cognitive complaints. However, clinicians who recognize differences among the cognitive profiles of mood stabilizers and other medications relevant to bipolar disorder may be able to craft pharmacotherapy regimens that not only minimize adverse effects (e.g., cognitive dulling) but also potentially optimize attention and related neurocognitive functioning as feasible.

At issue remains the extent to which neurocognitive deficits that are intrinsic to bipolar disorder represent endophenotypic traits (discussed in Chapter 4 of this volume, "The Endophenotype Concept: Examples From Neuropsychological and Neuroimaging Studies of Bipolar Disorder"), which, by definition, may have little potential for alteration (short of genetic modification, and the revelation of novel treatment targets or pathways). Separately lies the phenomenon of iatrogenic cognitive problems

159

that may arise secondary to certain psychotropic medications (described in Chapter 7 of this volume) and their potential for pharmacological remediation. Clinicians must continually assess the risks and benefits of any treatment regimen, as well as the potential medical, psychiatric, or other causes of cognitive problems, before embarking on alternative or adjunctive medications with the hope of ameliorating cognitive complaints.

When evaluating the existing literature on pharmacological cognitive enhancement, one must recognize that the vast majority of clinical studies have focused on patients with schizophrenia, or on older adults with mild cognitive impairment who are at increased risk for Alzheimer's dementia, or on patients with frank Alzheimer's dementia or other progressive neurocognitive disorders. Although there is limited capacity to extrapolate from such populations to patients with bipolar disorder, one can examine general pharmacodynamic effects of specific psychoactive agents with respect to neurocognitive function. A first consideration involves the putative effects of psychotropic compounds at the cellular and neurophysiological level.

Neuroprotection

The concept of neuroprotection refers to therapeutic strategies aimed to protect against neuronal injury or degeneration (e.g., pharmacological protection against the effects of trauma, ischemia, or apoptosis) and may bear clinically on the mood-stabilizing properties of some anticonvulsants (particularly those capable of inhibiting excitatory amino acids such as glutamate) and other psychotropic compounds (Li et al. 2002). From among the three types of ionotropic (i.e., ligand-gated) glutamate receptors in the brain—that is, α-amino-3-hydroxy-5-methylisoxazole-4-propionic acid (AMPA, formerly known as quisqualate), kainate, and N-methyl-D-aspartate (NMDA)—the downregulation of non-NMDA receptors is thought to play an important role in neuronal viability and plasticity.

It remains largely speculative whether neuroprotection at the cellular level confers clinical benefit for either affective symptoms or neurocognitive functioning. Nevertheless, structural magnetic resonance imaging studies suggest that even brief exposure to lithium (≤ 4–8 weeks) in patients with bipolar disorder may lead to increases in overall gray matter by 3%–4% (Bearden et al. 2007, in press; Moore et al. 2000) and in hippocampal volume (Bearden et al., in press; Yucel et al. 2008). Moreover, prolonged lithium treatment can normalize the altered striatal shape and decreased anterior cingulate volume present in drug-naïve patients (Hwang et al. 2006; Sassi et al. 2004). Additionally, magnetic resonance spectroscopy studies have demonstrated increases in gray matter myo-inositol levels, accompanied by decreases in glutamate, glutamine, and γ-aminobutyric acid (GABA) concentrations in bipolar disorder patients treated with lithium

(Friedman et al. 2004). Such increases in gray matter volume are presumed to reflect increased dendritic arborization and neuropil density rather than new neuronal development. However, the clinical significance of such neurotropically associated volumetric increases remains unknown.

Research findings suggest that in comparison to healthy control subjects, patients with bipolar disorder experience neurodegeneration, based on observed low levels of neuronal viability markers in the frontal lobes (Cecil et al. 2002) and hippocampus (Bertolino et al. 2003; Deicken et al. 2003), reduced cerebral volumes of the cortex and hippocampus (DelBello et al. 2004; Sassi et al. 2004; Sharma et al. 2003), and reduced white matter volumes in cortical and subcortical structures (Haznedar et al. 2005; McIntosh et al. 2005). Complementary studies of postmortem brain tissue from patients with bipolar disorder have further revealed decreased cell density and cell size throughout the cortex and limbic system. Specifically, reduced neuronal size has been observed in the anterior cingulate cortex (Chana et al. 2003), orbitofrontal cortex (Cotter et al. 2005), hippocampus (Liu et al. 2007), and amygdala (Bezchlibnyk et al. 2007), and reduced neuron density has been reported in the anterior cingulate cortex (Benes et al. 2001; Bouras et al. 2001) and dorsolateral prefrontal cortex (Rajkowska et al. 2001). Similar decreases in glial density have been documented in postmortem frontal and temporal cortex from patients with bipolar disorder, as compared with healthy control subjects (Brauch et al. 2006; Ongur et al. 1998; Uranova et al. 2004). Considered together, these findings indicate that pathological changes are present in the brains of individuals with bipolar disorder and appear to reflect cellular damage or degeneration in specific regions that are critical to mood regulation and neurocognitive function.

At the cellular level, neurotoxicity may result from stress-related glucocorticoid secretion and the activity of excitatory amino acids such as glutamate, which cause cytoplasmic vacuolization and neuronal death—a phenomenon potentially countered by agents such as lithium, valproate, and carbamazepine (Bown et al. 2003). The related concept of apoptosis—programmed cell death—is also relevant to the possible neuroprotective effects of psychotropic agents, as noted in the case of the B-cell lymphoma 2 (Bcl-2) protein, which exerts cytoprotective and neurogenic effects induced by lithium (Chen et al. 2000).

A number of intracellular mechanisms have been suggested to contribute to the putative neuroprotective effects of psychotropic agents such as lithium or valproate, including inhibition of NMDA receptor–mediated calcium influx (Nonaka et al. 1998), inhibition of glycogen synthase kinase-3β (Chen et al. 1999a), activation of cell survival factors (e.g., phosphatidylinositol 3-kinase/Akt signaling pathway) (Chalecka-Franaszek and

Chuang 1999; Kang et al. 2003), and upregulation of neurotrophic factors such as brain-derived neurotrophic factor (BDNF) (Chen et al. 1999b; Manji et al. 2000).

Antidepressant drugs have been shown to promote cellular viability and support neuronal processes through similar mechanisms. In preclinical studies, multiple classes of antidepressant drugs have been found to promote the proliferation and survival of new neurons in the rodent hippocampus and frontal cortex (Kodama et al. 2004; Malberg et al. 2000), while also increasing expression of BDNF and the transcription factor cyclic adenosine monophosphate response element binding protein (CREB) (Nibuya et al. 1995, 1996). Furthermore, the antidepressant imipramine supports the differentiation of neural stem cells by activating the expression of BDNF (Peng et al. 2008), whereas desipramine prevents the apoptotic death of neural stem cells by upregulating Bcl-2 protein levels (Huang et al. 2007). As in the case of mood stabilizers, a link between these neurogenic actions and neurocognitive improvement in patients has not been firmly established; however, structural magnetic resonance imaging studies in depressed patients have revealed that antidepressant treatment may prevent hippocampal volume loss (Sheline et al. 2003). Treatment with selective serotonin reuptake inhibitors (SSRIs) in particular appears to also improve hippocampal-dependent declarative memory in patients with major depressive disorder, in comparison to nontreated patients and healthy control subjects (Vythilingam et al. 2004). Evidence from postmortem brain studies supports the implication of CREB and BDNF in this amelioration of function, as increased levels of these neurotrophic molecules have been observed in the cortex and hippocampus of depressed patients with a history of antidepressant treatment (Chen et al. 2001; Dowlatshahi et al. 1998).

Data suggest that at least some atypical antipsychotics have potential neurotrophic effects associated with antimanic efficacy in humans. For example, in a study of 20 first-episode manic adolescent patients, DelBello et al. (2006) used proton magnetic resonance spectroscopy to show that patients who remitted with olanzapine were more likely than nonremitters to demonstrate greater increases in levels of N-acetyl-aspartate (NAA)—a marker of neuronal viability—in the medial ventral prefrontal cortex (a region that includes the anterior cingulate gyrus and the orbital frontal cortex, areas relevant to executive function and to social cognition or emotion-related learning, respectively) (see Figure 8–1).

Table 8–1 summarizes the extent to which lithium and anticonvulsant drugs have been shown to exert neuroprotective effects. Note that the table includes a number of anticonvulsant agents for which mood-stabilizing properties have not been clearly demonstrated (e.g., topiramate, gabapentin, tiagabine, and levetiracetam) but nevertheless represent experimental

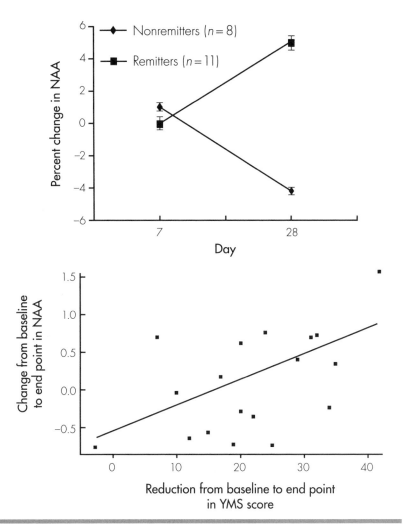

FIGURE 8–1. Increased neuronal viability and its association with improvement in mania symptoms during olanzapine treatment in adolescent mania.

NAA= *N*-acetyl-aspartate; YMS=Young Mania Scale.

Source. Reprinted from DelBello MP, Cecil KM, Adler CM, et al: "Neurochemical Effects of Olanzapine in First-Hospitalization Manic Adolescents: A Proton Magnetic Resonance Spectroscopy Study." *Neuropsychopharmacology* 31:1264–1273, 2006. Used by permission from Macmillan Publishers, Ltd.

TABLE 8–1. Putative neuroprotective effects of lithium and
anticonvulsant agents

Agent	Study	Findings
Carbamazepine	Hough et al. 1996	Inhibition of NMDA receptor–mediated calcium influx in cerebellar granule cells
	Mai et al. 2002	Facilitated activation of CREB
Divalproex	Chen et al. 1999b	Induction of Bcl-2
	Chen et al. 1999a	Inhibition of GSK-3β
	Nonaka et al. 1998	Inhibition of NMDA receptors
	Chen et al. 2006	Upregulation of BDNF
	Frey et al. 2006	
Gabapentin	Hara and Sata 2007	NMDA receptor blockade
	Sills 2006	Inhibition of voltage-gated calcium channels at the α₂δ subunit
	NA	Undemonstrated effects on BDNF or Bcl-2
Lamotrigine	Li et al. 2002 (review)	Reduced areas of neuronal death or neurotoxicity in animal models of ischemia or axotomy
	Mai et al. 2002	Undemonstrated effects on BDNF
	NA	Undemonstrated effects on Bcl-2
Levetiracetam	Wang et al. 2006	Reduced neuronal damage after subarachnoid hemorrhage and closed head injury in mice
	Cardile et al. 2003	Stimulates expression of BDNF and iNOS in rat cortical astrocyte cultures
Lithium	Chen et al. 1999b	Induction of Bcl-2
	Chen et al. 1999a	Inhibition of GSK-3β
	Frey et al. 2006	Upregulation of BDNF
	Fukumoto et al. 2001	Increased expression of BDNF in hippocampus, temporal cortex, and frontal cortex
	Mai et al. 2002	Facilitated activation of CREB
	Manji et al. 2000	Increased gray matter volume
	Nonaka et al. 1998	Inhibition of NMDA receptors
	Yucel et al., in press	Increased hippocampal volume
Tiagabine	Yang et al. 2000	Reduced neuronal damage after induced focal cerebral ischemia in animal models
	NA	Undemonstrated effects on BDNF or Bcl-2

TABLE 8–1. Putative neuroprotective effects of lithium and anticonvulsant agents *(continued)*

Agent	Study	Findings
Topiramate	Sfaello et al. 2005	In animal neonates, prevents loss of developing white matter from excito-toxicity caused by the AMPA/kainate glutamate agonist *S*-bromowillardiine
	Kudin et al. 2004	Calcium channel blockade in hippocampal mitochondria
	NA	Undemonstrated effects on BDNF or Bcl-2

Note. AMPA = α-amino-3-hydroxy-5-methylisoxazole-4-propionic acid glutamate receptor subtype; Bcl-2 = B-cell lymphoma 2 protein; BDNF = brain-derived neurotrophic factor; CREB = cyclic adenosine monophosphate response element binding protein; GSK-3β = glycogen synthase kinase-3 beta; iNOS = inducible nitric oxide synthase; NA = not applicable; NMDA = *N*-methyl-D-aspartate.

pharmacoltherapies relevant to bipolar disorder. Several of these compounds are discussed in detail in the following section. Figure 8–2 demonstrates neuroprotective effects associated with lithium or divalproex (valproate) on neuronal survival in vitro, and Figure 8–3 demonstrates increased anterior cingulate cortical volumes in patients with bipolar disorder treated with lithium in comparison to untreated patients and healthy control subjects.

Anticonvulsants

Lamotrigine

Unlike many other anticonvulsant agents that have psychotropic properties, lamotrigine has been shown through randomized prospective studies to have potential benefits with respect to cognitive function. Secondary analyses from the two pivotal FDA registration studies of lamotrigine for maintenance treatment of bipolar disorder found 81% improvement from baseline in global neurocognitive function following an index depressive episode and 35% improvement after an index manic episode (Khan et al. 2004). Improvements from baseline deficits were highly significant in both depressed and manic groups, and were evident during an initial open-label phase while the researchers were statistically controlling for potential confounding factors, such as change in mood, duration of illness, and duration of prior psychotropic medication use. Elsewhere, studies using functional magnetic resonance imaging suggest that lamotrigine use among stable bipolar patients appears associated with enhanced cortical function during working memory and facial affect recognition tasks, as demonstrated by in-

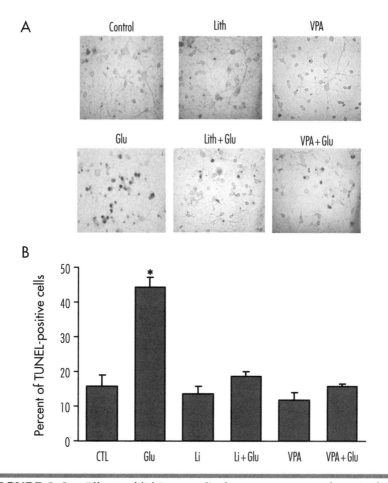

FIGURE 8–2.   Effects of lithium or divalproex on neuronal survival in vitro.

Effects of lithium (Lith) and valproate (VPA) on glutamate (Glu)-induced deoxyribonucleic acid fragmentation in primary cultured rat cerebral cortical cells. (A) Cells were pretreated with Lith (1 mmol/L) or VPA (0.6 mmol/L) for 1 week and then exposed to Glu at 100 μmol/L for 18 hours. (B) Deoxyribonucleic acid fragmentation was determined by TUNEL (terminal deoxynucleotidyltransferase-mediated deoxyuridine triphosphate nick end labeling) staining. Results are the mean ± standard error of mean ($n=6$).

*$P<0.01$ (one-way analysis of variance followed by the post hoc Dunnett's t test).

Source.   Reprinted from Shao L, Young LT, Wang JF: "Chronic Treatment With Mood Stabilizers Lithium and Valproate Prevents Excitotoxicity by Inhibiting Oxidative Stress in Rat Cerebral Cortical Cells." *Biological Psychiatry* 58:879–884, 2005. Used with permission from Elsevier Limited.

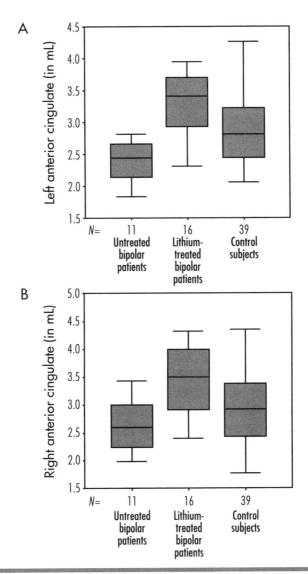

FIGURE 8–3. Effects of lithium on anterior cingulate cortical volume in patients with bipolar disorder.

Anterior cingulate volumes for untreated bipolar patients, lithium-treated bipolar patients, and healthy control subjects. (A) Untreated patients presented significantly reduced left anterior cingulate volume when compared with lithium-treated patients and healthy control subjects ($P<0.05$; analysis of covariance followed by post hoc testing with Sidak adjustment). (B) No significant differences in right anterior cingulate volume were found among the groups.

Source. Reprinted from Sassi RB, Brambilla P, Hatch JP, et al: "Reduced Left Anterior Cingulate Volumes in Untreated Bipolar Patients." *Biological Psychiatry* 56:467–475, 2004. Used with permission from Elsevier Limited.

creased activation in the prefrontal cortex and cingulate gyrus in bipolar patients who had received lamotrigine (Haldane et al. 2008).

Divalproex and Carbamazepine

In contrast to the neurocognitive improvement documented in individuals with bipolar disorder after lamotrigine therapy, subtle cognitive deficits have been noted in individuals treated with divalproex or carbamazepine— although it should be noted that few studies have examined the effects of these anticonvulsants on cognition in neuropsychiatric populations. In one series of cases, Stoll et al. (1996) found that a switch from lithium maintenance therapy to divalproex ameliorated patients' complaints of cognitive dulling and decreased creativity. However, a more recent screen of a larger subject pool revealed that bipolar patients taking divalproex or carbamazepine were impaired on measures of psychomotor speed, cognitive flexibility, and complex attention as compared with bipolar patients taking lamotrigine, oxcarbazepine, topiramate, or lithium (Gualtieri and Johnson 2006). Nevertheless, neuroprotective properties of divalproex have been identified in preclinical studies, indicating that the drug promotes the release of growth factors (e.g., BDNF) from cultured midbrain neurons (Chen et al. 2006) and is effective at preventing oxidative damage to cultured cortical neurons (Shao et al. 2005). These neuroprotective actions may be reflected in two recent neuroanatomical studies in which bipolar patients treated with divalproex or divalproex plus quetiapine displayed higher hippocampal NAA levels than untreated patients (Atmaca et al. 2007b) and showed increased anterior cingulate cortex volumes as compared with untreated patients (Atmaca et al. 2007a).

Pyrrolidone Derivatives (e.g., Levetiracetam)

Pyrrolidone derivatives, which include the anticonvulsant levetiracetam, represent a family of compounds thought to enhance learning and memory, as well as possible neuroprotective and anticonvulsant effects (Shorvon 2001). The first pyrrolidone described as having cognitive-enhancing or "nootropic" effects (Trofimov et al. 2005) was piracetam, which was followed by several additional compounds, including nefiracetam (Kitano et al. 2005), the peptide noopept (Trofimov et al. 2005), and the vinca alkaloid vinpocetine (Szatmari and Whitehouse 2003). Evidence to support the clinical efficacy of such agents in humans with cognitive impairment—mainly due to Alzheimer's or cerebrovascular-based dementias—appears largely inconclusive, and has not been adapted to other populations with cognitive complaints. In epilepsy patients, levetiracetam has been reported to improve attention and verbal fluency (Piazzini et al. 2006). In a review, Flicker and Grimley Evans (2004) determined that existing evidence from controlled trials was inconclusive to support the cognitive-enhancing properties of piracetam for individuals with dementia or minimal cognitive impairment. Although the thymoleptic effects of levetiracetam in bipolar disorder are not well established (Post et al. 2005), its cognitive effects appear at least benign, and further study of its possible nootropic effects appears warranted.

Atypical Antipsychotics

The capacity of atypical antipsychotics to increase extracellular dopamine in the medial and dorsolateral prefrontal cortex as well as the reward pathway (i.e., nucleus accumbens) (Kuroki et al. 1999) represents a viable pharmacological strategy to compensate for low attentional states, presumably mediated at least in part by mesocortical hypodopaminergic tone. Interest in the potential neurocognitive benefits of atypical antipsychotics for such disturbances has focused largely around negative symptom schizophrenia, although preliminary studies have also addressed the potential for agents such as olanzapine to improve amotivational and apathy states via this mechanism in mood disorders (Marangell et al. 2002). Furthermore, in contrast to first-generation antipsychotics such as haloperidol, most if not all atypical antipsychotics have been shown in preclinical studies to increase prefrontal cholinergic activity, which in turn, at least theoretically, leads to improvement in memory.

Notably, existing controlled trials using atypical antipsychotics in patients with schizophrenia or schizoaffective disorder report only relatively modest effect sizes, ranging from 0.13 to 0.43, in the magnitude of improvement in neurocognitive function (Bilder et al. 2002a; Harvey and Keefe 2001; Keefe et al. 2007b). In the National Institute of Mental Health's Clinical Antipsychotic Trials of Intervention Effectiveness (CATIE) schizophrenia study, small but significant benefits from baseline were seen in composite neurocognitive functioning, with similarity among all agents studied (i.e., olanzapine, risperidone, quetiapine, ziprasidone, and perphenazine) at 2 and 6 months (Keefe et al. 2007a). However, in the subgroup remaining in treatment at 18 months (37% of those initially studied at 2 months), perphenazine was associated with an unexpected, significantly better neurocognitive profile than any of the atypical agents. Among early psychosis patients in the CATIE study, similar modest but significant improvements in global cognitive function were observed after randomization to olanzapine, risperidone, or quetiapine, without observed differences among individual treatments (Keefe et al. 2007b). Also noteworthy was the observation that improved neurocognitive function predicted longer retention in the CATIE study protocol (Keefe et al. 2007a).

Findings from randomized trials that assessed the neurocognitive effects of atypical antipsychotics are summarized in Table 8–2 and described below.

TABLE 8–2. Comparative neurocognitive profiles among atypical antipsychotics in randomized studies

Agent	Study	Subjects and design	Findings
Olanzapine	Purdon et al. 2000	SZ outpatients taking OLZ ($n=21$) or RIS ($n=21$) or HAL ($n=23$) at 6, 30, and 54 weeks	OLZ>RIS=HAL on general cognitive index and on immediate recall and visual organization
	Bilder et al. 2002a	101 SZ or SzAff patients randomized to CLOZ, OLZ, RIS, or HAL for 14 weeks	OLZ=RIS>HAL in global neurocognitive function; CLOZ>HAL on motor function
	Keefe et al. 2007a	817 CATIE SZ subjects randomized to OLZ, PER, RIS, QUET, or ZIP	Small but significant improvement with all agents except ZIP ($P<0.006$) in global neurocognitive function at 2 and 6 months
	Lindenmayer et al. 2007	35 negative-symptom SZ patients randomized to OLZ versus HAL for 12 weeks	Significant improvements from baseline with OLZ in declarative verbal learning memory and motor functioning
Clozapine	Lee et al. 1994	36 treatment-resistant SZ patients taking CLOZ, 24 non-treatment-resistant SZ patients taking CLOZ, 23 non-treatment-resistant SZ patients taking conventional antipsychotics	CLOZ>conventional antipsychotics on improved attention and verbal fluency
Aripiprazole	Kern et al. 2006	168 SZ or SzAff patients randomized to ARI or OLZ for 26 weeks	Comparable improvements from baseline for both agents in general cognitive functioning but not executive functioning; improvement from baseline in verbal memory with ARI but not OLZ
Ziprasidone	Harvey et al. 2004	6-week multicenter double-blind randomized comparison of ZIP ($n=136$) and OLZ ($n=133$)	ZIP=OLZ in attention, memory, working memory, motor speed, and executive function

TABLE 8–2. Comparative neurocognitive profiles among atypical antipsychotics in randomized studies *(continued)*

Agent	Study	Subjects and design	Findings
Risperidone	Cuesta et al. 2001	9 chronic SZ patients taking RIS versus OLZ ($n=21$) or conventional antipsychotics ($n=8$) for 6 months	RIS>OLZ in fewer perseverative responses (WCST number of categories); no improvements in verbal fluency, nonverbal memory, or visuomotor function with any agents
	Reinares et al. 2000	Euthymic bipolar patients taking RIS ($n=11$) or HAL ($n=9$)	RIS>HAL in improving executive function
Quetiapine	Riedel et al., in press	8-week randomized comparison of QUET versus OLZ in 33 SZ patients	QUET>OLZ in improving reaction quality and attention
	Riedel et al. 2007	12-week randomized comparison of QUET versus RIS in 34 SZ patients	QUET=RIS in overall cognitive improvement; QUET>RIS in working memory, verbal memory, reaction quality, and attention

Note. ARI=aripiprazole; CATIE=Clinical Antipsychotic Trials of Intervention Effectiveness; CLOZ=clozapine; HAL=haloperidol; OLZ=olanzapine; PER=perphenazine; QUET=quetiapine; RIS=risperidone; SZ=schizophrenia; SzAff=schizoaffective; WCST=Wisconsin Card Sorting Test; ZIP=ziprasidone.

Olanzapine

Procholinergic, and thus possible procognitive, effects have been demonstrated in preclinical studies with both olanzapine and clozapine, specifically with respect to increased hippocampal acetylcholine release via blockade of terminal M_2 muscarinic autoreceptors (Johnson et al. 2005). Among outpatients with schizophrenia, use of olanzapine and risperidone has shown significant improvements from baseline in executive function, learning and memory, processing speed, attention/vigilance, verbal working memory, and motor functions (Keefe et al. 2006). In addition, a multisite Canadian study enrolling 65 outpatients with schizophrenia found that olanzapine was superior to risperidone or haloperidol on a general cognitive index and, more specifically, in immediate recall and visual organization (Purdon et al. 2000).

Clozapine

In addition to clozapine's putative effects on prefrontal dopamine turnover as a mechanism behind its cognitive benefits in schizophrenia, preclinical studies suggest the possibility of a beneficial cognitive effect related to its antagonism of H_1 histamine receptors (Roegge et al. 2007). Improvements in deficits associated with frontal lobe function in schizophrenia also appear to occur independent of any direct effect on regional cerebral blood flow (Zhao et al. 2006). From a pharmacogenetic perspective, improvement from baseline in attention and verbal fluency during clozapine treatment for schizophrenia has been associated with a specific functional polymorphism—the met/met homozygous and met/val heterozygous (as opposed to val/val homozygous) variants—of the gene encoding catechol O-methyltransferase (COMT) (Woodward et al. 2007), a key enzyme for dopamine and norepinephrine catabolism. Moreover, genetic variants of COMT represent viable markers that may confer susceptibility to neurocognitive dysfunction in both schizophrenia (Bilder et al. 2002b) and bipolar disorder (Burdick et al. 2007b; see also Chapter 4 of this volume). Randomized trials with clozapine, predominantly in chronic or refractory schizophrenia patients, point to the potential for improvements in elements of executive function, attention and recall, verbal fluency, and retrieval from reference memory (Buchanan et al. 1994; Hagger et al. 1993; Lee et al. 1994), as well as reaction time and accuracy of target detection (Galletly et al. 2000).

Aripiprazole

Because aripiprazole is a partial agonist of D_2 and D_3 dopamine receptors, there is compelling conceptual appeal in its potential to increase dopaminergic transmission in presumably hypodopaminergic brain regions (e.g., mesocortical tracts) in patients with diminished attention or negative symptoms. For that matter, this mechanism theoretically could suggest a possible broader benefit for aripiprazole to modulate central hypodopaminergic states, such as attention-deficit disorder, although empirical studies in this area have not been conducted.

In a 26-week open-label study of aripiprazole or olanzapine in 169 patients with schizophrenia or schizoaffective disorder, both agents yielded significant improvements from baseline in general cognitive functioning and verbal learning, but not in executive functioning (Kern et al. 2006). Verbal learning performance was significantly better with aripiprazole than olanzapine in the first 8 weeks of treatment as well as at week 26. Comparable improvements from baseline were seen with both agents in sustained attention, as measured by a continuous performance task.

Ziprasidone

During a 6-week randomized comparison of ziprasidone or olanzapine in hospitalized patients with schizophrenia or schizoaffective disorder, similar levels of improvement from baseline were seen in attention, memory, working memory, motor speed, and executive functioning (Harvey et al. 2004). A 6-month randomized comparison of these agents found similar degrees of normalization in executive function, verbal learning, and verbal fluency (Harvey et al. 2006). In the CATIE schizophrenia trial, improvement in a global cognitive battery among subjects taking ziprasidone was marginally significant ($P < 0.06$) (Keefe et al. 2007a). Harvey et al. (2004) noted that at least in the case of schizophrenia, between-group effect sizes for changes in neurocognitive function are relatively small between atypical antipsychotics such as ziprasidone and olanzapine.

Risperidone

In one of the few existing studies focusing on the cognitive effects of atypical antipsychotics specifically among individuals with bipolar disorder, Reinares et al. (2000) conducted a small but randomized comparison of risperidone versus haloperidol in 20 euthymic bipolar patients. Those taking risperidone demonstrated greater improvement in executive function.

Quetiapine

No clinical studies involving quetiapine have focused specifically on cognition in bipolar disorder. In 3-week studies of quetiapine use in patients with bipolar mania, somnolence was reported as an adverse drug effect in about one-third of subjects, presumably related to the drug's antihistamine effects. Nevertheless, cognitive complaints per se are not included among the common adverse effects listed in the manufacturer's package insert. Furthermore, as described in Table 8–2, schizophrenia patients taking quetiapine have been reported to demonstrate at least comparable if not greater improvement from baseline in overall cognitive function and subcomponent measures as compared with patients taking olanzapine or risperidone (Riedel et al. 2007, in press).

Antidepressants

Traditional antidepressants generally have not been used specifically for purposes of improving attention or other cognitive functions as separable entities from clinical depression, and their addition to mood-stabilizing agents may, in general, yield no greater efficacy than mood-stabilizing agents alone for acute bipolar depression (Sachs et al. 2007). It is worth noting, however, that noradrenergic-serotonergic mixed agonists, such as venlafaxine (Findling et al. 2007), or tricyclic antidepressants, such as desipramine, have previously demonstrated efficacy for treating symptoms of attention-deficit/hyperactivity disorder (ADHD) in children and adolescents (Spencer et al. 2002) and in adults (Wilens et al. 1996), although such studies have not been conducted in populations with dual-diagnosis ADHD and bipolar disorder. To the extent that noradrenergic antidepressants may pose a higher risk than other antidepressants for inducing mania or mood destabilization (Leverich et al. 2006), their use in patients with dual-diagnosis ADHD and bipolar disorder demands close monitoring for mood destabilization and the worsening of affective symptoms.

Similarly, the norepinephrine reuptake inhibitor atomoxetine is widely used as an alternative to psychostimulants in the treatment of ADHD and has at least theoretical relevance to the treatment of depression based on its catecholaminergic action (although randomized trials have failed to demonstrate its efficacy specifically for the treatment of depression in adolescents with comorbid ADHD [Bangs et al. 2007] or as adjunctive treatment in adults with unipolar depression who are partially responsive to sertraline [Michelson et al. 2007]). In the treatment of ADHD in children and adolescents with bipolar disorder, small open trials and case studies using atomoxetine have reported both the emergence (Henderson 2004) and the absence of emergence (Hah and Chang 2005) of mania or hypomania, again signaling the need for cautious observation when atomoxetine is used for ADHD features in patients with bipolar disorder.

Procholinergics

The use of cholinesterase inhibitors (e.g., donepezil) to increase central muscarinic and nicotinic acetylcholine transmission in hippocampal and cortical regions has an obvious rationale in Alzheimer's dementia and possibly in schizophrenia, insofar as the latter condition is thought to involve aberrant cortical cholinergic transmission. However, it is important to recognize that procholinergic pharmacological agents (e.g., cholinesterase inhibitors) may not necessarily lead to the enhancement of memory or other cognitive functions when the etiology of cognitive deficits is not clearly linked to cholinergic dysfunction. No published studies have yet been reported using procholinergic agents to counteract adverse cognitive effects of psychotropic medications such as topiramate. However, several clinical trials describe outcomes using cholinesterase inhibitors to target cognitive dysfunction in patients with bipolar disorder, schizophrenia, or schizoaffective disorder. Data also suggest that cholinergic enhancement (via donepezil) can improve verbal and visual episodic memory in healthy adults (Grön et al. 2005).

Donepezil

Possible thymoleptic effects of donepezil were initially described in a small pilot study of 11 treatment-resistant patients in mixed, hypomanic, or depressed illness phases (Burt et al. 1999), although a subsequent randomized trial failed to affirm efficacy in treatment-resistant mania (Eden Evins et al. 2006). Empirical efforts to counteract cognitive complaints using donepezil in psychiatric populations without dementia are scarce, and no randomized studies or large open trials exist specifically for this purpose among patients with bipolar disorder. A recent open trial of donepezil added to a variety of psychotropic agents resulted in global improvement among 39 of 58 (67%) private practice patients with bipolar disorder I, II, or not otherwise specified. Formal neurocognitive testing was not performed and perceived benefit was limited to non–bipolar I disorder patients (Kelly 2008). A 12-week placebo-controlled study of donepezil (5–10 mg/day) added to a variety of atypical antipsychotics for 250 patients with schizophrenia or schizoaffective disorder found no significant differences between active drug and placebo (Keefe et al., in press). A 3-month controlled trial also failed to demonstrate benefits for memory problems in patients with epilepsy (Hamberger et al. 2007). However, one small (*N*=6) open report described efficacy with donepezil to reduce topiramate-induced cognitive complaints in migraine sufferers (Wheeler 2006).

Rivastigmine

Rivastigmine, another cholinesterase inhibitor used in Alzheimer's dementia, has failed to demonstrate efficacy when compared with placebo among patients with schizophrenia in randomized trials measuring executive function, verbal skills, working memory, attention, and psychomotor speed (Kumari et al. 2006; Sharma et al. 2006). Studies in bipolar disorder have not been reported.

Galantamine

Galantamine reversibly inhibits acetylcholinesterase and is an allosteric modulator of cholinergic transmission. Results from a small number of open trials, primarily in patients with schizophrenia, suggest the potential for improvement from baseline in sustained or selective attention as well as psychomotor function when galantamine (dosed at 16 mg/day for up to 8 weeks) is added to atypical antipsychotics such as clozapine (Bora et al. 2005). A more recent and larger double-blind, placebo-controlled 12-week study of adjunctive galantamine in 86 patients with schizophrenia revealed no global improvement from baseline in cognitive performance but did point to significant improvement in processing speed—a measure sensitive to deficits, but also the measure that is most likely sensitive to detecting change over time (Buchanan et al. 2008). In patients with bipolar disorder, several published case reports suggest that galantamine use results in improvement in overall cognitive impairment (Schrauwen and Ghaemi 2006). Collectively, these early findings offer promise for galantamine as a viable potential strategy for cognitive enhancement in patients with bipolar disorder or schizophrenia.

α_7-Nicotinic Agonists

Functional synergy has been described between muscarinic and nicotinic receptors in the modulation of working memory and attention (Ellis et al. 2006). Consistent with observations that nicotine has modest positive neurocognitive effects in schizophrenia (Barr et al. 2008), results of a preliminary proof-of-concept placebo-controlled study indicate that administration of two single doses (75 or 100 mg) of the experimental α_7-nicotinic agonist DMXB-A within 24 hours was associated with clinically meaningful improvement from baseline in attention and overall neurocognitive function in schizophrenia patients with cognitive deficits (Olincy et al. 2006). The indirect nicotinic cholinergic agonism associated with atypical antipsychotics such as clozapine may similarly account for procognitive effects seen with such agents. Mice in which the α_7-nicotinic receptor gene has been knocked out phenotypically show impaired attention, suggesting a potentially important target for future drug development (Young et al. 2007).

Psychostimulants

Modafinil

The novel psychostimulant modafinil is thought to exert attentional and stimulant effects via direct activity at the dopamine transporter. In adults with schizophrenia, modafinil may improve attentional set shifting (Turner et al. 2004b), working memory (Spence et al. 2005), response inhibition

(Turner et al. 2004a), and executive function in those with poor baseline prefrontal executive function (Hunter et al. 2006). A study in 24 outpatients with schizophrenia or schizoaffective disorder found improvement in sedation and cognitive function (i.e., attention, working memory, executive function) with modafinil (up to 200 mg/day), but changes from baseline were no different from placebo (Sevy et al. 2005).

In healthy young adults, modafinil has been shown in a non-dosage-dependent fashion (i.e., 100–200 mg/day) to improve immediate verbal recall and short-term visual recognition memory, but no effect was evident on spatial working memory or verbal short-term memory (i.e., story recall) (Randall et al. 2005). However, earlier studies by the same investigators found either minimal effect on cognition in healthy, non-sleep-deprived, middle-aged volunteers (Randall et al. 2004) or a more robust effect on mood or anxiety than on cognition in healthy young volunteers (Randall et al. 2003). A placebo-controlled trial of modafinil (mean dosage 175 mg/day) added to mood stabilizers in nonpsychotic outpatients with bipolar depression showed significant improvement in depressive symptoms, with no significantly increased risk for inducing mania (Frye et al. 2007).

Amphetamine

Extrapolating from clinical observations in patients with frank attention-deficit disorder, clinicians often think of D-amphetamine or mixed amphetamine salts (e.g., amphetamine-dextroamphetamine) as potentially useful adjunctive pharmacotherapies to target "inattentiveness" as a freestanding symptom in patients with mood disorder. Indeed, amphetamine use has been shown to improve working memory and language production in healthy controls as well as schizophrenia patients (Barch and Carter 2005). For individuals with bipolar disorder, at least theoretical safety risks arise regarding the potential for amphetamines to induce mood destabilization, particularly given that D-amphetamine is commonly used to induce pharmacological mania in animal models. However, partly mitigating such concerns are data from child and adolescent studies of bipolar disorder with comorbid ADHD, in which no worsening of mania symptoms appears evident after adding amphetamine, mixed amphetamine salts, or methylphenidate to standard antimanic agents such as divalproex (Carlson et al. 2004; Scheffer et al. 2005). In clinical experience, relatively low dosages (e.g., 5–10 mg/day) of D-amphetamine added to traditional mood stabilizers are generally well tolerated and may be of value for symptom pictures involving psychomotor slowing, sedation, depressive features, and poor attention.

Notably, chronic amphetamine *abuse* has been associated with impaired working memory and executive dysfunction, even years after drug cessation (Ersche et al. 2006; Ornstein et al. 2000). Amphetamine abuse may cause neurotoxic effects on dopaminergic and serotonergic structures via oxidative stress, hyperthermia, excitotoxicity, and apoptosis (Cadet et al. 2007). Clinicians must determine a patient's candidacy for stimulant use on an individual basis, bearing in mind factors such as past or current substance abuse and the likelihood for misuse of stimulants, as well as the ability to minimize or eliminate other iatrogenic sources of cognitive dulling or impairment.

Methylphenidate

Controlled trials using methylphenidate in patients with bipolar disorder have not been reported. However, retrospective open-label reports of adding 5–40 mg/day of methylphenidate to mood-stabilizing agents (e.g., for depressive symptoms or for comorbid ADHD features) suggest relatively high degrees of safety and tolerability (Lydon and El-Mallakh 2006).

Other Dopamine Agonists

The antiparkinsonian D_2 and D_3 agonist pramipexole has been described in two preliminary placebo-controlled trials as possessing antidepressant properties in patients with bipolar depression (Goldberg et al. 2004; Zarate et al. 2004). Preliminary data from our group (Burdick et al. 2007a) support the utility of adjunctive pramipexole for improving attention, concentration, and visual search efficiency in the course of treatment for bipolar depression. Elsewhere, the D_1 agonist pergolide (Kimberg and D'Esposito 2003) and D_2 agonists such as bromocriptine (Kimberg et al. 1997) have been reported to exert at least modest enhancement of cognitive function in healthy control subjects. It is also noteworthy that the antiparkinsonian dopamine agonist amantadine appears to have minimal adverse cognitive effects, in contrast to anticholinergic antiparkinsonian agents such as benztropine (McEvoy 1987); hence, in the setting of cognitive complaints, amantadine may be a preferable agent to counteract antipsychotic-associated parkinsonism.

Other Pharmacological Agents

Limited data have addressed the potential neurocognitive benefits of several additional pharmacological agents. Most studies, however, pertain to the treatment of mild cognitive impairment (a likely precursor to dementia) or cognitive symptoms in unipolar depression rather than bipolar disorder.

Antiglutamatergic Agents

Memantine

Memantine, an NMDA receptor antagonist, represents a novel pharmacotherapy for the treatment of dementia. NMDA receptor–mediated long-term potentiation in the hippocampus represents a key neuropharmacological mechanism of learning and memory (see Chapter 3 of this volume, "Memory Deficits Associated With Bipolar Disorder"). Its potential utility for possible mood-stabilizing and cognitive-enhancing effects in bipolar disorder has been suggested from open-label self-report data in case reports (Teng and Demetrio 2006); however, affirmation is needed from larger-scale systematic or randomized trials. In major depression, memantine dosed from 5 to 20 mg/day has appeared no different from placebo with respect to acute antidepressant efficacy (Zarate et al. 2006).

Glycine

Agonism at the glycine modulatory site of the NMDA receptor represents a theoretically viable strategy to improve both cognitive and negative symptoms in schizophrenia patients, although the 16-week Cognitive and Negative Symptoms in Schizophrenia Trial (CONSIST; Buchanan et al. 2007) failed to identify improvement in any neurocognitive domains with glycine (target dosage of 60 mg/day) as compared with placebo. Studies of glycine augmentation in patients with bipolar disorder have not yet been reported.

D-Serine

D-serine is a ligand that potently activates NMDA receptors in the presence of glutamate (hence functioning in effect as an NMDA agonist). Although no studies have been reported on the possible cognitive effects of D-serine in patients with bipolar disorder, Tsai et al. (1998) added D-serine or placebo to existing conventional or atypical antipsychotics in a study of 31 patients with schizophrenia and found improvements from baseline in global cognitive function, as well as executive function in particular. Similarly, Heresco-Levy et al. (2005) found improvement in global cognitive function after adding D-serine to risperidone or olanzapine in 39 patients with schizophrenia. Whether similar results are likely to occur in patients with bipolar disorder or nonpsychotic mood disorders remains uncertain.

D-Cycloserine

The antituberculosis drug D-cycloserine (DCS) also is a selective partial agonist at the NMDA receptor glycine site. Despite promising findings from initial studies using DCS to treat negative symptoms in schizophrenia, dosages of 50 mg/day failed to demonstrate advantages over placebo in any neurocognitive domains among patients with schizophrenia studied in CONSIST (Buchanan et al. 2007). In patients with obsessive-compulsive disorder, administration of 125 mg of DCS 2 hours prior to exposure therapy was associated with greater efficiency and less distress than standard exposure therapy, suggesting the potential utility of DCS as a novel strategy to overcome interference from fear circuitry during paradigms of learning and memory as seen in psychotherapy (Kushner et al. 2007; for further discussion of fear-based learning and psychotherapy, see Chapter 6 of this volume, "Improving Psychotherapy Practice and Technique for Bipolar Disorder: Lessons From Cognitive Neuroscience").

Ampakines

AMPA receptor–positive modulators (ampakines) are an experimental class of drugs that have been shown in preliminary studies to enhance learning and memory. In one 4-week study of 105 outpatients with schizophrenia, augmentation of clozapine, olanzapine, or risperidone with the ampakine CX516 yielded little benefit with only small effect sizes (Goff et al. 2008). Further study is needed to estimate the likelihood with which agents in this family can offer potential benefit for baseline or iatrogenic cognitive complaints.

Acamprosate

Originally studied and used for the treatment of alcohol dependence, acamprosate binds to the type 5 metabotropic glutamate receptor (mGluR5), part of a receptor class that has been associated with motivation and the dopamine reward pathway. Another mGluR5 antagonist, 2-methyl-6-(phenylethynyl)-pyridine (MPEP), has demonstrated anxiolytic effects in rodent models of anxiety without impairing working memory or spatial learning (Ballard et al. 2005).

As a strategy for manipulating NMDA receptors, metabotropic glutamate receptor antagonists may offer a viable potential means for modifying cognitive dysfunction in primary psychotic disorders (Moghaddam 2004). However, in healthy adult volunteers, acamprosate dosed at 2 g/day for 7 days has been shown to impair working memory, delayed recall, and recognition tasks (Schneider et al. 1999).

Cyclooxygenase-2 Inhibitors

Because the activation of proinflammatory cytokines has been associated with cognitive impairment, nonsteroidal anti-inflammatory drugs have been suggested to potentially help reduce the risk for development of Alzheimer's dementia. Following such observations, the selective cyclooxygenase-2 (COX-2) inhibitors celecoxib and rofecoxib have been studied in otherwise healthy adults with mild neurocognitive impairment. Although use of these COX-2 inhibitors has not shown tangible improvement in patients with mild cognitive impairment or Alzheimer's dementia (Thal et al. 2005), preliminary evidence suggests that celecoxib may improve aspects of cognition when used in conjunction with an atypical antipsychotic for patients with schizophrenia (Müller et al. 2005). A rationale for using COX-2 inhibitors in the treatment of schizophrenia stems from interest in the potential involvement of inflammatory processes in schizophrenia, as well as an apparent neuroprotective effect of COX-2 inhibitors against glutamate-induced hippocampal neurotoxicity (Hewett et al. 2006). It remains to be demonstrated whether COX-2 inhibitors may hold value for intrinsic neurocognitive deficits in bipolar disorder or as a strategy to offset iatrogenic cognitive complaints in populations other than those with schizophrenia or dementia.

Serotonergic Agents

Buspirone

The density of serotonin type 1A (5-HT_{1A}) receptors in hippocampal regions has given rise to interest in their pharmacological perturbation to target memory and global cognition via 5-HT_{1A} partial agonism or antagonism. In addition to animal studies (Roth et al. 2004), a small clinical literature exists that supports a modest benefit in cognitive functioning among schizophrenia patients taking conventional antipsychotics with the addition of 5-HT_{1A} partial agonists such as tandospirone (Sumiyoshi et al. 2001) or buspirone (Sumiyoshi et al. 2007), although effects appear more robust with the former rather than latter agent. Buspirone has not been associated with adverse cognitive effects in healthy volunteers (Chamberlain et al. 2007).

Sibutramine

The presynaptic serotonin agonist sibutramine, studied as a single 20-mg dose in healthy adults, has been shown to improve attention, visual processing speed, and motor control (Wesnes et al. 2000). Limited data exist regarding the use of sibutramine for individuals with bipolar disorder, although its potential to counteract psychotropically induced weight gain has been described in preliminary studies (McElroy et al. 2007). Combinations of sibutramine with other serotonergic agents (e.g., SSRIs) are generally avoided in order to minimize the potential for serotonin syndrome.

Herbal, Hormonal, Nutritional, and Vitamin Remedies

Ginkgo Biloba

Although the potential mechanism of the leaf extract ginkgo biloba on central nervous system function is unknown, anecdotal reports initially described subjective improvement in memory and attention in healthy control subjects taking from 60 to 120 mg/day. However, double-blind controlled trials have yielded either negative findings compared with placebo (Burns et al. 2006) or transient (≤6 weeks) benefit in sustained attention and pattern recognition memory, without benefit in working memory, planning, or mental flexibility (Elsabagh et al. 2005). No adverse cognitive, behavioral, or emotional effects have been reported in mood disorder patients taking ginkgo biloba, although efficacy for cognitive complaints appears modest and inconsistent.

Omega-3 Fatty Acids

Omega-3 fatty acids (i.e., eicosapentaenoic acid [EPA]) have garnered interest in recent years based on preliminary (Stoll et al. 1999) though nonreplicated (Keck et al. 2006) suggestions of preventing or improving affective symptoms of bipolar disorder. Further theoretical interest stems from the potential of EPA to stabilize neuronal phospholipid membranes. Randomized studies of supplemental EPA (3 g/day) added to existing antipsychotic medications in schizophrenia patients with cognitive symptoms have yielded negative findings (Fenton et al. 2001). Despite the neurodevelopmental importance of such long-chain polyunsaturated fatty acids during embryogenesis, and the adverse effects of perinatal dietary deficiencies of EPA and docosahexaenoic acid (DHA) relative to normal neural development, supplemental EPA or DHA is not presently established as an evidence-based intervention for cognitive deficits in populations with psychiatric illness.

Estrogen

There is an extensive literature examining the extent to which estrogen replacement therapy may help to reduce the potential for cognitive decline associated with aging in postmenopausal women, likely by promoting neuronal sprouting in the hippocampus. In nondepressed postmenopausal women, estrogen has shown superiority to placebo for improving verbal and spatial working memory and errors of perseveration during verbal recall (Joffe et al. 2006), particularly when introduced early rather than late after menopause (MacLennan et al. 2006). However, controlled trials have yielded both negative and positive findings on the effects of estrogen with respect to both cognition and mood (Almeida et al. 2006; Rapp et al. 2003). There are presently no controlled or systematic studies of estrogen therapy to counteract cognitive complaints among individuals with bipolar disorder, and its use remains controversial in light of its observed potential to increase susceptibility to breast cancer (Chlebowski et al. 2003).

Vitamin E

Administration of vitamin E, which has antioxidant effects, has been suggested as a possible neuroprotective strategy to diminish neurocognitive impairment among older adults. One large, double-blind, multisite trial in adults with mild cognitive impairment above age 54 found better executive, language, and overall neurocognitive function over 18 months with vitamin E dosed daily at 2,000 IU, although there was no difference from adults administered placebo in the progression to frank Alzheimer's disease over 3 years (Peterson et al. 2005). Another study of healthy women above age 65 found no significant differences from placebo with 600 IU of vitamin E on alternate days (Kang et al. 2006). The potential utility and safety of supplemental vitamin E for cognitive deficits in nonelderly or nondementia patients with mood disorders have not received systematic study.

Taurine

The essential amino acid taurine has been regarded by some advocates as possessing cognitive-enhancement properties. Preliminary studies using commercially available preparations of taurine—often as a component ingredient of caffeinated beverages—suggest some degree of enhanced attention, verbal reasoning, reaction time, and overall well-being in healthy control subjects, without obvious adverse effects (Seidl et al. 2000; Warburton et al. 2001).

Conclusions

No single agent or class of psychotropic compounds has yet demonstrated substantial benefit for either enhancing cognitive function or reversing cognitive deficits in bipolar disorder. Existing treatments vary in the degrees to which they may exert at least modest (if not robust) cognitive efficacy. Concepts related to neuroprotection are of at least theoretical pharmacological importance, insofar as recurrent episodes in bipolar disorder may involve neurotoxic events that could be manifested by impaired cognitive function. Compared with clinical trials in schizophrenia, there has been remarkably little study of either beneficial or adverse cognitive effects of psychotropic agents specifically in patients with bipolar disorder. There is a compelling need for further investigation.

Take-Home Points

- Neurotrophic and neuroprotective effects have been demonstrated with lithium, divalproex, and some atypical antipsychotics, and may occur with other mood-stabilizing agents as a means to promote neuronal viability and counter possible neurodegenerative processes.

- Lamotrigine may enhance cortical function and can improve global cognitive function independent of mood benefits during treatment for bipolar depression.

- Atypical antipsychotics may help to improve attention by increasing prefrontal dopaminergic transmission, and may also have procholinergic effects (e.g., as occurs with olanzapine).

- Atypical antipsychotics have been associated with modest but significant improvement in overall cognitive function in patients with schizophrenia. Less is known about their potential cognitive benefits
specifically in patients with bipolar disorder, although controlled data
suggest that risperidone may improve executive function.

- An emerging literature supports the safety and efficacy of procholinergic agents to counteract at least some cognitive problems in patients
with bipolar disorder.

- Psychostimulants such as methylphenidate, modafinil, and amphetamine or mixed amphetamine salts may be of value when added to
mood-stabilizing agents for some patients with bipolar disorder as a
means to counteract problems with attention or subsidiary cognitive
functions. Clinicians must monitor potential risks for abuse potential or
mood destabilization.

- For cognitive enhancement in patients with bipolar disorder, there exist limited data supporting the use of currently available novel pharmacological strategies, including dopamine agonists (e.g., pramipexole),
antiglutamatergic agents (e.g., mementine), buspirone, and sibutramine. Systematic studies regarding the use of herbal, hormonal, nutri-
tional, or vitamin therapies to treat cognitive complaints have yielded
largely negative or, at best, inconsistent findings.

References

Almeida OP, Lautenschlager NT, Vasikaran S, et al: A 20-week randomized controlled trial of estradiol replacement therapy for women aged 70 years and older:
effect on mood, cognition and quality of life. Neurobiol Aging 27:141–149,
2006

Atmaca M, Ozdemir H, Cetinkaya S, et al: Cingulate gyrus volumetry in drug free
bipolar patients and patients treated with valproate or valproate and quetiapine.
J Psychiatr Res 41:821–827, 2007a

Atmaca M, Yildirim H, Ozdemir H, et al: Hippocampal ^{1}H MRS in patients with
bipolar disorder taking valproate versus valproate plus quetiapine. Psychol Med
37:121–129, 2007b

Ballard TM, Woolley ML, Prinssen E, et al: The effect of the mGlu5 receptor antagonist MPEP in rodent tests of anxiety and cognition: a comparison. Psychopharmacology (Berl) 179:218–229, 2005

Bangs ME, Emslie GJ, Spencer TJ, et al: Efficacy and safety of atomoxetine in adolescents with attention deficit/hyperactivity disorder and major depression.
J Child Adolesc Psychopharmacol 17:407–420, 2007

Barch DM, Carter CS: Amphetamine improves cognitive function in medicated individuals with schizophrenia and in healthy volunteers. Schizophr Res 77:43–58,
2005

Barr RS, Culhane JA, Jubelt LE, et al: The effects of transdermal nicotine on cognition in nonsmokers with schizophrenia and nonpsychiatric controls. Neuropsychopharmacology 33:480–490, 2008

Bearden CE, Thompson PM, Dalwani M, et al: Greater cortical gray matter density in lithium-treated patients with bipolar disorder. Biol Psychiatry 62:7–16, 2007

Bearden CE, Thompson PM, Dutton RA, et al: Three-dimensional mapping of hippocampal anatomy in unmedicated and lithium-treated patients with bipolar disorder. Neuropsychopharmacology (in press)

Benes FM, Vincent SL, Todtenkopf M: The density of pyramidal and nonpyramidal neurons in anterior cingulate cortex of schizophrenic and bipolar subjects. Biol Psychiatry 50:395–406, 2001

Bertolino A, Frye M, Callicott JH, et al: Neuronal pathology in the hippocampal area of patients with bipolar disorder: a study with proton magnetic resonance spectroscopic imaging. Biol Psychiatry 53:906–913, 2003

Bezchlibnyk YB, Sun X, Wang JF, et al: Neuron somal size is decreased in the lateral amygdalar nucleus of subjects with bipolar disorder. J Psychiatry Neurosci 32:203–210, 2007

Bilder RM, Goldman RS, Volavka J, et al: Neurocognitive effects of clozapine, olanzapine, risperidone, and haloperidol in patients with chronic schizophrenia or schizoaffective disorder. Am J Psychiatry 159:1018–1028, 2002a

Bilder RM, Volavka J, Czobor P, et al: Neurocognitive correlates of the COMT Val(158)Met polymorphism in chronic schizophrenia. Biol Psychiatry 52:701–707, 2002b

Bora E, Veznedaroqlu B, Kayahan B: The effect of galantamine added to clozapine on cognition in five patients with schizophrenia. Clin Neuropharmacol 28:139–141, 2005

Bouras C, Kovari E, Hof PR, et al: Anterior cingulate cortex pathology in schizophrenia and bipolar disorder. Acta Neuropathol (Berl) 102:373–379, 2001

Bown CD, Wang JF, Young LT: Attenuation of N-methyl-D-aspartate-mediated cytoplasmic vacuolization in primary rat hippocampal neurons by mood stabilizers. Neuroscience 117:949–955, 2003

Brauch RA, Adnan El-Masri M, Parker JC, et al: Glial cell number and neuron/glial cell ratios in postmortem brains of bipolar individuals. J Affect Disord 91:87–90, 2006

Buchanan RW, Holstein C, Breier A: The comparative efficacy and long-term effect of clozapine treatment on neuropsychological test performance. Biol Psychiatry 36:717–725, 1994

Buchanan RW, Javitt DC, Marder SR, et al: The Cognitive and Negative Symptoms in Schizophrenia Trial (CONSIST): the efficacy of glutamatergic agents for negative symptoms and cognitive impairment. Am J Psychiatry 164:1593–1602, 2007

Buchanan RW, Conley RR, Dickinson D, et al: Galantamine for the treatment of cognitive impairments in people with schizophrenia. Am J Psychiatry 165:82–89, 2008

Burdick KE, Braga RJ, Goldberg JF, et al: Cognitive dysfunction in bipolar disorder: future place of pharmacotherapy. CNS Drugs 21:971–981, 2007a

Burdick KE, Funke B, Goldberg JF, et al: COMT genotype increases risk for bipolar I disorder and influences neurocognitive performance. Bipolar Disord 9:370–376, 2007b

Burns NR, Bryan J, Nettelbeck T: Ginkgo biloba: no robust effect on cognitive abilities or mood in healthy young or older adults. Hum Psychopharmacol 21:27–37, 2006

Burt T, Sachs GS, Demopulos C: Donepezil in treatment-resistant bipolar disorder. Biol Psychiatry 45:959–964, 1999

Cadet JL, Krasnova IN, Jayanthi S, et al: Neurotoxicity of substituted amphetamines: molecular and cellular mechanisms. Neurotox Res 11:183–202, 2007

Cardile V, Pavone A, Gulino R, et al: Expression of brain-derived neurotropic factor (BDNF) and inducible nitric oxide synthase (iNOS) in rat astrocyte cultures treated with levetiracetam. Brain Res 976:227–233, 2003

Carlson PJ, Merlock MC, Suppes T: Adjunctive stimulant use in patients with bipolar disorder: treatment of residual depression and sedation. Bipolar Disord 6:416–420, 2004

Cecil KM, DelBello MP, Morey R, et al: Frontal lobe differences in bipolar disorder as determined by proton MR spectroscopy. Bipolar Disord 4:357–365, 2002

Chalecka-Franaszek E, Chuang DM: Lithium activates the serine/threonine kinase Akt-1 and suppresses glutamate-induced inhibition of Akt-1 activity in neurons. Proc Natl Acad Sci USA 96:8745–8750, 1999

Chamberlain SR, Müller U, Deakin JB, et al: Lack of deleterious effects of buspirone on cognition in healthy male volunteers. J Psychopharmacol 21:210–215, 2007

Chana G, Landau S, Beasley C, et al: Two-dimensional assessment of cytoarchitecture in the anterior cingulate cortex in major depressive disorder, bipolar disorder, and schizophrenia: evidence for decreased neuronal somal size and increased neuronal density. Biol Psychiatry 53:1086–1098, 2003

Chen B, Dowlatshahi D, MacQueen GM, et al: Increased hippocampal BDNF immunoreactivity in subjects treated with antidepressant medication. Biol Psychiatry 50:260–265, 2001

Chen G, Huang LD, Jiang YM, et al: The mood-stabilizing agent valproate inhibits the activity of glycogen synthase kinase-3. J Neurochem 72:1327–1330, 1999a

Chen G, Zeng WZ, Yuan PX, et al: The mood-stabilizing agents lithium and valproate robustly increase the levels of the neuroprotective protein bcl-2 in the CNS. J Neurochem 72:879–882, 1999b

Chen G, Rajkowska G, Du F, et al: Enhancement of hippocampal neurogenesis by lithium. J Neurochem 75:1729–1734, 2000

Chen PS, Peng GS, Li G, et al: Valproate protects dopaminergic neurons in midbrain neuron/glia cultures by stimulating the release of neurotrophic factors from astrocytes. Mol Psychiatry 11:1116–1125, 2006

Chlebowski RT, Hendrix SL, Langer RD, et al: Influence of estrogen plus progestin on breast cancer and mammography in healthy postmenopausal women. The Women's Health Initiative Randomized Trial. JAMA 289:3243–3253, 2003

Cotter D, Hudson L, Landau S: Evidence for orbitofrontal pathology in bipolar disorder and major depression, but not in schizophrenia. Bipolar Disord 7:358–369, 2005

Cuesta MJ, Peralta V, Zarzuela A: Effects of olanzapine and other atypical antipsychotics on cognitive function in chronic schizophrenia: a longitudinal study. Schizophr Res 48:17–28, 2001

Deicken RF, Pegues MP, Anzalone S, et al: Lower concentration of hippocampal N-acetylaspartate in familial bipolar I disorder. Am J Psychiatry 160:873–882, 2003

DelBello MP, Zimmerman ME, Mills NP, et al: Magnetic resonance imaging analysis of amygdala and other subcortical brain regions in adolescents with bipolar disorder. Bipolar Disord 6:43–52, 2004

DelBello MP, Cecil KM, Adler CM, et al: Neurochemical effects of olanzapine in first-hospitalization manic adolescents: a proton magnetic resonance spectroscopy study. Neuropsychopharmacology 31:1264–1273, 2006

Dowlatshahi D, MacQueen GM, Wang JF, et al: Increased temporal cortex CREB concentrations and antidepressant treatment in major depression. Lancet 352:1754–1755, 1998

Eden Evins A, Demopulos C, Nierenberg A, et al: A double-blind, placebo-controlled trial of adjunctive donepezil in treatment-resistant mania. Bipolar Disord 8:75–80, 2006

Ellis JR, Ellis KA, Bartholomeusz CF, et al: Muscarinic and nicotinic receptors synergistically modulate working memory and attention in humans. Int J Neuropsychopharmacol 9:175–189, 2006

Elsabagh S, Hartley DE, Ali O, et al: Differential cognitive effects of ginkgo biloba after acute and chronic treatment in healthy young volunteers. Psychopharmacology (Berl) 179:437–446, 2005

Ersche KD, Clark L, London M, et al: Profile of executive and memory function associated with amphetamine and opiate dependence. Neuropsychopharmacology 31:1036–1047, 2006

Fenton WS, Dickerson F, Boronow J, et al: A placebo-controlled trial of omega-3 fatty acid (ethyl eicosapentaenoic acid) supplementation for residual symptoms and cognitive impairment in schizophrenia. Am J Psychiatry 158:2071–2074, 2001

Findling RL, Greenhill LL, McNamara NK, et al: Venlafaxine in the treatment of children and adolescents with attention-deficit/hyperactivity disorder. J Child Adolesc Psychopharmacol 17:433–446, 2007

Flicker L, Grimley Evans G: Piracetam for dementia or cognitive impairment. Cochrane Database of Systematic Reviews, Issue 2, Article No: CD001011. DOI:10.1002/14651858.CD001011, 2004

Frey BN, Andreazza AB, Ceresér KM, et al: Effects of mood stabilizers on hippocampus BDNF levels in an animal model of mania. Life Sci 79:281–286, 2006

Friedman SD, Dager SR, Parow A, et al: Lithium and valproic acid treatment effects on brain chemistry in bipolar disorder. Biol Psychiatry 56:340–348, 2004

Frye MA, Grunze H, Suppes T, et al: A placebo-controlled evaluation of adjunctive modafinil in the treatment of bipolar depression. Am J Psychiatry 164:1242–1249, 2007

Fukumoto T, Morinobu S, Okamoto Y, et al: Chronic lithium treatment increases the expression of brain-derived neurotrophic factor in the rat brain. Psychopharmacology (Berl) 158:100–106, 2001

Galletly CA, Clark CR, McFarlane AC, et al: The effect of clozapine on speed and accuracy of information processing in schizophrenia. Prog Neuropsychopharmacol Biol Psychiatry 24:1329–1338, 2000

Goff DC, Lamberti JS, Leon AC, et al: A placebo-controlled add-on trial of the ampakine, CX516, for cognitive deficits in schizophrenia. Neuropsychopharmacology 33:465–472, 2008

Goldberg JF, Burdick KE, Endick CJ: Preliminary, randomized, double-blind, pla-cebo-controlled trial of pramipexole added to mood stabilizers for treatment-resistant bipolar depression. Am J Psychiatry 161:564–566, 2004

Grön G, Kirstein M, Thielscher A, et al: Cholinergic enhancement of episodic memory in healthy young adults. Psychopharmacology (Berl) 182:170–179, 2005

Gualtieri CT, Johnson LG: Comparative neurocognitive effects of 5 psychotropic anticonvulsants and lithium. MedGenMed 8:46, 2006

Hagger C, Buckley P, Kenny JT, et al: Improvement in cognitive functions and psy-chiatric symptoms in treatment-refractory schizophrenia patients receiving clozapine. Biol Psychiatry 34:702–712, 1993

Hah M, Chang K: Atomoxetine for the treatment of attention deficit/hyperactivity disorder in children and adolescents with bipolar disorders. J Child Adolesc Psychopharmacol 15:996–1004, 2005

Haldane M, Jogia J, Cobb A, et al: Changes in brain activation during working memory and facial recognition tasks in patients with bipolar disorder with la-motrigine monotherapy. Eur Neuropsychopharmacol 18:48–54, 2008

Hamberger MJ, Palmese CA, Scarmeas N, et al: A randomized, double-blind, pla-cebo-controlled trial of donepezil to improve memory in epilepsy. Epilepsia 48:1283–1291, 2007

Hara K, Sata T: Inhibitory effect of gabapentin on N-methyl-D-aspartate receptors expressed in *Xenopus* oocytes. Acta Anaesthesiol Scand 51:122–128, 2007

Harvey PD, Keefe RS: Studies of cognitive change in patients with schizophrenia following novel antipsychotic treatment. Am J Psychiatry 158:176–184, 2001

Harvey PD, Siu CO, Romano S: Randomized, controlled, double-blind, multi-center comparison of the cognitive effects of ziprasidone versus olanzapine in acutely ill inpatients with schizophrenia or schizoaffective disorder. Psycho-pharmacology (Berl) 172:324–332, 2004

Harvey PD, Bowie CR, Loebel A: Neuropsychological normalization with long-term atypical antipsychotic treatment: results of a six-month randomized, dou-ble-blind comparison of ziprasidone vs. olanzapine. J Neuropsychiatry Clin Neurosci 18:54–63, 2006

Haznedar MM, Roversi F, Pallanti S, et al: Fronto-thalamo-striatal gray and white matter volumes and anisotropy of their connections in bipolar spectrum ill-nesses. Biol Psychiatry 57:733–742, 2005

Henderson TA: Mania induction associated with atomoxetine. J Clin Psychophar-macol 24:567–568, 2004

Heresco-Levy U, Javitt DC, Ebstein R, et al: D-serine efficacy as add-on pharma-cotherapy to risperidone and olanzapine for treatment-refractory schizophre-nia. Biol Psychiatry 57:577–585, 2005

Hewett SJ, Silakova JM, Hewett JA: Oral treatment with rofecoxib reduces hippo-campal excitotoxic neurodegeneration. J Pharmacol Exp Ther 319:1219–1224, 2006

Hough CJ, Irwin RP, Gao XM, et al: Carbamazepine inhibition of N-methyl-D-as-partate-evoked calcium influx in rat cerebellar granule cells. J Pharmacol Exp Ther 276:143–149, 1996

Huang YY, Peng CH, Yang YP, et al: Desipramine activated Bcl-2 expression and inhibited lipopolysaccharide-induced apoptosis in hippocampus-derived adult neural stem cells. J Pharmacol Sci 104:61–72, 2007

Hunter HD, Ganesan V, Wilkinson ID, et al: Impact of modafinil on prefrontal executive function in schizophrenia. Am J Psychiatry 163:2184–2186, 2006

Hwang J, Lyoo IK, Dager SR, et al: Basal ganglia shape alterations in bipolar disorder. Am J Psychiatry 163:276–285, 2006

Joffe H, Hall JE, Gruber S, et al: Estrogen therapy selectively enhances prefrontal cognitive processes: a randomized, double-blind, placebo-controlled study with functional magnetic resonance imaging in perimenopausal and recently postmenopausal women. Menopause 13:411–422, 2006

Johnson DE, Nedza FM, Spracklin DK, et al: The role of muscarinic receptor antagonism in antipsychotic-induced hippocampal acetylcholine release. Eur J Pharmacol 506:209–219, 2005

Kang HJ, Noh JS, Bae YS, et al: Calcium-dependent prevention of neuronal apoptosis by lithium ion: essential role of phosphoinositide 3-kinase and phospholipase Cgamma. Mol Pharmacol 64:228–234, 2003

Kang JH, Cook N, Manson J, et al: A randomized trial of vitamin E supplementation and cognitive function in women. Arch Intern Med 166:2462–2468, 2006

Keck PE Jr, Mintz J, McElroy SL, et al: Double-blind, randomized, placebo-controlled trials of ethyl-eicosapentanoate in the treatment of bipolar depression and rapid cycling bipolar disorder. Biol Psychiatry 60:1020–1022, 2006

Keefe RS, Young CA, Rock SL, et al: One-year double-blind study of the neurocognitive efficacy of olanzapine, risperidone, and haloperidol in schizophrenia. Schizophr Res 81:1–15, 2006

Keefe RS, Bilder RM, Davis SM, et al: Neurocognitive effects of antipsychotic medications in patients with chronic schizophrenia in the CATIE trials. Arch Gen Psychiatry 64:633–647, 2007a

Keefe RS, Sweeney JA, Gu H, et al: Effects of olanzapine, quetiapine and risperidone on neurocognitive function in early psychosis: a randomized, double-blind, 52-week comparison. Am J Psychiatry 164:1061–1071, 2007b

Keefe RS, Malhotra AK, Meltzer HY, et al: Efficacy and safety of donepezil in patients with schizophrenia or schizoaffective disorder: significant placebo/practice effects in a 12-week, randomized, double-blind, placebo-controlled trial. Neuropsychopharmacology (in press)

Kelly T: Is donepezil useful for improving cognitive dysfunction in bipolar disorder? J Affect Disord 107:237–240, 2008

Kern RS, Green MF, Cornblatt BA, et al: The neurocognitive effects of aripiprazole: an open-label comparison with olanzapine. Psychopharmacology (Berl) 187:312–320, 2006

Khan DA, Ginsberg LD, Asnis GM, et al: Effect of lamotrigine on cognitive complaints in patients with bipolar I disorder. J Clin Psychiatry 65:1483–1490, 2004

Kimberg DY, D'Esposito M: Cognitive effects of the dopamine receptor agonist pergolide. Neuropsychologia 41:1020–1027, 2003

Kimberg DY, D'Esposito M, Farrah MJ: Effects of bromocriptine on human subjects depend on working memory capacity. Neuroreport 8:3581–3585, 1997

Kitano Y, Komiyama C, Makino M, et al: Effects of nefiracetam, a novel pyrrolidone-type nootropic agent, on the amygdala-kindled seizures in rats. Epilepsia 46:1561–1568, 2005

Kodama M, Fujioka T, Duman RS: Chronic olanzapine or fluoxetine administration increases cell proliferation in hippocampus and prefrontal cortex of adult rat. Biol Psychiatry 56:570–580, 2004

Kudin AP, Debska-Vielhaber G, Vielhaber S, et al: The mechanism of neuroprotection by topiramate in an animal model of epilepsy. Epilepsia 45:1478–1487,
2004

Kumari V, Aasen I, Ffytche D, et al: Neural correlates of adjunctive rivastigmine
treatment to antipsychotics in schizophrenia: a randomized, placebo-controlled, double-blind fMRI study. Neuroimage 29:545–556, 2006

Kuroki T, Meltzer HY, Ichikawa J: Effects of antipsychotic drugs on extracellular
dopamine levels in rat medial prefrontal cortex and nucleus accumbens. J Pharmacol Exp Ther 288:774–781, 1999

Kushner MG, Kim SW, Donahue C, et al: D-cycloserine augmented exposure therapy for obsessive-compulsive disorder. Biol Psychiatry 62:835–838, 2007

Lee MA, Thompson PA, Meltzer HY: Effects of clozapine on cognitive function in
schizophrenia. J Clin Psychiatry 55 (suppl B):82–87, 1994

Leverich GS, Altshuler LL, Frye MA, et al: Risk of switch in mood polarity to hypomania or mania in patients with bipolar depression during acute and contin-
uation trials of venlafaxine, sertraline, and bupropion as adjuncts to mood
stabilizers. Am J Psychiatry 163:232–239, 2006

Li X, Ketter TA, Frye MA: Synaptic, intracelluar, and neuroprotective mechanisms
of anticonvulsants: are they relevant for the treatment and course of bipolar disorders? J Affect Disord 69:1–14, 2002

Lindenmayer JP, Khan A, Iskander A, et al: A randomized controlled trial of olanzapine versus haloperidol in the treatment of primary negative symptoms and
neurocognitive deficits in schizophrenia. J Clin Psychiatry 68:368–379, 2007

Liu L, Schulz SC, Lee S, et al: Hippocampal CA1 pyramidal cell size is reduced in
bipolar disorder. Cell Mol Neurobiol 27:351–358, 2007

Lydon E, El-Mallakh RS: Naturalistic long-term use of methylphenidate in bipolar
disorder. J Clin Psychopharmacol 26:516–518, 2006

MacLennan AH, Henderson VW, Paine BJ, et al: Hormone therapy, timing of initiation, and cognition in women aged older than 60 years: the REMEMBER
pilot study. Menopause 13:28–36, 2006

Mai L, Jope RS, Li X: BDNF-mediated signal transduction is modulated by
GSK3beta and mood stabilizing agents. J Neurochem 82:75–83, 2002

Malberg JE, Eisch AJ, Nestler EJ, et al: Chronic antidepressant treatment increases
neurogenesis in adult rat hippocampus. J Neurosci 20:9104–9110, 2000

Manji HK, Moore GJ, Chen G: Lithium up-regulates the cytoprotective protein
Bcl-2 in the CNS in vivo: a role for neurotrophic and neuroprotective effects in
manic depressive illness. J Clin Psychiatry 61 (suppl 9):82–96, 2000

Marangell LB, Johnson CR, Kertz B, et al: Olanzapine in the treatment of apathy in
previously depressed participants maintained with selective serotonin reuptake
inhibitors: an open-label, flexible dose study. J Clin Psychiatry 63:391–395,
2002

McElroy SL, Frye MA, Altshuler LL, et al: A 24-week, randomized, controlled trial
of adjunctive sibutramine versus topiramate in the treatment of weight gain in
overweight or obese patients with bipolar disorders. Bipolar Disord 9:426–434,
2007

McEvoy JP: A double-blind cross-over comparison of antiparkinson drug therapy:
amantadine versus anticholinergics in 90 normal volunteers, with an emphasis
on differential effects on memory function. J Clin Psychiatry 48(suppl):20–23,
1987

McIntosh AM, Job DE, Moorhead TW, et al: White matter density in patients with schizophrenia, bipolar disorder and their unaffected relatives. Biol Psychiatry 58:254–257, 2005

Michelson D, Adler LA, Amsterdam JD, et al: Addition of atomoxetine for depression incompletely responsive to sertraline: a randomized, double-blind, placebo-controlled study. J Clin Psychiatry 68:582–587, 2007

Moghaddam B: Targeting metabotropic glutamate receptors for treatment of the cognitive symptoms of schizophrenia. Psychopharmacology (Berl) 174:39–44, 2004

Moore GJ, Bebchuk JM, Wilds IB, et al: Lithium-induced increase in human brain grey matter. Lancet 356:1241–1242, 2000

Müller N, Riedel M, Schwarz MJ, et al: Clinical effects of COX-2 inhibitors on cognition in schizophrenia. Eur Arch Psychiatry Clin Neurosci 255:149–151, 2005

Nibuya M, Morinobu S, Duman RS: Regulation of BDNF and trkB mRNA in rat brain by chronic electroconvulsive seizure and antidepressant drug treatments. J Neurosci 15:7539–7547, 1995

Nibuya M, Nestler EJ, Duman RS: Chronic antidepressant administration increases the expression of cAMP response element binding protein (CREB) in rat hippocampus. J Neurosci 16:2365–2372, 1996

Nonaka S, Hough CJ, Chuang DM: Chronic lithium treatment robustly protects neurons in the central nervous system against excitotoxicity by inhibiting *N*-methyl-D-aspartate receptor-mediated calcium influx. Proc Natl Acad Sci USA 95:2642–2647, 1998

Olincy A, Harris JG, Johnson LL, et al: Proof-of-concept trial of an alpha7 nicotinic agonist in schizophrenia. Arch Gen Psychiatry 63:630–638, 2006

Ongur D, Drevets WC, Price JL: Glial reduction in the subgenual prefrontal cortex in mood disorders. Proc Natl Acad Sci USA 95:13290–13295, 1998

Ornstein TJ, Iddon JL, Baldacchino AM, et al: Profiles of cognitive dysfunction in chronic amphetamine and heroin abusers. Neuropsychopharmacology 23:113–126, 2000

Peng CH, Chiou SH, Chen SJ, et al: Neuroprotection by imipramine against lipopolysaccharide-induced apoptosis in hippocampus-derived neural stem cells mediated by activation of BDNF and the MAPK pathway. Eur Neuropsychopharmacol 18:128–140, 2008

Peterson RC, Thomas RG, Grundman M, et al: Vitamin E and donepezil for the treatment of mild cognitive impairment. N Engl J Med 352:2379–2388, 2005

Piazzini A, Chifari R, Canevini MP, et al: Levetiracetam: an improvement of attention and of oral fluency in patients with partial epilepsy. Epilepsy Res 68:181–188, 2006

Post RM, Altshuler LL, Frye MA, et al: Preliminary observations on the effectiveness of levetiracetam in the open adjunctive treatment of refractory bipolar disorder. J Clin Psychiatry 66:370–374, 2005

Purdon SE, Jones BD, Stip ED, et al; for the Canadian Collaborative Group for Research in Schizophrenia: Neuropsychological change in early phase schizophrenia during 12 months of treatment with olanzapine, risperidone, or haloperidol. Arch Gen Psychiatry 57:249–258, 2000

Rajkowska G, Halaris A, Selemon LD: Reductions in neuronal and glial density characterize the dorsolateral prefrontal cortex in bipolar disorder. Biol Psychiatry 49:741–752, 2001

Randall DC, Shneerson JM, Plaha KK, et al: Modafinil affects mood, but not cognitive function, in healthy young volunteers. Hum Psychopharmacol 18:163–173, 2003

Randall DC, Fleck NL, Shneerson JM, et al: The cognitive-enhancing properties of modafinil are limited in non-sleep-deprived middle-aged volunteers. Pharmacol Biochem Behav 77:547–555, 2004

Randall DC, Viswanath A, Bharania P, et al: Does modafinil enhance cognitive performance in young volunteers who are not sleep deprived? J Clin Psychopharmacol 25:175–179, 2005

Rapp SR, Espeland MA, Shumaker SA, et al: Effect of estrogen plus progestin on global cognitive function in postmenopausal women: the Women's Health Initiative Memory Study: a randomized controlled trial. JAMA 289:2663–2672, 2003

Reinares M, Martinez-Aran A, Colom F, et al: Long-term effects of the treatment with risperidone versus conventional neuroleptics on the neuropsychological performance of euthymic bipolar patients [in Spanish]. Actas Esp Psiquiatr 28:231–238, 2000

Riedel M, Spellmann I, Strassnig M, et al: Effects of risperidone and quetiapine on cognition in patients with schizophrenia and predominantly negative symptoms. Eur Arch Psychiatry Clin Neurosci 257:360–370, 2007

Riedel M, Müller N, Spellmann I, et al: Efficacy of olanzapine versus quetiapine on cognitive dysfunctions in patients with an acute episode of schizophrenia. Eur Arch Psychiatry Clin Neurosci (in press)

Roegge CS, Perraut C, Hao X, et al: Histamine 1 receptor involvement in prepulse inhibition and memory function: relevance for the antipsychotic actions of clozapine. Pharmacol Biochem Behav 86:686–692, 2007

Roth BL, Hanizavareh SM, Blum AE: Serotonin receptors represent highly favorable molecular targets for cognitive enhancement in schizophrenia and other disorders. Psychopharmacology (Berl) 174:17–24, 2004

Sachs GS, Nierenberg AA, Calabrese JR, et al: Effectiveness of adjunctive antidepressant treatment for bipolar depression. N Engl J Med 356:1711–1722, 2007

Sassi RB, Brambilla P, Hatch JP, et al: Reduced left anterior cingulate volumes in untreated bipolar patients. Biol Psychiatry 56:467–475, 2004

Scheffer RE, Kowatch RA, Carmody T, et al: Randomized, placebo-controlled trial of mixed amphetamine salts for symptoms of comorbid ADHD in pediatric bipolar disorder after mood stabilization with divalproex sodium. Am J Psychiatry 162:58–64, 2005

Schneider U, Wohlfarth K, Schulze-Bonhage A, et al: Effects of acamprosate on memory in healthy young subjects. J Stud Alcohol 60:172–175, 1999

Schrauwen E, Ghaemi SN: Galantamine treatment of cognitive impairment in bipolar disorder: four cases. Bipolar Disord 8:196–199, 2006

Seidl R, Peryl A, Nicham R, et al: A taurine and caffeine containing drink stimulates cognitive performance and well-being. Amino Acids 19:635–642, 2000

Sevy S, Rosenthal MH, Alvir J, et al: Double-blind, placebo-controlled study of modafinil for fatigue and cognition in schizophrenia patients treated with psychotropic medications. J Clin Psychiatry 66:839–843, 2005

Sfaello I, Baud O, Arzimanoglou A, et al: Topiramate prevents excitotoxic damage in the newborn rodent brain. Neurobiol Dis 20:837–848, 2005

Shao L, Young LT, Wang JF: Chronic treatment with mood stabilizers lithium and valproate prevents excitotoxicity by inhibiting oxidative stress in rat cerebral cortical cells. Biol Psychiatry 58:879–884, 2005

Sharma T, Reed C, Aasen I, et al: Cognitive effects of adjunctive 24-weeks rivastigmine treatment to antipsychotics in schizophrenia: a randomized, placebo-controlled, double-blind investigation. Schizophr Res 85:73–83, 2006

Sharma V, Menon R, Carr TJ, et al: An MRI study of subgenual prefrontal cortex in patients with familial and non-familial bipolar I disorder. J Affect Disord 77:167–171, 2003

Sheline YI, Gado MH, Kraemer HC: Untreated depression and hippocampal volume loss. Am J Psychiatry 160:1516–1518, 2003

Shorvon S: Pyrrolidone derivatives. Lancet 358:1885–1892, 2001

Sills GJ: The mechanisms of action of gabapentin and pregabalin. Curr Opin Pharmacol 6:108–113, 2006

Spence SA, Green RD, Wilkinson ID, et al: Modafinil modulates anterior cingulate function in chronic schizophrenia. Br J Psychiatry 187:55–61, 2005

Spencer T, Biederman J, Coffey B, et al: A double-blind comparison of desipramine and placebo in children and adolescents with chronic tic disorder and comorbid attention-deficit/hyperactivity disorder. Arch Gen Psychiatry 59:649–656, 2002

Stoll AL, Locke CA, Vuckovic A, et al: Lithium-associated cognitive and functional deficits reduced by a switch to divalproex sodium: a case series. J Clin Psychiatry 57:356–359, 1996

Stoll AL, Severus WE, Freeman MP, et al: Omega 3 fatty acids in bipolar disorder: a preliminary double-blind, placebo-controlled trial. Arch Gen Psychiatry 56:407–412, 1999

Sumiyoshi T, Matsui M, Nohara S, et al: Enhancement of cognitive performance in schizophrenia by addition of tandospirone to neuroleptic treatment. Am J Psychiatry 158:1722–1725, 2001

Sumiyoshi T, Park S, Jayathilake K, et al: Effect of buspirone, a serotonin (1A) partial agonist, on cognitive function in schizophrenia: a randomized, double-blind, placebo-controlled study. Schizophr Res 95:158–168, 2007

Szatmari SZ, Whitehouse PJ: Vinpocetine for cognitive impairment and dementia. Cochrane Database of Systematic Reviews, Issue 1, Aricle No:CD003119. DOI: 10.1002/14651858.CD003119, 2003

Teng CT, Demetrio FN: Memantine may acutely improve cognition and have a mood stabilizing effect in treatment-resistant bipolar disorder. Rev Bras Psiquiatr 28:252–254, 2006

Thal LJ, Ferris SH, Kirby L, et al: A randomized, double-blind study of rofecoxib in patients with mild cognitive impairment. Neuropsychopharmacology 30:1204–1215, 2005

Trofimov SS, Voronina TA, Guzevatykh LS: Early postnatal effects of noopept and piracetam on declarative and procedural memory of adult male and female rats. Bull Exp Biol Med 139:683–687, 2005

Tsai G, Yang P, Chung LC, et al: D-serine added to antipsychotics for the treatment of schizophrenia. Biol Psychiatry 44:1081–1089, 1998

Turner DC, Clark L, Dowson J, et al: Modafinil improves cognition and response inhibition in adult attention-deficit/hyperactivity disorder. Biol Psychiatry 55:1031–1040, 2004a

Turner DC, Clark L, Pomarol-Clotet E, et al: Modafinil improves cognition and attentional set shifting in patients with chronic schizophrenia. Neuropsychopharmacology 29:1363–1373, 2004b

Uranova NA, Vostrikov VM, Orlovskaya DD, et al: Oligodendroglial density in the prefrontal cortex in schizophrenia and mood disorders: a study from the Stanley Neuropathology Consortium. Schizophr Res 67:269–275, 2004

Vythilingam M, Vermetten E, Anderson GM, et al: Hippocampal volume, memory, and cortisol status in major depressive disorder: effects of treatment. Biol Psychiatry 56:101–112, 2004

Wang H, Gao J, Lassiter TF, et al: Levetiracetam is neuroprotective in murine models of closed head injury and subarachnoid hemorrhage. Neurocrit Care 5:71–78, 2006

Warburton DM, Bersellini E, Sweeney E: An evaluation of a caffeinated taurine drink on mood, memory and information processing in healthy volunteers without caffeine abstinence. Psychopharmacology (Berl) 158:322–328, 2001

Wesnes KA, Garratt C, Wickens M, et al: Effects of sibutramine alone and with alcohol on cognitive function in healthy volunteers. Br J Clin Pharmacol 49:110–117, 2000

Wheeler SD: Donepezil treatment of topiramate-related cognitive dysfunction. Headache 46:332–335, 2006

Wilens TE, Biederman J, Prince J, et al: Six-week, double-blind, placebo-controlled study of desipramine for adult attention deficit hyperactivity disorder. Am J Psychiatry 153:1147–1153, 1996

Woodward ND, Jayathilake K, Meltzer HY: COMT val108/158met genotype, cognitive function, and cognitive improvement with clozapine in schizophrenia. Schizophr Res 90:86–96, 2007

Yang Y, Li Q, Wang CX, et al: Dose-dependent neuroprotection with tiagabine in a focal cerebral ischemia model in rat. Neuroreport 11:2307–2311, 2000

Young JW, Crawford N, Kelly JS, et al: Impaired attention is central to the cognitive deficits observed in alpha 7 deficient mice. Eur Neuropsychopharmacol 17:145–155, 2007

Yucel K, Taylor VH, McKinnon MC, et al: Bilateral hippocampal volume increase in patients with bipolar disorder and short-term lithium treatment. Neuropsychopharmacology 33:361–367, 2008

Zarate CA, Payne JL, Singh J, et al: Pramipexole for bipolar II depression: a placebo-controlled proof of concept study. Biol Psychiatry 56:54–60, 2004

Zarate CA, Singh JB, Quiroz JA, et al: A double-blind, placebo-controlled study of memantine in the treatment of major depression. Am J Psychiatry 163:153–155, 2006

Zhao J, He X, Liu Z, et al: The effects of clozapine on cognitive function and regional cerebral blood flow in the negative symptom profile schizophrenia. Int J Psychiatry Med 36:171–181, 2006

9

Cognitive Dysfunction in Children and Adolescents With Bipolar Disorder

Relative Contributions of Bipolar Disorder and Attention-Deficit/Hyperactivity Disorder

Paula K. Shear, Ph.D.
Melissa P. DelBello, M.D.

Despite historical controversy about the diagnostic specificity of childhood and adolescent bipolar disorder, there is strong evidence that this disorder affects children and adolescents with a prevalence rate similar to that found in adults (Lewinsohn et al. 1995) and that affected individuals demonstrate diagnostic stability over time (Geller et al. 2000). A sizable literature documents that in addition to their hallmark mood dysregulation, adults with bipolar disorder often demonstrate cognitive deficits that span a broad variety of functional domains (for reviews, see Bearden et al. 2001; Quraishi and Frangou 2002; and Chapters 1–5 of this book). Much less attention, however, has been paid to possible cognitive dysfunction in youth with bipolar disorder.

The presence of cognitive deficits is of important functional and perhaps prognostic significance in youth with bipolar disorder. Neuropsychological deficits are known to affect academic and vocational success (Lezak 1995), and early disruptions in classroom learning due to cognitive deficiencies may have long-term implications for future development. In addition, work in a variety of adult neuropsychiatric populations has demonstrated that cognitive deficits are important predictors of functional outcome. For example, in adults with schizophrenia, measures of cognitive abilities are stronger predictors of everyday functioning than are indices of psychiatric symptom severity (Green 1996; Green et al. 2000). Studies have begun to identify similar links between poorer functional outcome and neurocognitive impairment despite euthymia in patients with bipolar disorder (see Chapter 10, "Cognition and Functional Outcome in Bipolar Disorder"). Neuropsychological data inform our understanding of the neurophysiology of bipolar disorder, as deficits in specific cognitive domains are indicative of dysfunction in related neural networks.

In this chapter, we focus on research regarding neuropsychological functioning in youth with bipolar disorder. Because there is a high rate of co-occurring attention-deficit/hyperactivity disorder (ADHD) in youth with bipolar disorder and because co-occurring ADHD may affect the cognitive presentation of these patients, we pay particular attention to the potential differential cognitive effects of these two disorders. Finally, we discuss the functional and treatment implications of the cognitive trends identified in the existing literature. We emphasize at the outset that the existing cognitive data regarding youth with bipolar disorder are extremely limited. This area of study is undergoing rapid growth, and therefore it will be particularly important to integrate the work that is summarized here with future studies as they become available.

Diagnostic Issues

It is clear from the adult neuropsychological literature that certain clinical features of bipolar disorder are associated with differing cognitive presentations. For example, longer disease duration, a higher number of prior mood episodes (Lebowitz et al. 2001; McKay et al. 1995), and current abnormal mood state (Connelly et al. 1982; Fleck et al. 2005; Henry et al. 1973) are each known to negatively impact cognitive ability in adults. Before considering neuropsychological functioning in youth with bipolar disorder, then, it is important to highlight some of the clinical and diagnostic issues that can impact cognitive findings and may differentiate prepubescent and adolescent bipolar disorder from the more widely studied adult-onset disorder.

In terms of phenomenology, early-onset bipolar disorder often presents differently than adult-onset bipolar disorder. Specifically, compared with bipolar adults, bipolar youth more commonly exhibit chronic irritability, rapid cycling, and mixed (co-occurring manic and depressed) mood states, often in the absence of protracted euthymic periods between mood episodes (Findling et al. 2001; Pavuluri et al. 2005; Spencer et al. 2001). Thus, it is possible that reported cognitive findings in adults, which are most commonly derived from studies that recruit participants based on categorical classifications of hallmark mood state, may not translate precisely to the prototypical mood presentation in youth.

Additionally, and most important for the present discussion, compared with bipolar adults, children and adolescents with bipolar disorder more typically present with co-occurring disorders that are known to have direct effects on cognition. ADHD is one of the most common comorbid diagnoses in youth with bipolar disorder, with reported rates of attentional disorders in these patients that range from 30% to 98% (DelBello and Geller 2001; Geller and Luby 1997; Wozniak et al. 1995). This high co-occurrence of early-onset bipolar disorder and ADHD has been reported in several studies from different settings and samples; however, the relationship between these disorders remains unclear (DelBello et al. 2001). It has been proposed that high rates of comorbidity exist because pediatric mania with ADHD is a distinct form of early-onset bipolar disorder, because ADHD is a prodromal form of bipolar disorder, or simply because of misclassification due to the substantial symptom overlap between the two conditions (DelBello et al. 2001).

Because attentional complaints in themselves are nonpathognomonic—and in the case of bipolar mania and ADHD, may by definition appear indistinguishable—distinctions between the comorbidity and the differential diagnosis of ADHD and pediatric mania or hypomania require assessment of additional nonoverlapping symptoms. Geller et al. (1998a) identified five particular symptoms related to childhood or adolescent mania and hypomania that may be especially useful for discriminating mania or hypomania from ADHD: 1) elation, 2) grandiosity, 3) hypersexuality, 4) flight of ideas or racing thoughts, and 5) decreased need for sleep. In clinical experience, the first three of these may be especially important for diagnostic purposes. In addition, features such as psychosis or suicidality may be common in pediatric manifestations of bipolar disorder but are not indicative of ADHD.

Although there is indeed a marked degree of symptom overlap between ADHD and bipolar disorder, there is compelling evidence that this effect alone does not explain the high comorbidity. For example, Milberger et al. (1995) investigated whether ADHD and comorbid bipolar or major depressive disorder represented distinct disorders or were artifacts of diagnostic overlap. These authors reported that even after overlapping diagnostic criteria were accounted for statistically, 79% of the patients with major depressive disorder and 56% of those with bipolar disorder maintained their mood disorder diagnosis. These results are consistent with the findings of other studies in supporting the hypothesis that bipolar youth with ADHD have two distinct disorders (Biederman et al. 1998; Geller et al. 1998b). This diagnostic specificity is due in part to the fact that patients with bipolar disorder often demonstrate cardinal symptoms such as elevated mood, grandiosity, and hypersexuality that tend to be absent in individuals with ADHD alone (Geller et al. 1998a, 1998b). Further evidence of the separate contribution of ADHD comes from a study in which Faraone et al. (2001) assessed familial risk in children with ADHD with and without bipolar disorder and in healthy children; these authors concluded that ADHD with comorbid bipolar disorder is a distinct familial form of ADHD that is related to pediatric bipolar disorder. Thus, it is evident that examinations of cognitive functioning in youth with bipolar disorder must account for the potentially differential or additive effects of attentional disturbance in patients with these comorbid illnesses.

Several studies have demonstrated that ADHD is more common in prepubertal-onset bipolar disorder than in adolescent- or adult-onset bipolar disorder, suggesting that ADHD may be a developmental marker for early-onset bipolar illness. A complementary finding is that patients who have comorbid ADHD have a more severe course to their mood disorder (Nierenberg et al. 2005). Therefore, in addition to any possible additive contributions of the separate conditions of bipolar disorder and ADHD to cognitive functioning in comorbid patients, there is reason to hypothesize that these individuals may also be more vulnerable to cognitive losses because of a generally more severe disease course. A recent comparison of unmedicated children (ages 6–17 years) with ADHD who did or did not have comorbid bipolar disorder revealed strikingly few differences between both groups across multiple cognitive domains, with the notable exception of poorer performance on one measure of processing speed in the dual-diagnosis (bipolar and ADHD) group (Henin et al. 2007). For a comprehensive discussion of the co-occurrence of bipolar disorder and ADHD, the reader is referred to a review by Singh et al. (2006).

To summarize, the phenomenology of bipolar disorder in youth differs from that in adults along clinical dimensions that are known from adult neuropsychological work to be associated with changes in cognition. That is, above and beyond any developmental effects that may contribute to distinct patterns of cognitive performance in youth with bipolar disorder, the symptom presentation itself is likely to contribute to the presence of cognitive dysfunction that differs somewhat from the adult profiles. Furthermore, children and adolescents with bipolar disorder are highly likely to have comorbid ADHD that is not explicable solely on the basis of diagnostic overlap between the two conditions. This attentional disorder is itself typically associated with cognitive deficiencies, as discussed in a later section, "The Contribution of ADHD to Neuropsychological Functioning in Bipolar Disorder." In addition, there is evidence that comorbid bipolar disorder and ADHD may represent a more severe and an earlier-onset illness than bipolar disorder alone and may be most likely to occur together in younger children with bipolar disorder. Taken together, these findings suggest that it may be inaccurate to draw conclusions about neuropsychological functioning in child and adolescent patients by extrapolating from adult studies and also suggest the importance of parsing the relative contributions of bipolar disorder and ADHD to cognitive presentation in affected youth.

Neuropsychological Functioning

We begin with a general overview of cognitive findings in children and adolescents with bipolar disorder, to lay the foundation for a discussion of the small number of studies that have specifically addressed comorbidity between bipolar disorder and ADHD. Unless told otherwise, the reader should assume that the results being described compare patients with bipolar I disorder to psychiatrically healthy participants.

In terms of general intellectual functioning in youth with bipolar disorder, several investigators have found mild but statistically significant reductions in overall intelligence quotient (IQ) relative to psychiatrically healthy individuals (Doyle et al. 2005; Olvera et al. 2005), although this finding has not been universal (Robertson et al. 2003). Despite these statistically significant group findings, most reported mean IQs for bipolar patients are still within the average to low-average range of functioning relative to the general population; however, it must be emphasized that most neuropsychological studies exclude patients with low IQs, and thus the samples are not representative of the full distribution of individuals with bipolar disorder.

To illustrate an alternative approach, in a study of consecutive admissions to inpatient and day hospital programs in which there were not exclusions related to intellectual functioning, acutely ill children and adolescents with bipolar disorder at entry into the treatment programs had a mean Full Scale IQ of 75, a score that falls into the range of borderline intellectual functioning, and their Performance IQ scores were significantly impaired relative to a mixed group of patients with psychotic disorders, ADHD, conduct disorder, and oppositional defiant disorder (McCarthy et al. 2004). It is clear, therefore, that a subgroup of patients with bipolar disorder has more pronounced intellectual deficits. Future work will need to 1) clarify the effect of illness severity and chronicity on intelligence test performance, 2) examine whether the proportion of children and adolescents with bipolar disorder who have reduced intellectual functioning exceeds base rates in the general population, and 3) study potential medication effects.

In regard to specific cognitive domains, deficits in adults have been found to be most prominent in the areas of attention, working memory, verbal learning and memory, and executive functioning (Bearden et al. 2001; Quraishi and Frangou 2002). Because pediatric studies have tended to follow the adult literature, these are the cognitive domains that have been the focus of existing studies in youth as well.

As noted in Chapter 1, "Overview and Introduction: Dimensions of Cognition and Measures of Cognitive Function," cognitive abilities are to a certain degree hierarchical, in that impairment in a fundamental skill can lead to poor performance on tests that purport to measure a higher-level ability. To give an example from outside the bipolar disorder literature, it is challenging to assess verbal learning in individuals who have deficits in fundamental language production or comprehension, because successful performance on the memory tasks requires integrity of language skills in addition to the memory systems that are the target of the assessment. From this hierarchical perspective, attentional and working memory abilities are particularly important to other aspects of neuropsychological functioning, because deficits in these areas can compromise performance across diverse cognitive tasks. (*Working memory* refers to the ability to hold new information in mind and perform mental manipulations on that information.)

Multiple studies have demonstrated attentional disturbance in children and adolescents with bipolar disorder. Performance on digit span or spatial span tasks was impaired relative to controls or relative to published normative data in a combined group of children and adolescents who were euthymic or hypomanic (Dickstein et al. 2004), in a small group of unmedicated children with bipolar disorder (Castillo et al. 2000), in a combined group of children and adolescents with bipolar I or II disorder (Doyle et al. 2005), and in a group of incarcerated youth who had bipolar disorder and comorbid conduct disorder as well as other comorbidities (Olvera et al. 2005). The degree of impairment that symptomatic patients with bipolar disorder demonstrate on span tests is similar to that demonstrated by children with other severe mental illnesses (McCarthy et al. 2004).

On tests requiring sustained attention and vigilance over time, such as continuous performance tasks, deficits have been documented in symptomatic patients (Doyle et al. 2005; McClure et al. 2005a; Warner et al. 2005) as well as in those with euthymic mood (Pavuluri et al. 2006b), but no performance discrepancy has been found between euthymic patients and patients in a manic or mixed mood state or between medicated patients and unmedicated patients (Pavuluri et al. 2006b). A conflicting finding is that euthymic older adolescents and young adults were reported to have normal performance on a test of sustained attention; however, these patients endorsed a disproportionate number of complaints about attentional and general cognitive abilities in their daily lives (Robertson et al. 2003), suggesting a subjective impairment not captured by the laboratory measure of attention. Working memory ability has been found to be impaired in pediatric patients with bipolar disorder (Olvera et al. 2005), again with no difference in impairment level across mood states or medication conditions (Pavuluri et al. 2006b). Thus, there is strong evidence that attentional abilities are impaired in children and adolescents with bipolar disorder, and the few studies that have examined working memory have found performance decrements. No existing studies have focused on patients with bipolar depression, but deficits do appear to be present with equal magnitude in both euthymic and manic or mixed mood states. Therefore, it must be considered that performance on all tasks that require a strong attentional component, particularly sustained attention over time, may be affected in these patients.

Returning to the idea of hierarchical cognitive abilities, together with attention and working memory, the domains of expressive and receptive language, visuospatial perception and construction, and motor ability are foundational to many higher-order cognitive processes and are required to successfully perform many neuropsychological tasks. These abilities have not been well studied in children and adolescents with bipolar disorder. The few reports that are available indicate preserved language (Castillo et al. 2000), visuospatial ability (Castillo et al. 2000; Pavuluri et al. 2006b), and motor skills (Dickstein et al. 2004; Pavuluri et al. 2006b). It must be emphasized that extremely few studies have assessed these domains and some of the sample sizes are quite modest.

Several studies have addressed memory functioning in youth with bipolar disorder. Verbal memory impairment has been consistently identified, although the magnitude of the deficits tends to be small. On a verbal list learning task, patients demonstrated reduced acquisition of new information and impaired recognition of the list; however, there was no deficit in the learning slope over repeated trials, and retention across a delay interval was within normal limits (Glahn et al. 2005; McClure et al. 2005b). In other words, the patients were somewhat slower at learning new verbal information, but once the information was encoded, it was retained to a normal degree. Their strategies of organizing verbal material on the list were normal (e.g., categorizing words for more efficient encoding) (Glahn et al.

2005), suggesting an active learning strategy. Another study showed a trend toward a significant deficit in verbal list learning (Doyle et al. 2005). It must be emphasized that the learning deficiencies were quite modest in these studies, and in at least one case, the significant group differences may have been most reflective of the above-average performance in the controls rather than deficient performance in the patients. Verbal memory impairment has also been reported on a task that requires immediate and delayed memory for stories (McClure et al. 2005b; Olvera et al. 2005), suggesting that bipolar disorder is associated with verbal memory deficits both when material is relatively unstructured semantically (verbal list learning) and when it is semantically structured (stories). Consistent with these data, patients were substantially impaired on a composite measure that averaged performance across multiple different verbal memory measures (Pavuluri et al. 2006b).

Several studies have examined the degree to which disease or treatment factors may impact verbal learning and memory ability in pediatric bipolar patients. McClure et al. (2005b), studying both euthymic and symptomatic children and adolescents, reported that deficits in verbal list learning and story memory relative to controls were apparent only in the symptomatic patients and not in the euthymic group; these authors did not identify a significant medication effect on verbal memory. In contrast, Pavuluri et al. (2006b) found equally impaired performance on a battery of verbal memory tasks in unmedicated manic patients and in medicated euthymic patients. Glahn et al. (2004) compared verbal memory performance across groups of patients with bipolar I, bipolar II, and bipolar disorder not otherwise specified; the authors reported that verbal list learning performance differed from a comparison sample only in the bipolar I group, a finding that highlights the importance of studying diagnostically homogeneous groups of patients. Thus, the existing studies have inconsistent findings with regard to the presence or absence of memory problems in euthymic individuals, as well as with regard to the influence of mood state on performance, but there is a relative consensus that children and adolescents with bipolar disorder, as a group, demonstrate mild verbal memory impairment.

Visual memory has been less studied in youth with bipolar disorder, perhaps because cognitive findings in this domain in adults have been quite mixed and generally nonsignificant. The results of the few studies that have focused on visual memory in children and adolescents have been inconsistent. Some authors have reported significant deficits in pattern recognition memory (Dickstein et al. 2004) and memory for faces (Castillo et al. 2000; Olvera et al. 2005). In contrast, there are reports of intact performance in spatial recognition memory (Dickstein et al. 2004), in facial memory and memory for designs (McClure et al. 2005b), and on a composite measure of multiple visual memory tests (Pavuluri et al. 2006b). More research is indicated to clarify the nature and degree of any visual memory changes associated with bipolar disorder.

Executive functioning refers to a broad category of abilities, which include planning, problem solving, conceptualization, reasoning, goal-directed behavior, and inhibitory control. The existing studies that have examined executive functioning in youth with bipolar disorder have had somewhat mixed results, although the majority have identified deficits. Several investigators have employed sorting tasks, which require conceptualization and mental flexibility, and have reported deficits in groups with bipolar disorder (Dickstein et al. 2004; Olvera et al. 2005; Warner et al. 2005), as well as in youth (McDonough-Ryan et al. 2001) and young adults (Meyer et al. 2004) who were genetically at risk to develop bipolar disorder by virtue of having a parent with the disorder. Meyer et al. (2004) reported the interesting longitudinal finding that all genetically at-risk participants in their sample who demonstrated both attentional disturbance on neuropsychological testing and impaired card sorting performance as youth went on to develop bipolar disorder by young adulthood, a result that illustrates the potential prognostic importance of cognitive data.

In terms of other executive functioning findings, there are reports that youth with bipolar disorder exhibit impairment on a composite of multiple executive functioning measures (Pavuluri et al. 2006b), on tasks requiring the inhibition of an overlearned verbal response (Doyle et al. 2005), and on caregiver reports of everyday behaviors that are dependent on executive functioning abilities (Shear et al. 2002; Warner et al. 2005). Motor inhibition is reportedly intact both in euthymic bipolar patients and in those who are symptomatic (McClure et al. 2005a).

One study reported impaired executive functioning performance both in euthymic bipolar patients and in those with manic or mixed symptoms (Pavuluri et al. 2006b), and another study found euthymic patients to be impaired on a measure of response flexibility (McClure et al. 2005a). In contrast, however, Dickstein et al. (2004) reported that euthymic and hypomanic youth performed within normal limits on a problem-solving and reasoning task that requires the manipulation of disks to form towers of predetermined patterns, and Robertson et al. (2003) reported normal performance on a card sorting task by a euthymic bipolar group.

Thus, the preponderance of evidence suggests that executive functioning is impaired in bipolar youth and that such deficits may predate the onset of illness and serve as genetic risk markers. Nevertheless, study findings among euthymic bipolar children and adolescents remain mixed. It should be emphasized that *executive functioning* refers to a broad range of skills that are mediated by distinct brain regions; therefore, it is not necessarily expected that patients with a given disorder will perform uniformly across all types of executive functioning tasks.

In addition to demonstrating deficits on tests of specific cognitive abilities, children and adolescents with bipolar disorder are also often impaired in their academic achievement. The most common finding is relative weakness in arithmetic ability (Pavuluri et al. 2006a), which is evident even during periods of normal mood (Lagace et al. 2003; Robertson et al. 2003) and in children and adolescents who are at genetic risk to develop bipolar xdisorder (McDonough-Ryan et al. 2002). However, this deficit was not observed in one small group of medication-free latency-aged children (Castillo et al. 2000). Academic problems have also been identified in reading skills (Pavuluri et al. 2006a), although this finding has not always been replicated (Lagace et al. 2003). Regarding the degree of magnitude of these academic difficulties, one group of older adolescents in remission was found to be delayed an average of 2 years in their mathematical competence, with 30% of the sample of 44 patients reporting having failed a mathematics class in the previous year (Lagace et al. 2003). Parents report a high frequency of reading and mathematics difficulties in their children and adolescents with bipolar disorder (Pavuluri et al. 2006a), and patients with bipolar disorder frequently require placement in tutoring or special education programs (Doyle et al. 2005; Pavuluri et al. 2006a). These patients' psychiatric symptomatology, rather than their cognitive abilities per se, may of course play a role in the need for special school services. Not surprisingly, however, there is empirical evidence of an association between neuropsychological functioning and academic achievement in this population; specifically, attentional ability is predictive of mathematics achievement, and a combination of attentional, working memory, visual memory, and executive functioning indices is predictive of reading and writing skills (Pavuluri et al. 2006a).

Finally, in addition to reports of demonstrated deficits in these traditional domains of cognitive functioning, there is a small literature that has examined bipolar patients' performance on tasks that require affective processing. Despite the normal ability of youth with bipolar disorder to perform facial recognition tasks (Castillo et al. 2000; Olvera et al. 2005), these patients demonstrate deficits in their ability to correctly identify the affect that is conveyed by the facial expression of others (McClure et al. 2003, 2005b) and their ability to judge socially appropriate language in various situations (McClure et al. 2005a). Pilot work from our laboratory suggests that adolescents with bipolar disorder are also impaired in their ability to identify the emotion conveyed in adults' speech (Foster et al. 2007).

In summary of the discussion thus far, the limited existing literature suggests that children and adolescents with bipolar disorder relatively consistently exhibit deficits in attention, verbal learning and memory, and executive functioning. Results are more mixed in terms of the presence or absence of visual memory disturbance. The few existing studies of social cognition suggest that these patients are impaired in their ability to process the affective component of facial expressions, voice quality, and the linguistic demands of various social situations. Many of the identified deficits are rather subtle, and results are particularly inconsistent in euthymic patient samples. Investigators have failed to identify significant relationships between the severity of cognitive dysfunction and the severity of psychiatric symptomatology (Dickstein et al. 2004; Glahn et al. 2005; Pavuluri et al. 2006b; Shear et al. 2002); that is, as a group, bipolar youth are at increased risk for experiencing cognitive dysfunction, but there is no evidence at this time that cognitive impairment increases further as symptom severity increases. There is also no evidence from studies that medications typically used to treat pediatric bipolar disorder significantly impact neurocognitive function (McClure et al. 2005b; Pavuluri et al. 2006b), although this issue has not been assessed as extensively in children or adolescents as in adults (see Chapter 7, "Adverse Cognitive Effects of Psychotropic Medications") and awaits further study.

Together, these findings are consistent with reports of cognitive dysfunction in adults with bipolar disorder (as detailed more extensively in Chapters 1–5 of this book) making it tempting to speculate that bipolar disorder affects cognition similarly during childhood, adolescence, and adulthood. Although a similar neurocognitive profile may exist between bipolar youth and adult patients, a number of limitations in the current pediatric literature complicate interpretation of the findings and are related to the phenomenological differences among adult, child, and adolescent presentations of illness. The vast majority of existing studies include heterogeneous groups of pre- and postpubescent participants but fail to perform analyses of potential age effects in the data (bearing in mind also that age effects might not be linear). Therefore, it is not clear whether cognitive deficits are present across the full developmental range that is being studied. Similarly, many samples are not well characterized in terms of mood state or are collapsed into one group of participants despite their being in heterogeneous mood states, making it challenging to map the pediatric findings onto results from state-specific adult studies. Also, although it is of clear theoretical and clinical interest to understand the nature of cognitive functioning in specific, well-characterized mood syndromes, the phenomenological studies reviewed above indicate that many youth with bipolar disorder experience rather chronic mood abnormalities; from this perspective, it will be important for studies to address the cognitive effects of the subsyndromal mood alterations that are typical in many of these patients between full mood episodes.

Most prominent among the limitations of translating from the adult literature to the child and adolescent literature on cognitive dysfunction in bipolar disorder are differences in prevalence rates for certain Axis I comorbidities in bipolar youth (e.g., ADHD) versus adults (e.g., substance use disorders). Thus, many of the studies that purport to examine cognitive functioning in youth with bipolar disorder are essentially examining a complex amalgam of various diagnostic combinations. Although ADHD is by no means the only comorbidity exhibited by youth with bipolar disorder, comorbid ADHD is of particular interest to cognitive studies because of the diagnostic complexities (as reviewed in an earlier section, "Pediatric and Adolescent Bipolar Disorder: Diagnostic Issues") and because ADHD is itself clearly associated with cognitive deficits. We turn now to a discussion of the available literature that describes the extent to which the cognitive deficits we have reviewed thus far are explicable on the basis of comorbid ADHD.

The Contribution of ADHD to Neuropsychological Functioning

Research has repeatedly shown that individuals who have ADHD as their primary diagnosis demonstrate impairment on tasks requiring attention, inhibitory processes, self-regulation, and executive functioning, although more recent conceptual models rely less on the study of individual cognitive domains and emphasize instead integration of diverse functions (Barkley et al. 1992; Hervey et al. 2004; Nigg 2005; Willcutt et al. 2005). Because of the high comorbidity between childhood and adolescent bipolar disorder and ADHD, it is of considerable interest to understand the degree to which the cognitive deficits that have been attributed to bipolar disorder can be explained by co-occurring ADHD.

Only a handful of studies have addressed the differentiation versus comorbidity of bipolar disorder and ADHD in children and adolescents and their points of overlap with respect to cognitive symptoms. Although the majority of these studies report disproportionate cognitive deficits associated with comorbid ADHD, not all studies agree. Several factors complicate interpretation of the various studies, including the diversity of cognitive measures employed; the fact that most of these studies sampled both prepubescent and postpubescent individuals—populations that have differing risks for ADHD; and the fact that few authors have described the observed ADHD symptoms in a comprehensive way. Specifically, there is little documentation of ADHD subtypes in the comorbid samples, despite evidence that patients with different subtypes may exhibit differing cognitive presentations (Faraone et al. 1998; Nigg 2005).

Two studies of bipolar youth have attempted to control for ADHD by statistically removing the effect of the comorbid diagnostic classification rather than examining the magnitude of the effect on cognition. Using this methodology in a group of children and adolescents with bipolar I or II disorder in varying mood states, Doyle et al. (2005) reported that deficits in sustained attention, working memory, and processing speed persisted. Similarly, Olvera et al. (2005) found working memory deficits in a small group of incarcerated youth with bipolar disorder and comorbid conduct disorder, again after controlling for ADHD. It should be noted that this type of statistical control is a conservative method of examining the cognitive effects of bipolar disorder, as it likely reduces the magnitude of that effect. Despite this conservative approach, these studies support an independent contribution of bipolar disorder to cognitive dysfunction, above and beyond the effects of comorbid ADHD.

Some studies have directly compared patients with and without comorbid ADHD. Dickstein et al. (2004) studied a combined group of euthymic and hypomanic bipolar children and adolescents who were asked to complete a computerized battery designed to assess a broad variety of cognitive functions; these authors did not identify significant differences in performance between those patients with and without comorbid ADHD. In contrast, McClure et al. (2005a), whose sample included euthymic bipolar children and adolescents, as well as others in abnormal mood states, reported that, relative to healthy controls, patients with comorbid ADHD (but not those without comorbidity) demonstrated a significant but clinically subtle reduction in their ability to learn verbal word lists and stories. In a separate study, this research group demonstrated poorer social cognition in bipolar patients with comorbid ADHD on tasks requiring awareness of appropriate language in various social situations and the identification of emotional facial expressions (McClure et al. 2005b).

In an effort to parse the effects of medication status, mood state, and ADHD comorbidity, Pavuluri et al. (2006b) studied children and adolescents who were either medicated and in a euthymic mood state or unmedicated and in a manic mood state. Regardless of mood state or medication status, patients with comorbid ADHD were found to be more impaired than those with bipolar disorder alone on tasks requiring attention, executive functioning, and visual memory abilities. These authors later showed that the cognitive dysfunction they identified in pediatric patients with bipolar disorder was significantly associated with impaired academic achievement to a similar degree in those individuals with and without comorbid ADHD (Pavuluri et al. 2006a). That is, deficient academic achievement is related to the severity of cognitive dysfunction irrespective of whether or not the presence of ADHD contributes to the magnitude of the cognitive deficits.

In work from our laboratory examining comorbidity, we have focused specifically on pubescent and postpubescent adolescents, in order to minimize variability due to developmental effects. In one such study, we found that adolescents with bipolar disorder in manic or mixed mood states were rated by their caregivers as being impaired in the degree to which they demonstrated behaviors in their everyday lives that are associated with executive dysfunction. (These data were gathered with a self-report instrument called the Behavior Rating Inventory of Executive Function [BRIEF; Gioia et al. 2000], which asks questions about behaviors such as keeping school materials organized or interrupting conversations, behaviors that have been judged by a consensus of experts to likely reflect executive functioning skills.) Each of the adolescents in the sample who had bipolar disorder without ADHD demonstrated clinically significant elevations on scales measuring behavioral regulation and metacognition. Those patients with comorbid ADHD, however, were disproportionately impaired relative to those without comorbidity. Thus, based on caregiver ratings, executive dysfunction in daily life occurred in manic adolescents with bipolar disorder at a clinically significant level even in the absence of ADHD, and comorbid ADHD (in this study primarily ADHD, combined type) was associated with substantially more severe deficits (Shear et al. 2002). Similarly, we have pilot data to suggest that small groups of manic adolescents with bipolar disorder and comorbid ADHD (again, primarily combined type) performed significantly more poorly than those with bipolar disorder alone on tests of sequencing, working memory, and inhibition of an overlearned response (Shear et al. 2004). Corroborative evidence of functional brain differences between adolescents with bipolar disorder alone and those with comorbid ADHD comes also from a functional magnetic resonance imaging study that revealed activation of alternative neural pathways in bipolar adolescents with comorbid ADHD, specifically during the completion of an attentional task. Bipolar adolescents who had comorbid ADHD were more likely than adolescents with bipolar disorder alone to show reduced activation of prefrontal cortex in the presence of increased activation of posterior parietal and temporal cortical regions (Adler et al. 2005).

In a complementary study utilizing independent samples of patients, we compared performance on a battery of laboratory-based tests of executive functioning as well as on the BRIEF in three groups of adolescents: those with ADHD alone, those with manic or mixed-state bipolar disorder plus ADHD, and psychiatrically healthy subjects without a family history of mood or psychotic disorder. The comorbid group was significantly more impaired than the ADHD group on measures of attention, working memory, and behavioral regulation (Warner et al. 2005). Taken together, the results of this study and our previous reports on bipolar adolescents with and without comorbid ADHD provide evidence that 1) executive functioning is impaired in manic and mixed-state adolescents with bipolar disorder even in the absence of comorbid ADHD; 2) the degree of impairment in adolescents with bipolar disorder and comorbid ADHD exceeds that seen in adolescents with ADHD alone; and 3) patients with bipolar disorder and comorbid ADHD are disproportionately impaired in executive functioning and working memory compared with bipolar patients without ADHD.

Clinical Implications

It is important to emphasize that no existing neuropsychological test or series of tests can be used in isolation to make a diagnosis of ADHD or bipolar disorder or to differentiate between ADHD and bipolar disorder in individual cases; rather, these diagnoses are made exclusively on the basis of history and psychiatric symptomatology. The presence of cognitive, particularly attentional and inhibitory, disturbance on formal testing can indeed serve as corroborative evidence when patients meet diagnostic criteria for ADHD; however, it is not uncommon for individuals who meet diagnostic criteria to perform better cognitively in the structured setting of a neuropsychological evaluation that involves one-on-one interactions with an examiner than they do when there are fewer external constraints in their everyday lives. Stated differently, the presence of cognitive dysfunction on formal testing may corroborate diagnostic impressions, but the absence of marked disturbance on a neuropsychological evaluation should not necessarily be taken as negative diagnostic evidence. Additionally, as the existing literature demonstrates, there is considerable overlap of the cognitive deficits present in bipolar disorder with or without ADHD; therefore, neuropsychological testing alone cannot serve as a clinical index of the presence or absence of this comorbidity.

Nonetheless, findings from the existing neuropsychological literature have important clinical implications for clinicians who work with children and adolescents with bipolar disorder. The research suggests that, even when euthymic, these patients may experience impaired attention, working memory, verbal learning and memory, and executive function, as well as difficulties in academic achievement. Existing reports suggest that many of these cognitive impairments are subtle, although in some samples the degree of attentional and executive functioning disturbance is of clear clinical significance. Even mild cognitive deficiencies have been shown to be related to functional losses (Lezak 1995), and mnemonic and executive functioning deficits of the type that have been identified in bipolar youth strongly correlate with outcome in patients with psychiatric disorders (Green 1996) as well as in other clinical populations (Cahn et al. 1998).

These cognitive deficits are identifiable in groups of patients with bipolar disorder even in the absence of comorbid ADHD, and the preponderance of the evidence suggests that those individuals with comorbid ADHD demonstrate more severe cognitive dysfunction.

Therefore, clinicians need to be alert to the possibility that youth with bipolar disorder may be experiencing, in addition to their cardinal mood symptoms, cognitive problems that are associated with functional compromise and that may not be ameliorated completely by the remission of affective symptoms. To reiterate, childhood and adolescent bipolar disorder is not associated with a single pattern of neuropsychological dysfunction that affects all patients uniformly, so it is imperative to take a careful history of cognitive complaints on an individual basis, and it may be helpful to consider seeking a formal neuropsychological assessment if there is concern about substantial cognitive dysfunction (see Chapter 12, "Summary and Assessment Recommendations for Practitioners"). Comprehensive care of bipolar patients, particularly those with comorbid ADHD, may potentially require education of the family about neuropsychological dysfunction, work with patients and their families that targets compensation for cognitive deficits, and consideration of accommodations in the classroom and in vocational settings. See Table 9–1 for selected points that should be considered in the clinical assessment of children and adolescents with bipolar disorder.

Finally, from the standpoint of pharmacotherapy, the scarcity of empirical intervention studies of children or adolescents with a dual diagnosis of bipolar disorder and ADHD limits the extent to which broad generalizations can be drawn about the safety and efficacy of traditional therapeutics for either disorder. Nonetheless, a randomized trial in symptomatic subjects ages 6–17 years diagnosed with both bipolar mania and ADHD demonstrated little effect on ADHD symptoms with the use of a mood-stabilizing agent (i.e., divalproex), but substantial improvement occurred in ADHD symptoms—and no significant worsening of mania symptoms—with the subsequent addition of mixed amphetamine salts (dosed at 5 mg twice daily) (Scheffer et al. 2005). Also, retrospective findings by our group suggest that children and adolescents with bipolar disorder are more likely to have had an earlier age at onset when histories of stimulant treatment are present (DelBello et al. 2001), independent of the presence of comorbid ADHD (DelBello et al. 2001). Because stimulants show a relatively rapid onset of action to treat ADHD symptoms (on the order of days), clinicians can gauge the likelihood of improvement relatively quickly. Thus, the literature would most compellingly support a sequenced approach to pharmacotherapy in which antimanic agents are used before stimulants, both to minimize the potential for subsequent mood destabilization and to allow for the possibility that nonspecific cognitive symptoms may be ame-

TABLE 9–1.   Clinical assessment tips for evaluating cognitive problems in children and adolescents with suspected bipolar disorder

Consider the following questions:

- Was there prepubescent onset of the mood disorder (associated with a more severe course of mood symptoms)?
- Are there first-degree relatives with bipolar disorder or highly recurrent depression (associated with increased incidence of mood disorder in the patient being evaluated)?
- Is there evidence that attention-deficit/hyperactivity disorder is co-occurring with the mood symptoms (associated with more pronounced cognitive deficits than in bipolar disorder alone)?
- Is there a history of delay in reaching developmental milestones (associated with general intellectual decrements)?
- How well does the child perform academically? Is there a history of poor grades or difficulty with specific academic subjects such as math or reading? (These academic problems may be associated with a learning disorder, particularly if certain academic areas are markedly impaired in comparison to others.)
- In older adolescents, is there a history of difficulty in fulfilling work obligations because of cognitive problems?
- Are there reported impairments in the cognitive domains that are most commonly found to be affected in childhood and adolescent bipolar disorder, including attention, the ability to hold information in mind and manipulate it, the capacity to organize and problem solve, and the ability to learn and remember new information?
- Is there evidence of difficulty interpreting other people's emotional expressions accurately or making appropriate social judgments?

If there is concern about significant cognitive dysfunction, the patient should be referred for neuropsychological testing.

liorated at least in part by mood stabilizers. The persistence of attention problems in likely dual-diagnosis bipolar-ADHD children and adolescents would favor the addition (rather than the avoidance) of stimulants, with close observation for changes in clinical state.

Conclusions

ADHD is a common comorbid condition in children with bipolar disorder. Its differentiation from bipolar disorder hinges on recognizing the symptoms of both disorders that are nonoverlapping, as well as recognizing differences in their longitudinal course and response to pharmacotherapy. No specific neuropsychological test has been established to validate the existence of ADHD, and its diagnosis remains based on history and clinical interview. Because cognitive problems may exist in children or adolescents with bipolar disorder, a diagnosis of comorbid ADHD cannot be based solely on the presence of impaired attention, distractibility, or poor executive control in the context of untreated affective symptoms. The nature of cognitive problems in pediatric bipolar disorder generally appears similar to that seen in adults with bipolar disorder with respect to domains of attention and executive function, as well as verbal memory, although further research is needed to better define the scope of neurocognitive deficits in children or adolescents versus adults with bipolar disorder. Sequential treatments that first aim to stabilize mood, followed by adjunctive stimulants or other medications for ADHD if cognitive problems persist, may help to clarify diagnostic uncertainties as well as provide an evidence-based pharmacological approach.

Take-Home Points

- Compared with adult patients with bipolar disorder, bipolar youth more often demonstrate chronic irritability, rapid cycling, and mixed mood states without clear intermorbid euthymia.

- Pediatric bipolar disorder may be differentiable from ADHD based on noncognitive symptoms of mania, such as elation, hypersexuality, and grandiosity, as well as non-ADHD symptoms such as psychosis or suicidality.

- The existing research suggests that children or adolescents with bipolar disorder manifest similar cognitive deficits to those seen in adults. These include problems with attention (including sustained attention and vigilance), problems with aspects of executive function (e.g., conceptualization and mental flexibility), and modest but significant deficits in verbal memory. Language, visuospatial ability, and motor skills seem generally intact, based on limited studies to date.

- ADHD arises as a comorbid condition in a substantial majority of children with bipolar disorder and could represent a subtype of familial, early-onset bipolar illness.

- In youth diagnosed with bipolar disorder and ADHD, each condition likely contributes independently to the composite observable cognitive deficits. Dual-diagnosis youth may be especially prone to academic difficulties (especially in mathematics), executive dysfunction, and problems with affective processing.

- When symptoms of inattention and/or hyperactivity persist despite adequate mood stabilization in bipolar children and adolescents, pharmacotherapy with adjunctive stimulants for ADHD generally appears to be effective and well tolerated.

References

Adler CM, DelBello MP, Mills NP, et al: Comorbid ADHD is associated with altered patterns of neuronal activation in adolescents with bipolar disorder performing a simple attention task. Bipolar Disord 7:577–588, 2005

Barkley RA, Grodzinsky G, DuPaul GJ: Frontal lobe functions in attention deficit disorder with and without hyperactivity: a review and research report. J Abnorm Child Psychol 20:163–188, 1992

Bearden CE, Hoffman KM, Cannon TD: The neuropsychology and neuroanatomy of bipolar affective disorder: a critical review. Bipolar Disord 3:106–150, 2001

Biederman J, Russell R, Soriano J, et al: Clinical features of children with both ADHD and mania: does ascertainment source make a difference? J Affect Disord 51:101–112, 1998

Cahn DA, Sullivan EV, Shear PK, et al: Differential contributions of cognitive and motor component processes to physical and instrumental activities of daily living in Parkinson's disease. Arch Clin Neuropsychol 13:575–583, 1998

Castillo M, Kwock L, Courvoisie H, et al: Proton MR spectroscopy in children with bipolar affective disorder: preliminary observations. AJNR Am J Neuroradiol 21:832–838, 2000

Connelly EG, Murphy DL, Goodwin FK, et al: Intellectual function in primary affective disorder. Br J Psychiatry 140:633–636, 1982

DelBello MP, Geller B: Review of studies of child and adolescent offspring of bipolar parents. Bipolar Disord 3:325–334, 2001

DelBello MP, Soutullo SC, Hendricks W, et al: Prior stimulant treatment in adolescents with bipolar disorder: association with age at onset. Bipolar Disord 3:53–57, 2001

Dickstein DP, Treland JE, Snow J, et al: Neuropsychological performance in pediatric bipolar disorder. Biol Psychiatry 55:32–39, 2004

Doyle AE, Wilens TE, Kwon A, et al: Neuropsychological functioning in youth with bipolar disorder. Biol Psychiatry 58:540–548, 2005

Faraone SV, Biederman J, Weber W, et al: Psychiatric, neuropsychological, and psychosocial features of DSM-IV subtypes of attention-deficit/hyperactivity disorder: results from a clinically referred sample. J Am Acad Child Adolesc Psychiatry 37:185–193, 1998

Faraone SV, Biederman J, Monuteaux MC: Attention deficit hyperactivity disorder with bipolar disorder in girls: further evidence for a familial subtype? J Affect Disord 64:19–26, 2001

Findling RL, Gracious BL, McNamara NK, et al: Rapid, continuous cycling and psychiatric co-morbidity in pediatric bipolar I disorder. Bipolar Disord 3:202–210, 2001

Fleck DE, Shear PK, Strakowski SM: Processing efficiency and sustained attention in bipolar disorder. J Int Neuropsychol Soc 11:49–57, 2005

Foster MK, Shear PK, DelBello MP: Visual and auditory perception of emotion in adolescents with bipolar disorder. Poster presented at the annual conference of the American Psychological Association. San Francisco, CA, August 2007

Geller B, Luby J: Child and adolescent bipolar disorder: a review of the past 10 years. J Am Acad Child Adolesc Psychiatry 36:1168–1176, 1997

Geller B, Warner K, Williams M, et al: Prepubertal and young adolescent bipolarity versus ADHD: assessment and validity using the WASH-U-KSADS, CBCL, and TRF. J Affect Disord 51:93–100, 1998a

Geller B, Williams M, Zimerman B, et al: Prepubertal and early adolescent bipolarity differentiate from ADHD by manic symptoms, grandiose delusions, ultra-rapid or ultradian cycling. J Affect Disord 51:81–91, 1998b
Geller B, Zimerman B, Williams M, et al: Six-month stability and outcome of a prepubertal and early adolescent bipolar disorder phenotype. J Child Adolesc Psychopharmacol 10:165–173, 2000
Gioia GA, Isquith PK, Guy SC, et al: Behavior Rating Inventory of Executive Function. Odessa, FL, Psychological Assessment Resources, 2000
Glahn DC, Bearden CE, Niendam TA, et al: The feasibility of neuropsychological endophenotypes in the search for genes associated with bipolar affective disorder. Bipolar Disord 6:171–182, 2004
Glahn DC, Bearden CE, Caetano S, et al: Declarative memory impairment in pediatric bipolar disorder. Bipolar Disord 7:546–554, 2005
Green MF: What are the functional consequences of neurocognitive deficits in schizophrenia? Am J Psychiatry 153:321–330, 1996
Green MF, Kern RS, Braff DL, et al: Neurocognitive deficits and functional outcome in schizophrenia: are we measuring the "right stuff"? Schizophr Bull 26:119–136, 2000
Henin A, Mick E, Biederman J, et al: Can bipolar disorder–specific neuropsychological impairments in children be identified? J Consult Clin Psychol 75:210–220, 2007
Henry GM, Weingartner H, Murphy DL: Influence of affective states and psychoactive drugs on verbal learning and memory. Am J Psychiatry 140:966–971, 1973
Hervey AS, Epstein JN, Curry JF: Neuropsychology of adults with attention-deficit/ hyperactivity disorder: a meta-analytic review. Neuropsychology 18:485–503, 2004
Lagace DC, Kutcher SP, Robertson HA: Mathematics deficits in adolescents with bipolar I disorder. Am J Psychiatry 160:100–104, 2003
Lebowitz BK, Shear PK, Steed MA, et al: Verbal fluency in mania: relationship to number of manic episodes. Neuropsychiatry Neuropsychol Behav Neurol 14:177–182, 2001
Lewinsohn PM, Klein DN, Seeley JR: Bipolar disorders in a community sample of older adolescents: prevalence, phenomenology, comorbidity, and course. J Am Acad Child Adolesc Psychiatry 34:454–463, 1995
Lezak M: Neuropsychological Assessment. New York, Oxford University Press, 1995
McCarthy J, Arrese D, McGlashan A, et al: Sustained attention and visual processing speed in children and adolescents with bipolar disorder and other psychiatric disorders. Psychol Rep 95:39–47, 2004
McClure EB, Pope K, Hoberman AJ, et al: Facial expression recognition in adolescents with mood and anxiety disorders. Am J Psychiatry 160:1172–1174, 2003
McClure EB, Treland JE, Snow J, et al: Deficits in social cognition and response flexibility in pediatric bipolar disorder. Am J Psychiatry 162:1644–1651, 2005a
McClure EB, Treland JE, Snow J, et al: Memory and learning in pediatric bipolar disorder. J Am Acad Child Adolesc Psychiatry 44:461–469, 2005b
McDonough-Ryan P, DelBello M, Shear PK, et al: Neuropsychological functioning in children of parents with bipolar disorder. Paper presented at the annual meeting of the American Psychological Association, San Francisco, CA, August 2001

McDonough-Ryan P, DelBello M, Shear PK, et al: Academic and cognitive abilities in children of parents with bipolar disorder: a test of the nonverbal learning disability model. J Clin Exp Neuropsychol 24:280–285, 2002

McKay AP, Tarbuck AF, Shapleske J, et al: Neuropsychological function in manic-depressive psychosis: evidence for persistent deficits in patients with chronic, severe illness. Br J Psychiatry 167:51–57, 1995

Meyer SE, Carlson GA, Wiggs EA, et al: A prospective study of the association among impaired executive functioning, childhood attentional problems, and the development of bipolar disorder. Dev Psychopathol 16:461–476, 2004

Milberger S, Biederman J, Faraone SV, et al: Attention deficit hyperactivity disorder and comorbid disorders: issues of overlapping symptoms. Am J Psychiatry 152:1793–1799, 1995

Nierenberg AA, Miyahara S, Spencer T, et al: Clinical and diagnostic implications of lifetime attention-deficit/hyperactivity disorder comorbidity in adults with bipolar disorder: data from the first 1000 STEP-BD participants. Biol Psychiatry 57:1467–1473, 2005

Nigg JT: Neuropsychologic theory and findings in attention-deficit/hyperactivity disorder: the state of the field and salient challenges for the coming decade. Biol Psychiatry 57:1424–1435, 2005

Olvera RL, Semrud-Clikeman M, Pliszka SR, et al: Neuropsychological deficits in adolescents with conduct disorder and comorbid bipolar disorder: a pilot study. Bipolar Disord 7:57–67, 2005

Pavuluri MN, Birmaher B, Naylor MW: Pediatric bipolar disorder: a review of the past 10 years. J Am Acad Child Adolesc Psychiatry 44:846–871, 2005

Pavuluri MN, O'Connor MM, Harral EM, et al: Impact of neurocognitive function on academic difficulties in pediatric bipolar disorder: a clinical translation. Biol Psychiatry 60:951–956, 2006a

Pavuluri MN, Schenkel LS, Aryal S, et al: Neurocognitive function in unmedicated manic and medicated euthymic pediatric bipolar patients. Am J Psychiatry 163:286–293, 2006b

Quraishi S, Frangou S: Neuropsychology of bipolar disorder: a review. J Affect Disord 72:209–226, 2002

Robertson HA, Kutcher SP, Lagace DC: No evidence of attentional deficits in stabilized bipolar youth relative to unipolar and control comparators. Bipolar Disord 5:330–339, 2003

Scheffer RE, Kowatch RA, Carmody T, et al: Randomized, placebo-controlled trial of mixed amphetamine salts for symptoms of comorbid ADHD in pediatric bipolar disorder after mood stabilization with divalproex sodium. Am J Psychiatry 162:58–64, 2005

Shear PK, DelBello MP, Rosenberg HL, et al: Parental reports of executive dysfunction in adolescents with bipolar disorder. Child Neuropsychol 8:285–295, 2002

Shear PK, DelBello MP, Rosenberg HL, et al: Cognitive functioning in manic adolescents with bipolar disorder: contribution of comorbid ADHD. Paper presented at the annual meeting of the International Neuropsychological Society, Baltimore, MD, February 2004

Singh MK, DelBello MP, Kowatch RA, et al: Co-occurrence of bipolar and attention-deficit hyperactivity disorders in children. Bipolar Disord 8:710–720, 2006

Spencer TJ, Biederman J, Wozniak J, et al: Parsing pediatric bipolar disorder from its associated comorbidity with the disruptive behavior disorders. Biol Psychiatry 49:1062–1070, 2001

Warner J, DelBello MP, Shear PK, et al: Executive functioning deficits in youth with comorbid bipolar disorder+ADHD: are they additive? Paper presented at the annual meeting of the International Neuropsychological Society, St. Louis, MO, February 2005

Willcutt EG, Doyle AE, Nigg JT, et al: Validity of the executive function theory of attention-deficit/hyperactivity disorder: a meta-analytic review. Biol Psychiatry 57:1336–1346, 2005

Wozniak J, Biederman J, Kiely K, et al: Mania-like symptoms suggestive of childhood-onset bipolar disorder in clinically referred children. J Am Acad Child Adolesc Psychiatry 34:867–876, 1995

10

Cognition and Functional Outcome in Bipolar Disorder

Ivan J. Torres, Ph.D.
Colin M. DeFreitas, M.A.
Lakshmi N. Yatham, M.B.B.S., F.R.C.P.C.,
M.R.C.Psych.

The major theme of this book is that neurocognitive impairment represents a core symptom of bipolar disorder. Moreover, because clinical neuropsychological tests traditionally have been developed and validated to detect and measure brain dysfunction, the implication is that the measured cognitive deficits reflect underlying brain impairment. Understanding of the psychosocial, functional, adaptive, or real-life implications of these cognitive impairments, however, has lagged for several reasons. First, as alluded to above, neuropsychological tests have been validated primarily to identify brain dysfunction rather than to predict "real world" functioning. Second, there are many potential spheres of functioning that constitute psychosocial, real-world, or functional outcome, and potential outcome measures of psychosocial function are numerous and diverse. Third, the understanding of associations between cognitive deficits and functional outcome requires measurement at both of these levels, which makes research in this area more difficult than studies looking exclusively at cognitive deficits associated with the disorder.

Our purpose in this chapter is to review the emerging literature on the relationship between cognitive impairment and psychosocial functional outcome in patients with bipolar disorder. This is a critically important area of study, as the delineation or prediction of functional capacity is arguably the most clinically useful information that can be obtained from neuropsychological assessment of the individual patient. We begin with a brief summary of cognitive deficits in bipolar disorder and of functional impairments associated with the illness. This is followed by a review of studies investigating the association between cognitive function and psychosocial functioning in bipolar disorder. We touch on several key issues relevant to the topic, including the diversity of potential outcome measures, the influence of symptoms on the cognition–psychosocial function relationship in bipolar disorder, and the relevance of increased understanding of this relationship to the practicing clinician. We also summarize findings in schizophrenia for comparative purposes.

Cognitive Deficits

It has long been recognized that cognitive deficits are present in bipolar disorder during acute manic and depressive episodes (Goodwin and Jamison 2007). A considerable number of studies have subsequently been conducted in asymptomatic patients to determine whether the cognitive deficits persist in the euthymic state and thus represent trait features of the illness. Two recent meta-analyses confirmed that relative to healthy controls, euthymic bipolar patients demonstrate significant cognitive deficits in the broad areas of memory (verbal learning and recall), executive function (attentional shifting, auditory working memory, mental flexibility, response inhibition, verbal fluency), and sustained attention and visual motor speed (Robinson et al. 2006; Torres et al. 2007). Although deficits in these broad functions are typically medium to large in magnitude, patients do not show significant deficits in global estimates of intellectual functioning based on single-word reading or vocabulary skill. Thus, there appears to be some specificity to the cognitive impairment demonstrated by euthymic patients with bipolar disorder. Despite the possibility that variables such as medication status and residual affective symptomatology may have some impact on cognitive function in euthymic patients, these variables are not likely to fully account for the deficits described in these patients (Altshuler et al. 2004; Deckersbach et al. 2004; Kieseppä et al. 2005; Martinez-Aran et al. 2004a, 2004b; Thompson et al. 2005; see also Chapter 7, "Adverse Cognitive Effects of Psychotropic Medications").

Psychosocial Function

Traditionally, bipolar disorder has been associated with an episodic rather than chronic course (Kraepelin 1921). However, research over the last

30 years has consistently revealed diminished occupational, educational, psychosocial, and residential functioning that persists long past symptomatic recovery in a significant proportion of bipolar patients (Tohen et al. 2000; Zarate et al. 2000). Tsuang et al. (1979) assessed functional outcome 30 years after initial presentation in a sample of 100 bipolar patients and found that 28% were incapacitated and unable to work at all, while 27% lived in a psychiatric hospital or nursing home; these percentages were significantly higher than those of normal controls. Despite changes in treatment practices, more recent follow-up studies have mirrored these earlier data (Dion et al. 1988; Strakowski et al. 1998; Tohen et al. 2000). A review of studies on psychosocial outcome in patients with bipolar disorder revealed that 30%–60% of individuals failed to regain full functioning in occupational and social domains (MacQueen et al. 2001). Thus, although medication improves symptoms, such treatment is more limited in affecting functional outcome (Gitlin et al. 1995; Harrow et al. 1990). In addition, reduced functioning is consistent across bipolar I and II disorders (Judd et al. 2005) and across cultures (Jiang 1999; Kebede et al. 2006).

Research has provided some idea of the time course of functional impairment in bipolar disorder. Illness onset appears to be associated with a decline in functioning. For some patients, this reduced functioning persists. In a 2-year follow-up study, Harrow et al. (1990) reported a clear decline from premorbid levels in occupational functioning in 36% of bipolar patients. Likewise, patients at 5-year follow-up were more likely than healthy relatives to report declines in job status and income, and less likely to report improvements (Coryell et al. 1993). Although on average, patients recover functioning somewhat from 6-month to 4-year follow-up (Tohen et al. 1990), the majority of patients (about 75%) remain below premorbid levels of functioning at 1-year follow-up (Conus et al. 2006; Keck et al. 1998). Tsuang et al.'s (1979) finding of poor outcome 30 years after illness onset suggests that a subgroup of patients never recovers premorbid levels of functioning.

Identified correlates of poor functional outcome include increased severity of depressive and, to a lesser extent, manic symptoms (Bauer et al. 2001; Judd et al. 2005); the presence of psychosis (Harrow et al. 1990; Tohen et al. 1990; but not Keck et al. 2003); and age at onset and childhood psychopathology (Carlson et al. 2002). However, the presence of symptoms is not sufficient to explain poor functional outcome, as functioning is disrupted even during asymptomatic periods (Judd et al. 2005; Laroche et al. 1995). Given the extent of psychosocial impairment in bipolar disorder, it is not surprising that patients with the illness also report marked reductions on ratings of quality of life (Michalak et al. 2005; Yatham et al. 2004).

Relationship Between Cognitive Deficits and Psychosocial Functioning

Despite increased understanding regarding 1) the nature and severity of cognitive impairment and 2) the functional deficits in bipolar disorder, considerably less research has been conducted assessing the relationship between cognitive impairment and psychosocial function (Green 2006; Zarate et al. 2000). Nevertheless, in recent years, several such studies have emerged and have provided some insight into the potential cognitive basis of functional impairments in bipolar disorder. Importantly, the majority of studies in this area have examined patients in the remitted or euthymic state; this strategy offers a stringent test of whether cognitive deficits indeed indicate something about the real-world functioning of patients with bipolar disorder. The study of asymptomatic patients necessarily truncates the range of severity of cognitive and functional impairments, thus making it more difficult to detect correlations between cognition and psychosocial function, if such correlations exist. If cognitive deficits are found to be linked to functional impairments when patients are asymptomatic, functional impairments are more likely to be associated with trait or persistent neurocognitive deficits than with fluctuating or state-dependent deficits.

The preliminary studies that have been conducted vary considerably with regard to the instruments used to assess neuropsychological and functional status, as well as the bipolar sample characteristics. Table 10–1 summarizes studies that have investigated cognitive and functional status concurrently, and is organized according to the type of functional outcome measure used. This list includes studies that have employed measures of global functional status with the Global Assessment of Functioning (GAF) Scale (American Psychiatric Association 2000), studies using other global assessment scales, and studies evaluating specific aspects of psychosocial function, namely employment or occupational status.

Global Psychosocial Function Measured With the GAF

The most frequently used scale in studies evaluating the relationship between cognition and psychosocial function is the GAF or its predecessor, the Global Assessment Scale (Endicott et al. 1976). The GAF has been incorporated into DSM since 1987, when DSM-III-R was published (American Psychiatric Association 1987). The GAF requires the clinician to rate the patient's gross psychological, social, and occupational functioning on a scale from 0 to 100. Because the scale requires the rater to consider psychological or mental symptoms but to exclude physical or medical factors in generating functional ratings, the scale is weighted toward measuring dysfunction associated with mental disorder (Goldman et al. 1992). Thus, the scale requires the rater to make the difficult discrimination between dysfunction associated with mental problems and that related to physical problems. Nevertheless, the common use of this scale is owing to its simplicity, brevity, and integration into DSM diagnostic axes.

In the majority of studies that have used fairly comprehensive neuropsychological batteries covering multiple cognitive domains, findings point to an association between GAF scores and memory, as well as between GAF scores and several aspects of executive function (Martinez-Aran et al. 2002, 2004a, 2004b; Torrent et al. 2006). The only study that failed to find a relationship between GAF and cognitive scores employed only screening measures of gross cognitive ability rather than tests of specific cognitive domains, a procedure that may account for the negative findings (Gildengers et al. 2004). The association between global psychosocial functioning and executive and memory functioning has also been observed on other clinician rating scales that are similar to the GAF in that they give weight to the presence of psychological symptoms (Atre-Vaidya et al. 1998), thus providing some convergent support for the GAF studies findings, which were largely conducted by the same research group. The association between memory and psychosocial functioning is most frequently reported for verbal memory tasks, but this may be a function of the infrequent study of nonverbal memory. The specific nature of the association between psychosocial functioning and executive ability remains less clear, because positive findings are observed on a wide range of tasks measuring verbal fluency, attentional shifting, and auditory working memory. To summarize, the cognitive tests associated with global functional measures that emphasize psychological functioning are highly consistent with the cognitive deficits (i.e., in memory and executive function) described in an earlier section, "Cognitive Deficits in Bipolar Disorder," for euthymic patients with bipolar disorder.

Other Global Psychosocial Function Measures

A significant number of studies have been conducted using a range of other global measures of psychosocial functioning. Although these measures vary according to format (clinician administered vs. patient self-report) and brevity (single scale rating vs. summary score based on comprehensive or structured interview), the measures discussed in this section do not give preferential weight to the presence of psychological symptoms. Rather, these scales allow for consideration of multiple sources of functional impairment, including medical or physical factors. These alternatives to the GAF offer the potential to provide a purer index of functional status that is less influenced by a particular etiology such as mental disorder. Similar to the GAF, however, the measures discussed in this section are also based on global scores derived from functional ratings across multiple specific areas

TABLE 10–1. Neuropsychological functions associated with global and specific measures of psychosocial functioning in bipolar disorder

Study	Population sample	Functional measure	Neuropsychological tests/Findings
Global function (using GAF)			
Martinez-Aran et al. 2004a	40 euthymic	GAF	Exec (WCST, Stroop, fluency, **SpanB**, TMT), vMem, SpanF, Vocab
Martinez-Aran et al. 2004b	108 bipolar mixed	GAF	Exec (**WCST, Stroop, fluency, SpanB, TMT**), vMem, **nvMem**, Vocab
Martinez-Aran et al. 2002	49 euthymic	GAF	Exec (WCST, fluency [trend], TMT), Span, Vocab
Torrent et al. 2006	38 bipolar I euthymic	GAF	Exec (WCST, Stroop, fluency, **SpanB, TMT**), vMem, SpanF, Vocab
	33 bipolar II euthymic	GAF	Exec (WCST, Stroop, fluency, SpanB, **TMT**), vMem, SpanF, Vocab
Gildengers et al. 2004	18 euthymic, >60 years old	GAS	MMSE, DRS, EXIT
Atre-Vaidya et al. 1998	25 Veterans Affairs patients	IRS	Exec (fluency), **vMem**, Ravens, Vocab, DRS
Other global function			
Depp et al. 2006	54 bipolar	QWB	**DRS**
	Mid–late age	SF-36 Mental (self)	DRS
Olley et al. 2005	15 bipolar I euthymic	SOFAS	Exec (Stroop, fluency, **ID-ED**, SOC, TOM)
		LFQ (self)	Exec (Stroop, fluency, ID-ED, SOC, TOM)
Atre-Vaidya et al. 1998	13 community	SSIM	Exec (**fluency**), **vMem**, Ravens Progressive Matrices, Vocab, DRS
Laes and Sponheim 2006	27 bipolar	Social Adjustment Scale–II	Exec (fluency, **TOL**), **vMem (trend)**, CPT, BD, Vocab

TABLE 10–1. Neuropsychological functions associated with global and specific measures of psychosocial functioning in bipolar disorder *(continued)*

Study	Population sample	Functional measure	Neuropsychological tests/Findings
Harmer et al. 2002	20 euthymic	SASS (self)	Facial emotion recognition
Zubieta et al. 2001	15 bipolar I euthymic with history of prior psychosis	SOFAS	Exec (WCST, **Stroop**, fluency), **vMem**, nvMem, Span, TOVA, Psychomotor speed (Bead-Tap Test)
Specific psychosocial function			
Dickerson et al. 2004	117 bipolar	Employment status	Exec (**LettNum**), **TMTA**, WAIS Information subtest, **RBANS**
Martinez-Aran et al. 2004b	108 bipolar mixed	Occupational function	Exec (WCST, Stroop, **fluency**, SpanB, TMT), **vMem**, nvMem, Vocab
Torrent et al. 2006	33 bipolar II euthymic	Occupational adaptation	Exec (WCST, Stroop, fluency, SpanB, **TMT**), vMem, SpanF, Vocab

Note. Cognitive tasks in boldface are those that were reported to be significantly associated with psychosocial function. All psychosocial function measures were clinician administered except when followed by "(self)," which indicates a self-report instrument. BD=Block Design; CANTAB=Cambridge Neuropsychological Test Automated Battery; CPT=Continuous Performance Test; DRS=Dementia Rating Scale; Exec=executive function; EXIT=Executive Interview; GAF=Global Assessment of Functioning; GAS=Global Assessment Scale; ID-ED=Intradimensional/Extradimensional task (from CANTAB); SOC=Stockings of Cambridge (from CANTAB); IRS=Impairment Rating Scale; LettNum=Letter Number Sequencing; LFQ=Life Functioning Questionnaire; MMSE=Mini-Mental State Examination; QWB=Quality of Well-Being Scale; SASS=Social Adaptation Self-Evaluation Scale; SF-36=Medical Outcomes Study Short-Form Health Survey; SOFAS=Social and Occupational Functional Assessment Scale; SSIM=Structured and Scaled Interview for Maladjustment; nvMem=nonverbal memory; RBANS=Repeatable Battery for the Assessment of Neuropsychological Status; Span=Digit Span; SpanB=Digit Span Backward; SpanF=Digit Span Forward; TMT=Trail Making Test; TMTA=Trail Making Test—Part A; TOL=Tower of London; TOM=theory of mind; TOVA=Test of Variables of Attention; vMem=verbal memory; Vocab=vocabulary; WCST=Wisconsin Card Sorting Test.

such as employment, family relationships, social functioning, and other similar domains. The middle section of Table 10–1 summarizes the various neuropsychological studies of bipolar disorder that have included more etiology-neutral measures of global psychosocial functioning.

It is most informative to first consider the studies that have measured multiple cognitive domains, because these studies have the potential to detect associations between specific cognitive abilities and functional outcome. Of the three studies using such neuropsychological batteries, global functioning was associated with verbal memory and some aspect of executive function in all studies (Atre-Vaidya et al. 1998; Laes and Sponheim 2006; Zubieta et al. 2001). In a study restricted to a battery of tests of executive function, Olley et al. (2005) reported an association between attentional-shifting aspects of executive function and a clinician-rated measure of psychosocial function, but not between executive function and a self-report scale. Interestingly, findings have been reported elsewhere to suggest that discrepancies between self-reported and objective measures of functional outcome may be frequent in patients with bipolar disorder but rarer in patients with unipolar depression (Goldberg and Harrow 2005).

Two studies employed either gross cognitive screening measures or a single test of specific cognitive ability (facial emotion processing), thus limiting the ability to assess the influence of multiple cognitive domains such as memory or executive functioning (Depp et al. 2006; Harmer et al. 2002). These latter studies generally failed to identify a correlation between neuropsychological functioning and functional status in bipolar disorder. In sum, the results in this section converge with those observed in studies employing the GAF. Global psychosocial function appears to be robustly associated with verbal memory functioning. Moreover, a relationship between global function and executive functioning is frequently reported, although the exact nature of the specific executive deficit that predicts psychosocial functioning is less clear.

One interesting observation is that in all studies that employed a self-report rather than a clinician-rated measure of global functioning, there was no association between cognitive ability and functional status. Although this may be partly explained by the failure to measure executive function or memory directly in most of these studies (Depp et al. 2006; Harmer et al. 2002), this explanation cannot account for negative findings in the study that did measure functions such as executive ability (Olley et al. 2005). The latter study is particularly informative because in addition to failing to observe a relationship between executive function and global functioning on a self-report measure, Olley et al. did report an association between executive function and a clinician-administered measure of global functional outcome. What may account for a failure to observe an association between cognitive function and functional status when using self-report global functional mea-sures? One possibility is that patients' self-ratings of functional status may be distorted by diminished insight into their illness or into the limitations im-posed by their illness. The possibility that self-ratings of functional capacity may be less accurate or valid than clinician ratings may be responsible for the absence of correlation between cognition and patient-rated functional sta-tus. Emerging data indeed suggest that diminished insight is prevalent in pa-tients with bipolar disorder (Amador et al. 1994). Moreover, like other aspects of neuropsychological functioning, poor insight appears to involve state and trait components and may itself be associated with poor functional outcome (Ghaemi and Rosenquist 2004; Varga et al. 2006). Another pos-sible reason for the discrepant findings between self-report and clinician-rated measures is that different aspects of function may be tapped by each class of functional measures, and this variation may account for the differen-tial association with cognitive function. Clearly, more studies with multiple functional outcome measures are required to further evaluate this possibility.

Specific Psychosocial (Occupational) Function

The final set of studies reviewed in Table 10–1 includes those that have in-vestigated the relationship between cognitive ability and functional capac-ity in a specific domain, occupational functioning (Dickerson et al. 2004; Martinez-Aran et al. 2004b; Torrent et al. 2006). Two studies by the same research group evaluated this relationship using a full neuropsychological battery. In one study, patients with good occupational functioning in the previous 3 years showed better executive function (fluency) and verbal memory scores than patients classified as having poor occupational func-tioning (Martinez-Aran et al. 2004b). Torrent et al. (2006) reported poorer executive functioning (attentional shifting), but not memory, in a sample of bipolar II patients with poor occupational status, relative to those with high occupational status. In a large sample, Dickerson et al. (2004) di-vided their sample into three groups based on occupational status (no work, part-time work, full-time work) and found that gross cognitive, memory, working memory, and attention scores predicted occupational group. These findings resulted despite the use of a limited screening cog-nitive battery. Although limited in number, these preliminary studies sup-port a significant association between cognitive functioning and work status. Moreover, these positive associations are most commonly observed on tests of verbal memory and various measures of executive function.

Influence of Symptoms

Because the majority of studies in Table 10–1 evaluated patients in the eu-thymic state, it can be reasoned that the cognitive correlates of poor psychosocial function most likely represent trait-related neuropsychological disturbance. However, it is possible that some of the cognitive correlates of functional impairment may be driven by dysfunction associated with residual affective or other psychiatric symptoms. After all, as reviewed earlier in this chapter, psychosocial functioning in patients with bipolar disorder has been linked to the presence of various affective and psychotic symptoms (Harrow et al. 2000; Judd et al. 2005). To evaluate the effect of both cognitive and psychiatric symptom variables on psychosocial functioning, several of the studies listed in Table 10–1 assessed the relative influence of both neuropsychological and symptom variables on functional status through multiple regression analysis. After covarying for psychiatric symptoms, Dickerson et al. (2004) found an independent association between general cognitive ability (Repeatable Battery for the Assessment of Neuropsychological Status score) and employment status. Similarly, even after controlling for the influence of current depressive or manic symptoms, Martinez-Aran et al. (2004b) found that memory deficits were associated with psychosocial functioning. Torrent et al. (2006), even after controlling for the effect of affective symptoms and other clinical variables, found that psychosocial functioning was associated with diminished executive function in the form of reduced attentional shifting capacity in a sample of patients with bipolar II disorder. In contrast to these data, Laes and Sponheim (2006) found that when controlling for psychotic symptoms, memory deficits were no longer associated with impaired psychosocial functioning in bipolar disorder. However, the authors did not run this analysis using measures of executive function, which showed the strongest correlation with psychosocial functioning. Taken together, these data indicate that the associations between cognitive functioning and psychosocial functioning cannot be fully attributed to residual affective and psychiatric symptomatology.

Summary of Cognitive and Psychosocial Findings

Investigations of the association between cognitive impairment and psychosocial function in bipolar disorder represent an area of increasing interest and a literature in its early stages. Inspection of Table 10–1 reveals that most studies in this area have investigated relatively small patient samples. There is also tremendous diversity among the cognitive tasks and psychosocial functioning measures that have been utilized, as well as variation in the sample characteristics of the bipolar samples studied. Despite these observations, several preliminary conclusions can be made based on the existing literature. First, the balance of the data does support a significant association between cognition and psychosocial functioning. Second, this relationship is most consistently observed on functions that have been most frequently associated with impairment in bipolar disorder, namely memory ability and executive functioning. The memory findings appear to be the most consistently reported, but this may be due in part to the fact that similar tasks (e.g., word list learning) are used across most studies. The specific executive skills that predict psychosocial functioning in bipolar disorder remain to be fully elucidated, and this is partly due to the use of a wide range of measures of executive function across studies. Nevertheless, the most frequently observed correlates of psychosocial functioning include attentional shifting, verbal fluency, and auditory working memory variables. Third, the association between cognition and psychosocial function is present when considering both global aspects of psychosocial function and functioning in specific domains such as employment or occupational status.

It should be emphasized that the studies reviewed in Table 10–1 obtained measures of cognition and psychosocial function concurrently, a practice that may increase the likelihood of detecting cognition-function correlations. A recent study, however, investigated the association between each of six domains of cognitive function at baseline (attention, working memory, ideational fluency, verbal knowledge, nonverbal functions, learning) and functional status after 1 year in a sample of 78 patients with bipolar disorder (Jaeger et al. 2007). After controlling for baseline and follow-up residual symptoms, two domains (attention, ideational fluency) were found to be predictive of functional outcome. The fact that the cognition–functional status relationship was present even after a 1-year interval underscores the robustness of the association, as well as increases the likelihood that it reflects trait-related cognitive impairment independent of fluctuating symptoms.

Findings in Schizophrenia

Because the research area relating neuropsychological functioning to psychosocial functioning is further developed in schizophrenia than in bipolar disorder, and because of the overlap in cognitive deficits reported in both disorders, it is useful to compare the emerging research findings in bipolar disorder with those in schizophrenia (Green 2006). Research in schizophrenia has revealed a variety of neurocognitive deficits that appear largely stable across the life span (Kurtz 2005). In a review and meta-analysis of neurocognitive deficits and functional outcome in schizophrenia, Green et al. (2000) concluded that there was a robust association between these domains of function, that global measures of neurocognition account for 20%–60% of the variance in functional outcome, and that reported associations between symptoms and functional outcome across the literature are weaker than cognition–functional outcome links. The relationship be-

tween neurocognition and functional outcome holds longitudinally, so
that measures of neurocognition predict functioning 6 months later
(Green et al. 2004). In terms of particular cognitive domains, it appears
that measures of secondary verbal memory, executive ability (verbal fluency, card sorting), and psychomotor ability or reaction time most frequently are associated with ratings of community functioning and daily
activities (Green et al. 2000). Thus, on the surface, there appears to be considerable overlap in the findings for both disorders despite the fact that
cognitive impairments are recognized to be more severe in schizophrenia
than in bipolar disorder (Altshuler et al. 2004; Krabbendam et al. 2005).

A small number of studies have directly investigated the association between cognition and psychosocial outcome in samples of patients with
schizophrenia or bipolar disorder in order to identify potential differences
in cognition–psychosocial function relationships between groups. Laes and
Sponheim (2006) reported that verbal memory predicted functional outcome over and above the effects of general cognition in patients with
schizophrenia, and that psychotic symptoms were also related to outcome
beyond the effects of cognition; in contrast, verbal memory did not have
this predictive power in patients with bipolar disorder, and the influence of
psychotic symptoms was minimal. Martinez-Aran et al. (2002) reported
that clinical symptom variables but not executive function were associated
with functional outcome in patients with bipolar disorder, whereas symptoms and executive deficits were related to functional outcome in patients
with schizophrenia. This latter study, however, did not include memory
measures. These preliminary data suggest that the association between
cognition (or symptoms) and psychosocial function may be more robust in
schizophrenia than in bipolar disorder. However, it is too early to tell
whether there are meaningful differences between bipolar disorder and
schizophrenia in the association between cognitive function and functional
outcome. Even if differences were evident, it is unclear whether this might
merely reflect differences in the magnitude of cognitive impairment between the two disorders (Krabbendam et al. 2005), which could influence
the sensitivity to detect cognition-function associations in either disorder.
At a broader level, it should not be surprising, and perhaps should be expected, that cognitive deficits associate with psychosocial function regardless of the etiology of the disorder under study.

Clinical Application of Findings

The evidence of cognitive impairment in bipolar disorder and its link to
psychosocial functioning provides important clinical implications for the
assessment and treatment of the individual patient. Knowledge of existing
cognitive limitations can be utilized to quantify and predict difficulties that

patients are likely to experience in real-world functioning. Results from neuropsychological assessment may thus be particularly useful to help anticipate or predict functional limitations in newly diagnosed patients with bipolar disorder. The time of initial illness onset typically occurs during a period in life when patients are heavily engaged in academic, early occupational, and interpersonal and social roles that have the potential to be diminished by cognitive impairment. Detection of neuropsychological impairments at this important life stage can facilitate the identification and isolation of specific cognitive targets for treatment via medical, psychological, or rehabilitative and compensational treatments. Neuropsychological assessment at this time may also provide useful baseline cognitive data that can serve as a basis to compare future changes in cognitive status that may result from intervening treatments, illness progression, comorbidity variables, or other sources of functional change.

The present analysis also provides some direction regarding the specific cognitive functions that are associated with functional outcome and that should thus be evaluated in the course of neuropsychological evaluation. Although it would be most useful to obtain a comprehensive evaluation, this may not always be possible given resource and time restrictions. At the very least, an evaluation should include measures of verbal and nonverbal memory function, the former including a task assessing verbal list learning. Another important area that should be assessed is the domain of executive function, via tasks such as verbal fluency, auditory working memory, and attentional and mental set shifting. Also, it appears prudent to include measures of attention and sustained attention or vigilance, given the sensitivity of these measures to bipolar disorder (Clark and Goodwin 2004). The use of brief mental status or screening cognitive instruments has a very limited utility in this context for several reasons. As this review reveals, cognitive screening measures were typically less associated with psychosocial function than were more psychometrically sound measures of specific cognitive ability such as memory, likely as a function of diminished sensitivity to impairment in the former measures (e.g., de Jager et al. 2002). Finally, the most useful neuropsychological findings are most likely to be those that reflect trait-related or symptom-invariant deficits. Thus, patients should be evaluated during asymptomatic or euthymic periods, rather than in the midst of an acute mood or psychotic episode.

In addition to predicting deficits in everyday functioning that may arise from cognitive impairments, neuropsychological evaluation may provide beneficial information that helps explain the source of functional impairment. For example, in patients with clear and documented psychosocial impairments, neuropsychological evaluation can help sort out whether problems arise from cognitive impairment or other factors. For individuals who indeed demonstrate impairments, a richer understanding of each patient's cognitive weakness as well as strengths can direct the patient toward appropriate treatments, development of compensational strategies based on cognitive strengths, or other rehabilitative interventions formulated to help optimize functioning. In other instances, findings of intact cognitive functioning can help point to other factors that are playing a primary role in the genesis of psychosocial dysfunction. These factors may include situational or other stressors, affective symptoms, interpersonal conflicts, comorbidity, or numerous other factors. In turn, this increased understanding of the source of psychosocial disability can lead to selection of more appropriate treatments.

Conclusions

In many regards, research on the association between cognitive and psychosocial functioning in bipolar disorder is still in its infancy. Nevertheless, it is increasingly clear that an important determinant of psychosocial disability is underlying cognitive impairment. The demonstrated link between cognitive impairment and global and specific psychosocial disability provides further empirical evidence for the utility of neuropsychological assessment in the context of bipolar disorder and psychiatric illness in general. Although the relevance and utility of neuropsychological assessment have long been recognized in the fields of neurology and neurosurgery, the importance of such assessment to psychiatry has only more recently been discussed (Keefe 1995).

Despite the initial strides in connecting cognitive deficits to psychosocial functioning, there is considerably less understanding of the processes or mechanisms that may link cognitive deficits to poor psychosocial functioning in bipolar disorder. This is partly owing to the fact that with some exceptions, research in this area has largely proceeded on an empirically rather than theoretically driven basis. As reviewed by Green et al. (2000), much work is needed to identify factors or variables that may mediate the link between cognition and psychosocial function in schizophrenia, such as learning ability/potential, social cognition, or other constructs. Such variables may also be relevant to bipolar disorder, although preliminary evidence indicates that learning potential and emotional face processing may not be obvious mediators of psychosocial outcome (Harmer et al. 2002; Laes and Sponheim 2006). Additionally, the relationship between psychosocial dysfunction and other concepts such as poor insight or metacognition deserves further study in bipolar disorder (Varga et al. 2006). Finally, given the variable findings with regard to executive function correlates of psychosocial outcome, there is a need for further specification of executive function components that may correspond to specific aspects of psychosocial dysfunction. By providing a better theoretical framework and understanding of the mechanisms underlying psychosocial dysfunction in bipolar disorder, the next wave of studies may identify more specific targets for treatment or remediation.

Take-Home Points

- Impaired psychosocial functioning is evident in a substantial proportion of individuals with bipolar disorder, even in the absence of affective symptoms.

- Overall functioning, as measured on the Global Assessment of Functioning Scale (GAF), has been shown to correlate with memory and components of executive function in individuals with bipolar disorder. When assessment scales other than the GAF are used, global functional impairment has also been linked with verbal memory deficits. At 1-year follow-up, data show that functional impairment may be predicted by baseline deficits in attention and ideational fluency.

- Cognitive deficits have been more robustly associated with objective, clinician-based assessments of impaired psychosocial functioning than with patients' self-reported assessments of functional status.

- Intact occupational functioning is associated with intact verbal memory and executive function (notably, fluency and attentional shifting).

- Links between psychosocial impairment and cognitive function in patients with bipolar disorder remain robust after controlling in multivariate models for the influence of affective or other psychiatric symptoms.

- Baseline assessment of attention, verbal and nonverbal memory (i.e., verbal list learning), and executive function may help to establish a benchmark for longitudinal assessment and anticipate the likelihood of functional impairment even after resolution of symptoms from an index affective episode.

- Neuropsychological assessment can also play a role in explaining the source of psychosocial impairment and help direct treatment and rehabilitation.

References

Altshuler LL, Ventura J, van Gorp WG, et al: Neurocognitive function in clinically stable men with bipolar I disorder or schizophrenia and normal control subjects. Biol Psychiatry 56:560–569, 2004

Amador XF, Flaum M, Andreasen NC, et al: Awareness of illness in schizophrenia and schizoaffective and mood disorders. Arch Gen Psychiatry 51:826–836, 1994

American Psychiatric Association: Diagnostic and Statistical Manual of Mental Disorders, 3rd Edition, Revised. Washington, DC, American Psychiatric Association, 1987

American Psychiatric Association: Diagnostic and Statistical Manual of Mental Disorders, 4th Edition, Text Revision. Washington, DC, American Psychiatric Association, 2000

Atre-Vaidya N, Taylor MA, Seidenberg M, et al: Cognitive deficits, psychopathology, and psychosocial functioning in bipolar mood disorder. Neuropsychiatry Neuropsychol Behav Neurol 11:120–126, 1998

Bauer MS, Kirk GF, Gavin C, et al: Determinants of functional outcome and healthcare costs in bipolar disorder: a high-intensity follow-up study. J Affect Disord 65:231–241, 2001

Carlson GA, Bromet EJ, Driessens C, et al: Age at onset, childhood psychopathology, and 2-year outcome in psychotic bipolar disorder. Am J Psychiatry 159:307–309, 2002

Clark L, Goodwin GM: State- and trait-related deficits in sustained attention in bipolar disorder. Eur Arch Psychiatry Clin Neurosci 254:61–68, 2004

Conus P, Cotton S, Abdel-Baki A, et al: Symptomatic and functional outcome 12 months after a first episode of psychotic mania: barriers to recovery in a catchment area sample. Bipolar Disord 8:221–231, 2006

Coryell W, Scheftner W, Keller M, et al: The enduring psychosocial consequences of mania and depression. Am J Psychiatry 150:720–726, 1993

Deckersbach T, Savage CR, Reilly-Harrington N, et al: Episodic memory impairment in bipolar disorder and obsessive-compulsive disorder: the role of memory strategies. Bipolar Disord 6:233–244, 2004

de Jager CA, Milwain E, Budge M: Early detection of isolated memory deficits in the elderly: the need for more sensitive neuropsychological tests. Psychol Med 32:483–491, 2002

Depp CA, Davis CE, Mittal D, et al: Health-related quality of life and functioning of middle-aged and elderly adults with bipolar disorder. J Clin Psychiatry 67:215–221, 2006

Dickerson FB, Boronow JJ, Stallings CR, et al: Association between cognitive functioning and employment status of persons with bipolar disorder. Psychol Serv 55:54–58, 2004

Dion GL, Tohen M, Anthony WA, et al: Symptoms and functioning of patients with bipolar disorder six months after hospitalization. Hosp Community Psychiatry 39:652–657, 1988

Endicott J, Spitzer RL, Fleiss JL, et al: The Global Assessment Scale: a procedure for measuring overall severity of psychiatric disturbance. Arch Gen Psychiatry 33:766–771, 1976

Ghaemi SN, Rosenquist KJ: Is insight in mania state-dependent? a meta-analysis. J Nerv Ment Dis 192:771–775, 2004

Gildengers AG, Butters MA, Seligman K, et al: Cognitive functioning in late-life bipolar disorder. Am J Psychiatry 161:736–738, 2004

Gitlin MJ, Swendsen J, Heller TL, et al: Relapse and impairment in bipolar disorder. Am J Psychiatry 152:1635–1640, 1995

Goldberg JF, Harrow M: Subjective life satisfaction and objective functional outcome in bipolar and unipolar mood disorders: a longitudinal analysis. J Affect Disord 89:79–89, 2005

Goldman HH, Skodol AE, Lave TR: Revising Axis V for DSM-IV: a review of measures of social functioning. Am J Psychiatry 149:1148–1156, 1992

Goodwin FK, Jamison KR: Manic-Depressive Illness: Bipolar Disorder and Recurrent Depression, 2nd Edition. New York, Oxford University Press, 2007

Green MF: Cognitive impairment and functional outcome in schizophrenia and bipolar disorder. J Clin Psychiatry 67:3–8, 2006

Green MF, Kern RS, Braff DL, et al: Neurocognitive deficits and functional outcome in schizophrenia: are we measuring the "right stuff"? Schizophr Bull 26:119–136, 2000

Green MF, Kern RS, Heaton RK: Longitudinal studies of functional outcome in schizophrenia: implications for MATRICS. Schizophr Res 72:41–51, 2004

Harmer CJ, Grayson L, Goodwin GM: Enhanced recognition of disgust in bipolar illness. Biol Psychiatry 51:298–304, 2002

Harrow M, Goldberg JF, Grossman LS, et al: Outcome in manic disorders: a naturalistic follow-up study. Arch Gen Psychiatry 47:665–671, 1990

Harrow M, Grossman LS, Herbener ES, et al: Ten-year outcome: patients with schizoaffective disorders, schizophrenia, affective disorders and mood-incongruent psychotic symptoms. Br J Psychiatry 177:421–426, 2000

Jaeger J, Berns S, Loftus S, et al: Neurocognitive test performance predicts functional recovery from acute exacerbation leading to hospitalization in bipolar disorder. Bipolar Disord 9:93–102, 2007

Jiang HK: A prospective one-year follow-up study of patients with bipolar affective disorder. Zhonghua Yi Xue Za Zhi (Taipei) 62:477–486, 1999

Judd LL, Akiskal HS, Schettler PJ, et al: Psychosocial disability in the course of bipolar I and II disorders: a prospective, comparative, longitudinal study. Arch Gen Psychiatry 62:1322–1330, 2005

Kebede D, Alem A, Shibire T, et al: Symptomatic and functional outcome of bipolar disorder in Butajira, Ethiopia. J Affect Disord 90:239–249, 2006

Keck PE Jr, McElroy SL, Strakowski SM, et al: 12-month outcome of patients with bipolar disorder following hospitalization for a manic or mixed episode. Am J Psychiatry 155:646–652, 1998

Keck PE Jr, McElroy SL, Havens JR, et al: Psychosis in bipolar disorder: phenomenology and impact on morbidity and course of illness. Compr Psychiatry 44:263–269, 2003

Keefe RS: The contribution of neuropsychology to psychiatry. Am J Psychiatry 152:6–15, 1995

Kieseppä T, Tuulio-Henriksson A, Haukka J, et al: Memory and verbal learning functions in twins with bipolar-I disorder, and the role of information-processing speed. Psychol Med 35:205–215, 2005

Krabbendam L, Arts B, van Os J, et al: Cognitive functioning in patients with schizophrenia and bipolar disorder: a quantitative review. Schizophr Res 80:137–149, 2005

Kraepelin E: Manic-Depressive Insanity. Edinburgh, UK, Livingstone, 1921

Kurtz MM: Neurocognitive impairment across the lifespan in schizophrenia: an update. Schizophr Res 74:15–26, 2005

Laes JR, Sponheim SR: Does cognition predict community function only in schizophrenia? a study of schizophrenia patients, bipolar affective disorder patients, and community control subjects. Schizophr Res 84:121–131, 2006

Laroche I, Hodgins S, Toupin J: Correlations between symptoms and social adjustment in patients suffering from schizophrenia or major affective disorder. Can J Psychiatry 40:27–34, 1995

MacQueen GM, Young LT, Joffe RT: A review of psychosocial outcome in patients with bipolar disorder. Acta Psychiatr Scand 103:163–170, 2001

Martinez-Aran A, Penadés R, Vieta E, et al: Executive function in patients with remitted bipolar disorder and schizophrenia and its relationship with functional outcome. Psychother Psychosom 71:39–46, 2002

Martinez-Aran, A, Vieta E, Colom F, et al: Cognitive impairment in euthymic bipolar patients: implications for clinical and functional outcome. Bipolar Disord 6:224–232, 2004a

Martinez-Aran A, Vieta E, Reinares M, et al: Cognitive function across manic or hypomanic, depressed, and euthymic states in bipolar disorder. Am J Psychiatry 161:262–270, 2004b

Michalak EE, Yatham LN, Lam RW: Quality of life in bipolar disorder: a review of the literature. Health and Quality of Life Outcomes [Epub] 3:72, 2005

Olley AL, Malhi GS, Bachelor J, et al: Executive functioning and theory of mind in euthymic bipolar disorder. Bipolar Disord 7 (suppl 5):43–52, 2005

Robinson LJ, Thompson JM, Gallagher P, et al: A meta-analysis of cognitive deficits in euthymic patients with bipolar disorder. J Affect Disord 93:105–115, 2006

Strakowski SM, Keck PE Jr, McElroy SL, et al: Twelve month outcome after a first hospitalization for affective psychosis. Arch Gen Psychiatry 55:49–55, 1998

Thompson JM, Gallagher P, Hughes JH, et al: Neurocognitive impairment in euthymic patients with bipolar affective disorder. Br J Psychiatry 186:32–40, 2005

Tohen M, Waternaux CM, Tsuang MT: Outcome in mania: a 4-year prospective follow-up of 75 patients utilizing survival analysis. Arch Gen Psychiatry 47:1106–1111, 1990

Tohen M, Hennen J, Zarate CM, et al: Two-year syndromal and functional recovery in 219 cases of first-episode major affective disorder with psychotic features. Am J Psychiatry 157:220–228, 2000

Torrent C, Martinez-Aran A, Daban C, et al: Cognitive impairment in bipolar II disorder. Br J Psychiatry 189:254–259, 2006

Torres IJ, Boudreau VG, Yatham LN: Neuropsychological functioning in euthymic bipolar disorder: a meta-analysis. Acta Psychiatr Scand 116(suppl):17–26, 2007

Tsuang MT, Woolson RF, Fleming JA: Long-term outcome of major psychoses. Arch Gen Psychiatry 39:1295–1301, 1979

Varga M, Magnusson A, Flekkoy K, et al: Insight, symptoms and neurocognition in bipolar I patients. J Affect Disord 91:1–9, 2006

Yatham LN, Lecrubier Y, Fieve RR, et al: Quality of life in patients with bipolar I depression: data from 920 patients. Bipolar Disord 6:379–385, 2004

Zarate CA Jr, Tohen M, Land M, et al: Functional impairment and cognition in bipolar disorder. Psychiatr Q 71:309–329, 2000

Zubieta JK, Huguelet P, O'Neil RL, et al: Cognitive function in euthymic bipolar I disorder. Psychol Res 102:9–20, 2001

11

Cognition Across the Life Span

Clinical Implications for Older Adults With Bipolar Disorder

Eduard Vieta, M.D., Ph.D.
Anabel Martinez-Aran, Ph.D.
Joseph F. Goldberg, M.D.

In this chapter, we address illness characteristics that affect cognition over the life span of patients with bipolar disorder. Previous chapters have touched on neurobiological factors associated with cognitive dysfunction in bipolar disorder, such as functional neuroanatomical anomalies or genetic underpinnings. Here, we consider the totality of both neurobiological and clinical correlates of neurocognitive dysfunction, with particular emphasis on their manifestations throughout the life span—from prodromal phases though the aging process. Despite the limited breadth of literature regarding geriatric bipolar disorder in general, we review existing data on age-inappropriate cognitive decline in older adults with bipolar disorder.

As described more fully in Chapter 10 of this volume, "Cognition and Functional Outcome in Bipolar Disorder," the association between psychopathological symptoms and functional disability may be less robust than generally thought, but by contrast, persistent cognitive deficits may be more closely linked to social and occupational functioning—as seen in other severe psychiatric disorders such as schizophrenia (Carpenter and Strauss 1991). The association between affective symptoms and impaired functioning is overestimated by most clinicians, when cognitive deficits more likely constitute better predictors of poor outcome (Jaeger and Berns 1999; Jaeger et al. 2007). For this reason, it is important that mental health professionals pay close attention to cognitive complaints in patients with bipolar disorder. More suitable pharmacological and psychological interventions are needed to improve cognitive impairment and, consequently, functional outcome, as described further in this chapter.

Factors Associated With Poor Cognitive Functioning

In this section, we summarize a number of factors that, directly or indirectly, may influence cognitive functioning in bipolar disorder.

Premorbid Deficits

There is little empirical data from which to determine how common it is for cognitive deficits to arise in individuals before the onset of bipolar disorder because very few studies have been carried out with high-risk populations. One notable observation, described from the Israeli Draft Board Registry, has been that premorbid intellectual and reading comprehension skills among adolescents who were later hospitalized for nonpsychotic bipolar mania appear indistinguishable from those who remained psychiatrically healthy (Reichenberg et al. 2002). By contrast, adolescents who subsequently developed schizophrenia showed marked impairment across multiple intellectual and comprehension measures. Similarly, in the Maudsley Family Study, premorbid intelligence quotient (IQ) was found to be lower among individuals who later developed schizophrenia, but not bipolar disorder, as compared with healthy controls (Toulopoulou et al. 2006).

Precisely what characteristics best define the prodromal phase of bipolar disorder remain at issue, and the extent to which cognitive manifestations of illness may be evident before, or alongside, the first emergence of affective signs in high-risk individuals is largely unknown (Correll et al. 2007).

Genetic Contributions

Support for a genetic contribution to cognitive dysfunction in bipolar disorder is found in a study by Decina et al. (1983), in which children of bipolar probands had significantly higher Verbal IQ (VIQ) than Performance IQ (PIQ) scores as measured by the Wechsler Intelligence Scale for Children—Revised. Cornblatt et al. (1989, 1992) studied children with an affectively ill parent and observed some degree of attentional impairment using a continuous performance test. Nevertheless, consistent with the findings in affected adults, the deficits in affective-risk children were of lesser magnitude than those of schizophrenia-risk children, not stable over time, and not directly related to later behavioral disturbances. Winters et al. (1981) found that the high-risk children showed increased reaction time on a visual search task but did not demonstrate dysfunctions in other cognitive domains. Finally, McDonough-Ryan et al. (2002) reported a significantly higher incidence of VIQ-PIQ discrepancy in subjects at high risk for bipolar disorder than in healthy controls. Moreover, the high-risk group performed worse than healthy controls on measures of reading, spelling, and arithmetic.

Psychotic Symptoms

As noted in Chapter 5 of this volume, "The Impact of Mood, Anxiety, and Psychotic Symptoms on Cognition in Patients With Bipolar Disorder," the presence of psychotic symptoms, or specifically the previous history of psychotic symptoms, appears to be associated with poorer cognitive functioning in patients with bipolar disorder (Daban et al. 2006; Martinez-Aran et al. 2004b; Rocca et al. 2008), although not all studies agree (Selva et al. 2007). Albus et al. (1996) studied first-episode patients with and without psychotic symptoms. Those patients with psychotic symptoms showed poorer performance on cognitive measures, independent of diagnosis (unipolar disorder, bipolar disorder, schizophrenia). Consistent with these findings, Martinez-Aran et al. (2008) observed that bipolar patients with a prior history of psychotic symptoms were more impaired on verbal memory functioning than patients without such a history. In contrast, current evidence indicates that in schizophrenia, cognitive dysfunction is a more stable trait and is associated with negative and disorganized syndromes rather than with positive symptoms. Further investigation of the impact of psychotic symptoms on neurocognition is warranted, as research on this issue in bipolar disorder is limited.

Bipolar Subtype

Most of what is known about cognition in bipolar disorder across the life span is derived from studies focused on bipolar I patients or mixed samples of bipolar I and II subjects. Only Harkavy-Friedman et al. (2006) and Torrent et al. (2006) have included pure bipolar II samples in their studies of cognitive function. The former study focused specifically on suicide attempters and found that both bipolar I and bipolar II patients performed significantly worse than healthy controls on a wide range of neurocognitive measures. Moreover, although performance on most measures was comparable between bipolar I and bipolar II subjects, it was significantly poorer for bipolar II than bipolar I subjects on a psychomotor task and on a measure of selective attention/inhibition (Harkavy-Friedman et al. 2006). In contrast, Torrent et al. (2006) reported that although bipolar II patients were impaired on an executive function task, the Wisconsin Card Sorting Test, bipolar I subjects were generally more impaired than patients with bipolar II disorder. The extent to which differences in cognitive function between bipolar I patients and bipolar II patients may relate to a history of psychotic symptoms (which are by definition absent in bipolar II disorder) is still a matter of debate; however, cognitive problems may be more inclusive of the bipolar spectrum phenotype. Taylor Tavares et al. (2007) found that moderately depressed, unmedicated bipolar II patients appeared cognitively intact relative to a comparison group of unmedicated unipolar depressed patients, with the latter group demonstrating pervasive executive dysfunction (i.e., impairments in spatial working memory, attentional set shifting, decision making, and impulsivity), suggesting that these cognitive deficits are not "specific" to the bipolar spectrum.

Subclinical Symptomatology

There is evidence that many patients with bipolar disorder are symptomatic most of the time, despite adequate treatment (Fava 1996, 1997, 1999; Judd et al. 2002). However, in many studies, patients are simply described as euthymic, as recovered, or as ambulatory outpatients. The presence of subsyndromal symptoms appears to influence the general level of functioning in these patients (Fava 1999; Kessing 1998; Martinez-Aran et al. 2004a, 2004b). Residual depressive symptomatology, which is very common, may be easily confused with negative symptoms (e.g., apathy, abulia, anhedonia) and appears to be correlated with social maladjustment (Bauwens et al. 1991) and cognitive impairment (Kessing 1998; Martinez-Aran et al. 2000, 2002). Some authors suggest that it is difficult to assess subclinical symptoms (Ferrier et al. 1999); therefore, only a few studies have included measures of the extent of subclinical depressive symptoms at the time of neuropsychological assessment (Abas et al. 1990; Kessing 1998; McKay et al. 1995; Trichard et al. 1995). The presence of subsyndromal or persistent residual depressive symptoms has been shown to be associated with more difficulties in social and occupational functioning (Altshuler et al. 2002, 2006; Ferrier et al. 1999); however, the direction of causality is not clear because it is feasible that patients with significant psychosocial problems are more likely to develop depressive symptoms (Altshuler et al. 2002).

Hormonal Factors

Hypercortisolemia can occur in the depressed and manic phases of bipolar disorder. Some studies have suggested that high levels of cortisol may produce damage to the hippocampus, even after the acute episode has resolved. Hippocampal dysfunction, if present, could partially explain the impaired performance found in neuropsychological measures of declarative learning and memory (Altshuler 1993; van Gorp et al. 1998). The hippocampus provides negative feedback to the hypothalamic-pituitary-adrenal axis and has an important role in declarative memory, emotional processing, and vulnerability to stress in patients with mood disorders (Brown et al. 1999). Nevertheless, a study on the neurocognitive performance of euthymic bipolar patients did not find any association between cognitive measures and hypercortisolemia (Thompson et al. 2005).

Prohaska et al. (1996) found that subclinically hypothyroid subjects who were medicated with lithium displayed a consistent, but nonsignificant, pattern of worse performance on measures of verbal learning and memory than euthyroid subjects. Tremont and Stern (1997) obtained similar results and observed that cognitive side effects improved in patients treated with thyroxine. Performance on these measures was more highly correlated with serum thyrotropin levels than with serum lithium levels.

Therefore, hormonal factors may be associated with neurocognitive dysfunction, and these relationships warrant further empirical investigation. Cognitive dysfunctions may be markers of vulnerability to bipolar disorder relapse (Fava 1999) and may shed light on neurobiological disturbances present during the euthymic state (Vieta et al. 1997, 1999).

Amino Acids

Abnormal elevation of homocysteine, the homologue of cysteine and metabolite of methionine, has been implicated as a correlate of several cardiovascular, metabolic, and central nervous system disorders. Elevated levels of homocysteine have been associated with cognitive impairment in otherwise healthy older adults, and at least one recent report suggests that the presence of elevated homocysteine levels in euthymic bipolar disorder patients may, independent of age, be associated with overall cognitive deficits and, in particular, impairment in attention, language, and immediate recall (Dittmann et al. 2007). Given a growing interest in the role of homocysteine and folate metabolism in depression, it remains unknown whether L-methylfolate supplementation could exert a beneficial effect on cognitive problems associated with depression.

Also, as noted in Chapter 8 of this volume, "Pharmacological Strategies to Enhance Neurocognitive Function," supplemental oral intake of the sulfur amino acid taurine has been suggested by some investigators as a possible cognitive-enhancement strategy in healthy volunteers. We are unaware of known adverse cognitive consequences associated with taurine-deficient dietary intake, although the ability to conserve taurine in mammals appears to decline with advancing age.

Duration of Illness

Lifetime duration of bipolar disorder has been associated with cognitive dysfunction (Johnstone et al. 1985), and a negative impact on memory and executive functions has been found (van Gorp et al. 1998). Findings with respect to the impact of longer duration of illness on cognitive impairment are contradictory. In their systematic review, Robinson and Ferrier (2006) showed that five of 11 studies reported at least a significant relationship between chronicity of bipolar disorder and a cognitive measure. The length of illness negatively correlated with scores on tests of executive function (Clark et al. 2002; Thompson et al. 2005), psychomotor speed (Martinez-Aran et al. 2004a; Thompson et al. 2005), and verbal memory (Cavanagh et al. 2002; Clark et al. 2002; Deckersbach et al. 2004b; Martinez-Aran et al. 2004a). Proton magnetic resonance spectroscopy studies also have reported an asssociation between illness duration and hippocampal neuronal loss (as measured by N-acetylaspartate levels) (Deicken et al. 2003). Verbal memory is the cognitive domain that has been most consistently associated with duration of illness. In this regard, a higher number of past manic episodes was also associated with poorer performance on verbal memory measures. On the other hand, the other six studies that did not report positive findings comparing length of illness and cognitive functioning investigated smaller patient samples, suggesting that there could be a problem of statistical power.

Length of Time Euthymic

Duration of euthymia is the length of time an individual is in clinical remission before neuropsychological testing. None of the studies have reported any significant associations between duration of euthymia and performance on cognitive tests (Clark et al. 2002; El-Badri et al. 2001; MacQueen et al. 2001; Thompson et al. 2005).

Number of Episodes

Cognitive deficits in euthymic patients seem to be related to the frequency of episodes in both bipolar and unipolar patients (Kessing 1998), with manic episodes impacting neuropsychological impairment most extensively (Martinez-Aran et al. 2004b; Morice 1990; van Gorp et al. 1998). Moreover, as depicted in Figure 11–1, the risk of the eventual development of dementia in patients with either unipolar depression or bipolar disorder increases as a function of episode number. Patients with recurrent manic episodes have shown persistent impairment at follow-up (McKay et al. 1995), although research evidence is still limited. Number of episodes of either polarity has been associated with dimished verbal fluency in euthymic bipolar patients as compared with healthy controls (Rocca et al. 2008).

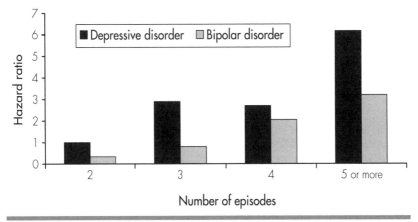

FIGURE 11–1. Risk of developing dementia increases with the number of episodes in patients with unipolar depression or bipolar disorder.

Hazard ratio: the rate of a diagnosis of dementia for patients with a given number of episodes compared with the rate for patients with one prior episode.

Source. Adapted from Kessing LV, Andersen PK: "Does the Risk of Developing Dementia Increase With the Number of Episodes in Patients With Depressive Disorder and in Patients With Bipolar Disorder?" *Journal of Neurology, Neurosurgery, and Psychiatry* 75:1662–1666, 2004.

Rapid cycling and severity of the episodes may also contribute to neurocognitive impairment (Johnson and Magaro 1987). Convincing correlations between cognitive impairment and number of episodes make a strong argument for improved long-term management of illness.

Robinson and Ferrier (2006) reported data from 13 studies that demonstrated a correlation between the number of affective episodes and performance on cognitive measures. Ten of these studies considered the impact of depressive and manic episodes separately.

Manic Episodes

Most studies that have assessed illness burden with cognitive function (7 of 10 reported by Robinson and Ferrier [2006]) have reported significant negative correlations between the number of past manic episodes and cognitive ability. The measures that were most strongly correlated with manic episodes were those involving verbal memory and executive function tasks. Poorer performance on verbal memory tasks was associated with a higher number of past manic episodes (Cavanagh et al. 2002; Clark et al. 2002; Deckersbach et al. 2004b; Martinez-Aran et al. 2004a; van Gorp et al. 1998). With regard to the complex domain of executive function, a relationship between impaired concept formation and more manic episodes

has also been observed (van Gorp et al. 1998; Zubieta et al. 2001), but
other measures of executive function do not appear to correlate with number of manic episodes. A single study has reported a similar relationship between performance on measures of visual memory and number of manic
episodes (Deckersbach et al. 2004a).

Depressive Episodes

Nearly half of the studies reviewed by Robinson and Ferrier (2006) reported significant relationships between past depressive episodes and cognitive performance. Despite the consistency of this finding, in a meta-
analysis conducted by Robinson et al. (2006), cognitive correlations with
depressive episodes were found to be weaker than those reported for manic
episodes. Significant relationships have been described for the number of
depressive episodes and executive function (Clark et al. 2002; Thompson
et al. 2005; Zubieta et al. 2001), verbal learning (Clark et al. 2002; Deckersbach et al. 2004b), visual memory (Deckersbach et al. 2004a; Mac-
Queen et al. 2001), and spatial working memory (Clark et al. 2002).

Number of Hospitalizations

Most studies have reported that bipolar patients with a higher number of
hospitalizations demonstrate poorer performance on cognitive measures.
Rubinsztein et al. (2000) described a relationship between visual memory
measures and the number of admissions, whereas Martinez-Aran et al.
(2004b) observed that the number of hospitalizations correlated with verbal memory performance. Thompson et al. (2005) reported relationships
between number of hospitalizations and several neuropsychological domains, including verbal fluency, spatial memory, psychomotor speed, and
executive function. In contrast, Zubieta et al. (2001) described a more specific pattern of relationship between executive functioning measures and
admissions for mania. In contrast, Clark et al. (2002) reported a relationship between cognitive performance on several tasks and admissions for
depressive episodes. It is likely that the number of hospital admissions constitutes an indirect measure of the severity of individual episodes as well as
of the course of illness.

Age at Illness Onset

A single study has reported a relationship between later age at onset of bipolar disorder and poorer performance on measures of psychomotor speed
and executive function (Martinez-Aran et al. 2004a). Several other studies
did not find a significant relationship between age at onset and cognitive
performance (Deckersbach et al. 2004a, 2004b; El-Badri et al. 2001;
Zubieta et al. 2001).

The Aging Process

Many older patients with bipolar disorder have concomitant neurological risk factors or illnesses. Although very few studies have focused on the neuropsychology of elderly adults with bipolar disorder, existing studies provide evidence of cognitive deterioration in the longitudinal assessment of older patients (Dhingra and Rabins 1991) and greater cognitive impairment in older than younger patients (Savard et al. 1980). Gildengers et al. (2004) reported that more than half of their elderly euthymic bipolar subjects exhibited significant deficits on neuropsychological tests compared with age- and education-matched healthy comparison subjects, especially on tasks requiring sustained attention and executive control of working memory. Martino et al. (2008) observed slower motor speed, poorer verbal memory, and more executive dysfunction in a group of 20 elderly adults with bipolar disorder compared with a group of healthy controls. Similarly, Young et al. (2006) compared a group of 70 older adults with bipolar disorder (mean age 68.9 years) to 37 older adults without bipolar disorder (mean age 74.8 years) and found the bipolar subjects to have lower total scores on the Mini-Mental State Examination (MMSE) (Folstein et al. 1975) and lower scores on the Mattis Dementia Rating Scale Initiation-Perseveration and Memory subscales (Jurica et al. 2001), independent of mania symptoms. By contrast, Depp and Jeste (2004) found little evidence for substantial global cognitive impairment, with only 6% of their sample falling below a commonly used cutoff for cognitive impairment on the Mattis Dementia Rating Scale.

The prevalence of dementia in older people with bipolar disorder has received inadequate attention. The incidence of concomitant dementia seems to be highly variable, ranging from 3% to 25%, within samples of inpatients with bipolar disorder (Broadhead and Jacoby 1990; Himmelhoch et al. 1980; Ponce et al. 1999; Stone 1989). In a comparison of older inpatients with unipolar and bipolar depression and younger patients with affective disorders, Burt et al. (2000) found that the older patients showed poorer performance on measures of delayed recall. Significantly worse cognitive performance was also observed in older bipolar patients than in unipolar patients (Savard et al. 1980). In contrast, compared with institutionalized patients with schizophrenia, institutionalized patients with chronic affective disorder had an impaired neuropsychological profile, with worse performance on the MMSE, word list learning, delayed recall, construction, and naming (Harvey et al. 1997). Another interesting finding, from a study by Kessing and Andersen (2004), suggests that the risk of developing dementia seems to increase with the number of episodes in unipolar depressive and bipolar affective disorders. On average, the rate of dementia tended to in-

crease 13% with every episode leading to hospital admission for unipolar patients and 6% with every episode leading to admission for bipolar patients.
Further research is needed to examine whether cognitive decline in bipolar
disorder is greater than that expected from normal aging, as some investigators have failed to find significant differences in the cognitive status of
first-episode and multiepisode bipolar patients (Nehra et al. 2006).

From the standpoint of clinical management, an abrupt deterioration in
a person's cognitive functioning—as with any acute mental status change—
should signal the need for an appropriate medical or neurological workup
to identify potential reversible causes of dementia or delirium. Typically,
this would include a complete neurological examination, as well as measurement of electrolytes, complete blood cell count, thyroid function tests,
measurement of serum B_{12} and folic acid levels, toxicology screen, rapid
plasma regain, HIV test (if risk factors are present), neuroimaging if indicated, and heavy metal screening if indicated (e.g., in the presence of a pe-
ripheral neuropathy or known toxic exposure). Before concluding that
newly observed cognitive decline in older adults with bipolar disorder is
age appropriate or attributable to bipolar disorder itself, clinicians must
remain alert to other potential neuropsychiatric etiologies of cognitive
dysfunction (see Chapter 12 of this volume, "Summary and Assessment
Recommendations for Practitioners").

Clinicians also must bear in mind that depression itself commonly presents with cognitive complaints, and efforts should be made to assure the
absence of clinical depression before ascribing problems with attention,
memory, or information processing to other potential causes. Clinically,
depressed patients may be more prone to express apathy or indifference
than to make efforts to conceal a cognitive deficit about which they may
have some awareness (e.g., by refusing to answer a question, labeling a
question as silly or irrelevant, or refusing to comply with formal testing).

It is often difficult to discriminate between cognitive deficits consistent
with depression and age-appropriate cognitive decline in older adults.
Consider the following example.

Case Vignette 1

A 78-year-old male retired professional with a history of bipolar II disorder,
hypertension, myocardial infarction with coronary artery stenting, chronic
renal insufficiency, and chronic intermittent alcohol abuse sought consultation for depression. He had twice previously undergone courses of bilateral electroconvulsive therapy (ECT), once 4 months ago and another time
4 years earlier for prior depressive episodes. He was now taking divalproex
750 mg/day with extended-release bupropion 300 mg/day. He conveyed
a helpless demeanor and described classic melancholic features with vegetative signs. His exam was notable for his blunted affect, monotonous and

at times halting speech, frequent sighing, and diffuse but mild psychomotor agitation. He had no tremor or focal neurological signs. There were no current or recent hypomanic signs, no suicidal features, and no clear delusions or hallucinations. However, his thought processes were notable for apparent instances of thought blocking, tangential and circumstantial thinking, and perseveration about his predicament and associated worries. His orientation and attention were intact, but he frequently answered "I don't know" in response to questions testing sustained concentration and both short- and long-term memory. His MMSE score was 26. He was euthyroid, with no remarkable laboratory abnormalities other than a serum creatinine level of 1.9 mg/dL and a serum valproic acid level of 62 μg/mL.

Notable in this case were the patient's lack of attempts to conceal memory or concentration problems and the general preservation of higher-order cognitive functions (i.e., attention), coupled with the presence of severe depression. Neurotoxicity from divalproex appeared unlikely, given his low therapeutic serum valproic acid level and the absence of focal neurological signs. The history of cardiovascular disease and alcohol abuse raised obvious concerns about cerebrovascular insufficiency that could predispose to dementia, and the potential cognitive aftereffects of bilateral ECT in an older adult with possible superimposed structural brain deficits due to chronic alcohol use or hypertension posed additional confounds for differential diagnosis. The frontal lobe features suggested by his perseveration were thought to reflect depression and/or cerebral microvascular disease. The distinction between bipolar depression with versus without underlying dementia could not be made in the presence of severe melancholia. Stimulant augmentation was considered but deemed a relative contraindication due to cardiovascular risk. The patient declined a recommendation for further ECT based on concerns about further cognitive worsening, and opted instead for augmentation of divalproex with olanzapine 2.5 mg/day, to target agitation and mood, as well as lamotrigine 12.5 mg/day (dosed with pharmacokinetic appreciation for divalproex cotherapy, as well as renal insufficiency), to target attention and depressive features.

Pharmacotherapy: Broad Considerations

There are no published studies that specifically address the cognitive effects of traditional mood stabilizers or related pharmacotherapies for older adult patients with bipolar disorder. All atypical antipsychotics marketed in the United States (including risperidone, olanzapine, quetiapine, aripiprazole, ziprasidone, and clozapine) have been identified by the U.S. Food and Drug Administration (FDA) as increasing the risk for sudden death when used in dementia-related psychosis; the risks stem from a variety of possible causes that include cardiovascular and cerebrovascular events, esophageal dysmotility, and falls. However, because most elderly dementia patients have a preexisting increased prevalence of cerebrovascular insufficiency or coronary artery disease, it is difficult to estimate with confidence the unique impact that atypical antipsychotics may contribute to this overall risk. No pharmacotherapy is presently approved by the FDA for the treatment of psychosis in elderly dementia patients (regardless of the presence of bipolar disorder), prompting the need for caution and deliberation among practitioners in choosing among the likely risks and benefits of existing treatment options.

In general, practitioners must recognize the need for potential dosage reductions with all renally excreted medications in patients with diminished renal function. Older adults taking lithium are at risk for elevated serum lithium levels in the presence of malnutrition or reduced sodium intake, or if lithium is coadministered with thiazide diuretics or angiotensin II receptor antagonists, tetracycline, cyclosporine, or nonsteroidal anti-inflammatory drugs (a relative contraindication with lithium). Although chronic lithium use has been associated with end-organ effects (notably, renal insufficiency) in a minority of individuals, the duration of lithium exposure has not been directly linked with cognitive decline. Notably, in a 6-year longitudinal study, Engelsmann et al. (1988) observed stable neuropsychological performance without cognitive deterioration in patients treated with lithium. As a separate matter, clinicians also should recognize that in the aftermath of acute lithium intoxication (e.g., overdose), neurotoxic effects of lithium (including cognitive disorganization) may persist for an extended period even after serum lithium levels become undetectable, because high lithium concentrations are retained in the central nervous system.

From the standpoint of drug safety, studies using divalproex off label to treat symptoms of agitation in elderly dementia patients have yielded mixed results (reviewed by Porsteinsson 2006), with some studies reporting a possible heightened risk for hyperammonemic encephalopathy (Beyenburg et al. 2007) and poor tolerability (due mainly to somnolence) if dosed above 1,000 mg/day in patients with Alzheimer's dementia (Profenno et al. 2005). A Cochrane Review does not recommend the use of divalproex for agitation associated with dementia based on then-current knowledge, but calls for further research in this area (Lonergan et al. 2004).

Studies using either divalproex or lithium for bipolar mania in older adults are scarce and limited mainly to case series or open-label retrospective reports. One retrospective study in acute mania found higher response rates with lithium when serum levels were ≥0.8 mEq/L, and an optimal antimanic response to divalproex when dosed to produce valproic acid levels above 65 μg/mL but below 90 μg/mL (Chen et al. 1999). There are presently no published data on the adverse cognitive effects of lithium, divalproex, or other anticonvulsants with demonstrated mood-stabilizing properties (i.e., carbamazepine or lamotrigine) specifically in older adults with bipolar disorder.

As noted in Chapter 8 of this volume, procholinergic agents such as donepezil or rivastigmine as well as the antiglutamatergic agent galantamine have demonstrated significant, albeit modest, improvements in overall cognitive function in patients with dementia. Such agents generally appear safe in older adults and may be of some value as a means to target cognitive impairment. Also as noted in Chapter 8, psychostimulants can sometimes prove useful in the management of impaired attention, and, in addition, clinicians have long used psychostimulants as an adjunctive strategy for anergic depression in older adults (e.g., methylphenidate begun at 2.5 mg/day and titrated to effect by increments of about 2.5 mg/day, in once- or twice-daily doses; however, given the potential for tachyarrhythmias, consultation with a cardiologist may be advisable in patients with a history of significant coronary heart disease). There is little evidence to suggest a substantial risk for induction of mania with stimulants in bipolar patients taking a traditional mood stabilizer (Lydon and El-Mallakh 2006), although in the absence of controlled trials, caution is warranted if using this strategy in elderly adults with bipolar disorder and cognitive decline.

Adverse Cognitive Effects of Medications: Longitudinal Considerations

Lithium, antidepressants, benzodiazepines, neuroleptics, and anticholinergics may affect motor speed and memory abilities in experimental conditions. However, the effect of pharmacological treatment is still uncertain from the perspective of bipolar patients showing deficits in neuropsychological function. Furthermore, the effect of pharmacological variables on neuropsychological performance is difficult to assess because most bipolar patients have combined treatment and variable dosage. Detailed reviews of the adverse and beneficial correlates of psychotropic medications for patients with bipolar disorder are provided in this volume in Chapter 7, "Adverse Cognitive Effects of Psychotropic Medications," and Chapter 8.

It seems probable that long-term neuroleptic treatment at least partially reverses attentional deficits and improves short-term verbal memory (Cassens et al. 1990; Spohn and Strauss 1989). Despite this long-term cognitive improvement, poorer neuropsychological performance is observed in patients with high dosages of neuroleptic and anticholinergic medications (Donnelly et al. 1982). Current reviews suggest that conventional neuroleptics do not cause cognitive deficits but also do little to improve them (Green 1998). As noted in Chapter 8, most studies on antipsychotic medications (whether conventional or atypical) have focused on samples of patients with schizophrenia, and the authors have often concluded that it is the illness itself, rather than antipsychotic treatment, that appears more responsible for information processing deficits. Similarly, in the case of bipolar disorder, it is likely that cognitive impairment, when evident, arises more proximally from the illness itself than from the effects of pharmacotherapy, whether short or long term.

Other Factors

Substance abuse, which is highly prevalent in individuals with bipolar disorder, clearly worsens the course of the illness and may also cause cognitive deficits. Van Gorp et al. (1998) found that bipolar patients with alcohol dependence showed significantly worse performance on measures of frontal lobe functioning (e.g., the Wisconsin Card Sorting Test) and on some measures of verbal memory (e.g., the California Verbal Learning Test) compared with bipolar patients without alcohol dependence and health-controls. As possible explanations, the authors suggested that alcohol may affect performance on tasks of set shifting and categorization, as well as memory functioning. Nevertheless, they also indicated that bipolar patients who abused alcohol may have had a more severe form of the illness, and added that more months of illness in this comorbid group could result in greater cognitive impairment. Memory function may also be influenced by sleep disturbances (Cipolli 1995), which are quite common in patients with bipolar disorder, even during remission periods. Verbal learning has been observed to be impaired after sleep deprivation in healthy young volunteers (Drummond et al. 2000).

Memory functioning has been studied among depressed patients, whose depression was characterized by physiological symptoms, such as loss of appetite and sleep disorders, but the connection between depressive symptoms and memory functioning was not convincing (Kalska et al. 1999). The effects of benzodiazepine hypnotics should be controlled for because of possible anterograde amnesia, daytime sedation, or rebound insomnia (Vogel 1992).

The effects of other clinical variables, such as insight, rapid cycling, medication adherence, and comorbid diseases, should also be investigated. Another relevant research area is premorbid personality traits.

Conclusions

The assessment of cognitive functioning in bipolar patients is relevant because of its potential to impact psychosocial functioning in these patients. Although poor functioning may previously have been attributed to clinical variables such as psychosis or depression, recent studies have suggested an important relationship between cognitive impairment and poor psychosocial functioning (Laes and Sponheim 2006; Martinez-Aran et al. 2004a, 2004b, 2007; Zubieta et al. 2001).

A poorer clinical course of illness may also have a negative impact on cognition such that a higher number of episodes (especially manic episodes), longer duration of illness, and an increased number of hospitalizations may be related to more severe cognitive impairment. Thus, the prevention of relapse is essential in reducing the negative impact of bipolar disorder on patients' cognitive functioning. These findings reinforce a neurodegenerative hypothesis—that cognitive dysfunctions may represent a consequence of the bipolar illness process. As such, it is important for clinicians to make every effort to improve the clinical course of patients by optimizing the pharmacological treatment and including psychoeducation for patients and their families. Bipolar patients with persistent cognitive impairment may also benefit from cognitive rehabilitation in order to improve not only cognitive functioning but also their general functioning, although more research is required to determine the most effective strategies.

Nevertheless, from a neurodevelopmental standpoint, some cognitive deficits may be present before illness onset, to some degree, and possibly in only a subgroup of bipolar patients. The relative contributions of genetic liability and disease-related factors (i.e., number of episodes, and subsyndromal or acute affective symptomatology) to cognitive course in patients with bipolar disorder are unknown. Longitudinal studies are needed to assess the evolution of cognitive impairment in bipolar patients, in order to determine the stability or progression of cognitive deficit, as affected by genetic and disease-related contributors. Regardless, early diagnosis and the potential for prophylactic treatment are critical in intervening to alleviate or ameliorate cognitive decline from baseline levels of function.

The causes of cognitive impairment in elderly patients with bipolar disorder are likely heterogeneous and include neurodevelopmental anomalies, multiple episodes, vascular disease, comorbid history of substance abuse or dependence, and side effects of medication, among other factors. Further research is needed to understand how bipolar disorder affects cognition in elderly patients and whether bipolar disorder is a risk factor for subsequent dementia.

Take-Home Points

- Multiple factors bear on cognitive function in patients with bipolar disorder, the most notable being genetic contributions, psychosis, affective symptoms, substance abuse, illness duration, and episode burden (especially number of manic episodes).

• The occurrence of multiple manic and depressive episodes appears correlated with cognitive impairment. However, it is unclear whether repeated affective episodes are further associated with a progressive worsening of cognitive deficits in bipolar disorder. Some studies suggest an increased risk for eventual dementia associated with an increasing number of lifetime affective episodes.

• Taken together, existing data suggest that individuals who are at high risk for bipolar disorder (including those with a family history) will require close monitoring for early signs of bipolar illness. Early intervention followed by psychoeducation for the patient and family very early in the course of the illness may help to indirectly slow the progression of cognitive deficits by effectively preventing relapse.

References

Abas MA, Sharakian BJ, Levy R: Neuropsychological deficits and CT scan changes in elderly depressives. Psychol Med 20:507–520, 1990

Albus M, Hubmann W, Wahlheim C, et al: Contrasts in neuropsychological test profile between patients with first-episode schizophrenia and first-episode affective disorders. Acta Psychiatr Scand 94:87–93, 1996

Altshuler L: Bipolar disorder: are repeated episodes associated with neuroanatomic and cognitive changes? Biol Psychiatry 33:563–565, 1993

Altshuler LL, Gitlin MJ, Mintz J, et al: Subsyndromal depression is associated with functional impairment in patients with bipolar disorder. J Clin Psychiatry 63:807–811, 2002

Altshuler LL, Post RM, Black DO, et al: Subsyndromal depressive symptoms are associated with functional impairment in patients with bipolar disorder: results of a large, multisite study. J Clin Psychiatry 67:1551–1560, 2006

Bauwens F, Tray A, Pardoen D, et al: Social adjustment of remitted bipolar and unipolar outpatients. Br J Psychiatry 159:239–244, 1991

Beyenburg S, Back C, Diederich N, et al: Is valproate encephalopathy under-recognised in older people? a case series. Age Ageing 36:344–346, 2007

Broadhead J, Jacoby R: Mania in old age: a first prospective study. Int J Geriatr Psychiatry 5:215–222, 1990

Brown ES, Rush AJ, McEwen BS: Hippocampal remodeling and damage by corticosteroids: implications for mood disorders. Neuropsychopharmacology 21:474–484, 1999

Burt T, Prudic J, Peyser S, et al: Learning and memory in bipolar and unipolar major depression: effects of aging. Neuropsychiatry Neuropsychol Behav Neurol 13:246–253, 2000

Carpenter WT, Strauss JS: The prediction of outcome in schizophrenia, IV: eleven year follow-up of the Washington IPSS cohort. J Nerv Ment Dis 179:517–525, 1991

Cassens G, Inglis AK, Appelbaum PS, et al: Neuroleptics: effects on neuropsychological function in chronic schizophrenic patients. Schizophr Bull 16:477–499, 1990

Cavanagh JTO, van Beck M, Muir W, et al: Case-control study of neurocognitive function in euthymic patients with bipolar disorder: an association with mania. Br J Psychiatry 180:320–326, 2002

Chen ST, Altshuler LL, Melnyk AA, et al: Efficacy of lithium vs. valproate in the treatment of mania in the elderly: a retrospective study. J Clin Psychiatry 60:181–186, 1999

Cipolli C: Symposium: cognitive processes and sleep disturbances: sleep, dreams and memory: an overview. J Sleep Res 4:2–9, 1995

Clark L, Iversen SD, Goodwin GM: Sustained attention deficit in bipolar disorder. Br J Psychiatry 180:313–319, 2002

Cornblatt BA, Winters L, Erlenmeyer-Kimling L: Attentional markers of schizophrenia: evidence from the New York High Risk Study, in Schizophrenia: Scientific Progress. Edited by Schulz SC, Taminga CA. New York, Oxford University Press, 1989, pp 83–92

Cornblatt BA, Lenzenweger MF, Dworkin RH, et al: Childhood attentional dysfunctions predict social deficits in unaffected adults at risk for schizophrenia. Br J Psychiatry Suppl 161:59–64, 1992

Correll CU, Penzer JB, Lencz T, et al: Early identification and high-risk strategies for bipolar disorder. Bipolar Disord 9:324–338, 2007

Daban C, Martinez-Aran A, Torrent C, et al: Specificity of cognitive deficits in bipolar disorder versus schizophrenia: a systematic review. Psychother Psychosom 75:72–84, 2006

Decina P, Kestenbaum CJ, Farber S, et al: Clinical and psychological assessment of children of bipolar probands. Am J Psychiatry 140:548–553, 1983

Deckersbach T, McMurrich S, Ogutha J, et al: Characteristics of non-verbal memory impairment in bipolar disorder: the role of encoding strategies. Psychol Med 34:823–832, 2004a

Deckersbach T, Savage CR, Reilly Harrington N, et al: Episodic memory impairment in bipolar disorder and obsessive-compulsive disorder: the role of memory strategies. Bipolar Disord 6:233–244, 2004b

Deicken RF, Peques MP, Anzalone S, et al: Lower concentration of hippocampal N-acetylaspartate in familial bipolar I disorder. Am J Psychiatry 160:873–882, 2003

Depp CA, Jeste DV: Bipolar disorder in older adults: a critical review. Bipolar Disord 6:343–367, 2004

Dhingra U, Rabins PV: Mania in the elderly: a 5–7 year follow-up. J Am Geriatr Soc 39:581–583, 1991

Dittmann S, Seemüller F, Schwarz MJ, et al: Association of cognitive deficits with elevated homocysteine levels in euthymic bipolar patients and its impact on psychosocial functioning: preliminary results. Bipolar Disord 9:63–70, 2007

Donnelly E, Murphy D, Goodwin F, et al: Intellectual function in primary affective disorder. Br J Psychiatry 140:633–636, 1982

Drummond SP, Brown GC, Gillin JC, et al: Altered brain response to verbal learning following sleep deprivation. Nature 403:605–606, 2000

El-Badri SM, Ashton CH, Moore PB, et al: Electrophysiological and cognitive function in young euthymic patients with bipolar affective disorder. Bipolar Disord 3:79–87, 2001

Engelsmann F, Katz J, Ghadirian AM, et al: Lithium and memory: a long-term follow-up study. J Clin Psychopharmacol 8:207–212, 1988

Fava GA: The concept of recovery in bipolar disorders. Psychother Psychosom 65:2–13, 1996

Fava GA: Conceptual obstacles to research progress in affective disorders. Psychother Psychosom 66:283–285, 1997

Fava GA: Subclinical symptoms in mood disorders: pathophysiological and therapeutic implications. Psychol Med 29:47–61, 1999

Ferrier IN, Stanton BR, Kelly TP, et al: Neuropsychological function in euthymic patients with bipolar disorder. Br J Psychiatry 175:246–251, 1999

Folstein MF, Folstein SE, McHugh PR: "Mini-Mental State." A practical method for grading the cognitive state of patients for the clinician. J Psychiatr Res 12:189–198, 1975

Gildengers AG, Butters MA, Seligman K, et al: Cognitive functioning in late-life bipolar disorder. Am J Psychiatry 161:736–738, 2004

Green MF: Schizophrenia From a Neurocognitive Perspective: Probing the Impenetrable Darkness. Needham Heights, MA, Allyn & Bacon, 1998

Harkavy-Friedman JM, Keilp JG, Grunebaum MF, et al: Are BPI and BPII suicide attempters distinct neuropsychologically? J Affect Disord 94:255–259, 2006

Harvey PD, Earle-Boyer EA, Wielgus MS, et al: Encoding, memory and thought disorder in schizophrenia and mania. Schizophr Bull 12:252–261, 1986

Harvey PD, Leff J, Trieman N, et al: Cognitive impairment in geriatric chronic schizophrenic patients: a cross-national study in New York and London. Int J Geriatr Psychiatry 12:1001–1007, 1997

Himmelhoch JM, Neil JF, May SJ, et al: Age, dementia, dyskinesias, and lithium response. Am J Psychiatry 137:941–945, 1980

Jaeger J, Berns S: Neuropsychological management, treatment and rehabilitation of psychiatric patients, in Assessment of Neuropsychological Functions in Psychiatric Disorders. Edited by Calev A. Washington, DC, American Psychiatric Press, 1999, pp 447–480

Jaeger J, Berns S, Loftus S, et al: Neurocognitive test performance predicts functional recovery from acute exacerbation leading to hospitalization in bipolar disorder. Bipolar Disord 9:93–102, 2007

Johnson MH, Magaro P: Effects of mood and severity on memory processes in depression and mania. Psychol Bull 101:28–40, 1987

Johnstone EC, Owens DGC, Frith CD, et al: Institutionalization and the outcome of functional psychoses. Br J Psychiatry 146:36–44, 1985

Judd LL, Akiskal HS, Schettler PJ, et al: The long-term natural history of the weekly symptomatic status of bipolar I disorder. Arch Gen Psychiatry 59:530–537, 2002

Jurica YJ, Leitten CL, Mattis S: Dementia Rating Scale-2: Professional Manual. Lutz, FL, Psychological Assessment Resources, 2001

Kalska H, Punamaki RL, Makinen-Pelli T, et al: Memory and metamemory functioning among depressed patients. Appl Neuropsychol 6:96–107, 1999

Kessing LV: Cognitive impairment in the euthymic phase of affective disorder. Psychol Med 28:1027–1038, 1998

Kessing LV, Andersen PK: Does the risk of developing dementia increase with the number of episodes in patients with depressive disorder and in patients with bipolar disorder? J Neurol Neurosurg Psychiatry 75:1662–1666, 2004

Laes JR, Sponheim SR: Does cognition predict community function only in schizophrenia? a study of schizophrenia patients, bipolar affective disorder patients, and community control subjects. Schizophr Res 84:121–131, 2006

Lonergan ET, Cameron M, Luxenberg J: Valproic acid for agitation in dementia. Cochrane Database of Systematic Reviews, Issue 2, Article No:CD003945. DOI: 10.1002/14651858.CD003945.pub2, 2004

Lydon E, El-Mallakh RS: Naturalistic long-term use of methylphenidate in bipolar disorder. J Clin Psychopharmacol 25:516–518, 2006

MacQueen GM, Young LT, Galway TM, et al: Backward masking task performance in stable, euthymic out-patients with bipolar disorder. Psychol Med 31:1269–1277, 2001

Martinez-Aran A, Vieta E, Colom F, et al: Cognitive dysfunctions in bipolar disorder: evidence of neuropsychological disturbances. Psychother Psychosom 69:2–18, 2000

Martinez-Aran A, Penadés R, Vieta E, et al: Executive function in patients with remitted bipolar disorder and schizophrenia and its relationship with functional outcome. Psychother Psychosom 71:39–46, 2002

Martinez-Aran A, Vieta E, Colom F, et al: Cognitive impairment in euthymic bipolar patients: implications for clinical and functional outcome. Bipolar Disord 6:224–232, 2004a

Martinez-Aran A, Vieta E, Reinares M, et al: Cognitive function across manic or hypomanic, depressed, and euthymic states in bipolar disorder. Am J Psychiatry 161:262–270, 2004b

Martinez-Aran A, Vieta E, Torrent C, et al: Functional outcome in bipolar disorder: the role of clinical and cognitive factors. Bipolar Disord 9:103–113, 2007

Martinez-Aran A, Torrent C, Tabares-Seisdedos R, et al: Neurocognitive impairment in bipolar patients with and without history of psychosis. J Clin Psychiatry 69:233–239, 2008

Martino DJ, Igoa A, Marengo E, et al: Cognitive and motor features in elderly people with bipolar disorder. J Affect Disord 105:291–295, 2008

McDonough-Ryan P, DelBello M, Shear PK, et al: Academic and cognitive abilities in children of parents with bipolar disorder: a test of the nonverbal learning disability model. J Clin Exp Neuropsychol 24:280–285, 2002

McKay AP, Tarbuck AF, Shapleske J, et al: Neuropsychological function in manic-depressive psychosis. Br J Psychiatry 167:51–57, 1995

Morice R: Cognitive inflexibility and pre-frontal dysfunction in schizophrenia and mania. Br J Psychiatry 157:50–54, 1990

Nehra R, Chakrabarti S, Pradhan BK, et al: Comparison of cognitive functions between first and multi-episode bipolar affective disorders. J Affect Disord 93:185–192, 2006

Ponce H, Kunik M, Molinari V, et al: Divalproex sodium treatment in elderly male bipolar patients. Journal of Geriatric Drug Therapy 12:55–63, 1999

Porsteinsson AP: Divalproex sodium for the treatment of behavioural problems associated with dementia in the elderly. Drugs Aging 23:877–886, 2006

Profenno LA, Jakimovich L, Holt CJ, et al: A randomized, double-blind, placebo-controlled pilot trial of safety and tolerability of two doses of divalproex sodium in outpatients with probable Alzheimer's disease. Curr Alzheimer Res 2:553–558, 2005

Prohaska ML, Stern RA, Nevels CT, et al: The relationship between thyroid status and neuropsychological performance in psychiatric outpatients maintained on lithium. Neuropsychiatry Neuropsychol Behav Neurol 9:30–34, 1996

Reichenberg A, Weiser M, Rabinowitz J, et al: A population-based cohort study of premorbid intellectual, language, and behavioral functioning in patients with schizophrenia, schizoaffective disorder, and nonpsychotic bipolar disorder. Am J Psychiatry 159:2027–2035, 2002

Robinson LJ, Ferrier IN: Evolution of cognitive impairment in bipolar disorder: a systematic review of cross-sectional evidence. Bipolar Disord 8:103–116, 2006

Robinson LJ, Thompson JM, Gallagher P, et al: A meta-analysis of cognitive deficits in euthymic patients with bipolar disorder. J Affect Disord 93:105–115, 2006

Rocca CC, Macedo-Soares MB, Gorenstein C, et al: Verbal fluency dysfunction in euthymic bipolar patients: a controlled study. J Affect Disord 107:187–192, 2008

Rubinsztein JS, Michael A, Paykel ES, et al: Cognitive impairment in remission in bipolar affective disorder. Psychol Med 30:1025–1036, 2000

Savard RJ, Rey AC, Post RM: Halstead-Reitan Category Test in bipolar and unipolar affective disorders. J Nerv Ment Dis 168:293–303, 1980

Selva G, Salazar J, Balanzá-Martínez V, et al: Bipolar I patients with and without a history of psychotic symptoms: do they differ in their cognitive functioning? J Psychiatr Res 41:265–272, 2007

Spohn HE, Strauss ME: Relation of neuroleptic and anticholinergic medication to cognitive functions in schizophrenia. J Abnorm Psychol 98:367–380, 1989

Stone K: Mania in the elderly. Br J Psychiatry 155:220–224, 1989

Taylor Tavares JV, Clark L, Cannon DM, et al: Distinct profiles of neurocognitive function in unmedicated unipolar depression and bipolar II depression. Biol Psychiatry 62:917–924, 2007

Thompson JM, Gallagher P, Hughes JH, et al: Neurocognitive impairment in euthymic patients with bipolar affective disorder. Br J Psychiatry 186:32–40, 2005

Torrent C, Martinez-Aran A, Daban C, et al: Cognitive impairment in bipolar II disorder. Br J Psychiatry 189:254–259, 2006

Toulopoulou T, Quraishi S, McDonald C, et al: The Maudsley Family Study: premorbid and current general intellectual function levels in familial bipolar disorder and schizophrenia. J Clin Exp Neuropsychol 28:243–259, 2006

Tremont G, Stern RA: Use of thyroid hormone to diminish the cognitive side effects of psychiatric treatment. Psychopharmacol Bull 33:273–280, 1997

Trichard C, Martinot JL, Alagille M, et al: Time course of prefrontal lobe dysfunction in severely depressed in-patients: a longitudinal neuropsychological study. Psychol Med 25:79–85, 1995

van Gorp WG, Altshuler L, Theberge DC, et al: Cognitive impairment in euthymic bipolar patients with and without prior alcohol dependence. Arch Gen Psychiatry 55:41–46, 1998

Vieta E, Gastó C, Martínez de Osaba MJ, et al: Prediction of depressive relapse in remitted bipolar patients using corticotrophin-releasing hormone challenge test. Acta Psychiatr Scand 95:205–211, 1997

Vieta E, Martínez-de-Osaba MJ, Colom F, et al: Enhanced corticotropin response to corticotropin-releasing hormone as a predictor of mania in euthymic bipolar patients. Psychol Med 29:971–978, 1999

Vogel G: Clinical uses and advantages of low doses of benzodiazepine hypnotics. J Clin Psychiatry 53:19–22, 1992

Winters KC, Stone AA, Weintraub S, et al: Cognitive and attentional deficits in children vulnerable to psychopathology. J Abnorm Child Psychol 9:435–453, 1981

Young RC, Murphy CF, Heo M, et al: Cognitive impairment in bipolar disorder in old age: literature review and findings in manic patients. J Affect Disord 92:125–131, 2006

Zubieta JK, Huguelet P, O'Neil RL, et al: Cognitive function in euthymic bipolar I disorder. Psychiatry Res 102:9–20, 2001

12

Summary and Assessment Recommendations for Practitioners

Joseph F. Goldberg, M.D.
Katherine E. Burdick, Ph.D.

Interest in the cognitive dysfunction associated with bipolar disorder has grown from efforts in basic science—notably, genetics and functional neuroanatomy— to the refinement of nosology and differential diagnosis to issues of practical clinical management. Throughout this book, we have sought to provide clinicians with a comprehensive overview of cognitive functioning in bipolar disorder, by integrating clinical and empirically based observations and recommendations with relevant scientific corollaries and applications from cognitive neuroscience. Although at first glance the clinical relevance of neurocognition in bipolar disorder may not be readily apparent—or may seem purely academic—the consequences of ignoring or misidentifying cognitive impairment bear on virtually all aspects of disease management and treatment, as well as on patients' quality of life and psychosocial functioning.

In this final chapter, we aim to distill major tenets from the foregoing chapters into their most basic elements from the standpoint of practical management issues for clinicians who evaluate and treat children, adolescents, adults, or older adults with bipolar disorder. Several initial key points merit emphasis at the outset.

- Cognitive impairment is common and observable in a majority of individuals with bipolar disorder during acute mood states. Moreover, specific deficits in attention, verbal memory, and executive function may be traitlike features evident across all mood states, with persistence during periods of euthymia.

- The genetic underpinnings of cognitive dysfunction in bipolar disorder are apparent from monozygotic twin studies as well as from documentation of trait deficits in unaffected first-degree relatives of bipolar probands. Molecular genetic studies also have increasingly turned to variations in neurocognitive function as a strategy for linking candidate genes with heritable traits transmitted within families of individuals with bipolar disorder.

- The magnitude and scope of cognitive deficits in bipolar disorder coalesce mainly around problems with attention, verbal memory, and executive function. Cognitive deficits do not appear to be as global, pervasive, or disabling in patients with bipolar disorder as in schizophrenia. They occur in patients with either bipolar I or bipolar II disorder and persist across all phases of illness, including euthymia. Cognitive impairment also appears to be independent of the presence or absence of psychosis, although patients with psychotic forms of bipolar disorder may show more verbal memory deficits than do those without a history of psychosis. Limited research also suggests that cognitive deficits may be more likely among those bipolar patients who are also prone to develop involuntary movement disorders after lithium and neuroleptic exposure, suggesting possible shared brain vulnerabilities to adverse neurological drug effects (Waddington et al. 1989).

- Racial or gender differences have not been identified in either global cognitive function or domains of neurocognition among subgroups with bipolar disorder.

- No longitudinal or progressive decline in cognitive functioning, as classically associated with Kraepelin's construct of dementia praecox, has been demonstrated for individuals with bipolar disorder. However, a history of multiple episodes (especially manias) appears correlated with the presence of cognitive deficits. In addition, there remains uncertainty about the potential for neurotoxic events or neurodegenerative processes to occur across protracted, multiple affective episodes, or from extended periods of untreated but symptomatic bipolar illness— the possible cognitive sequelae of which are largely unknown.

- Improvement in depressive symptoms appears to correlate with improvement in at least some cognitive domains, but relationships between affective or anxiety symptoms and cognition are complex and warrant independent monitoring and assessment.

- Isolated symptoms such as inattentiveness or distractibility are diagnostically nonspecific. They require contextual evaluation and corroboration with other affective and psychomotor manifestations of bipolar disorder.

• The extent to which cognitive deficits can reasonably be attributed to medications versus disease-specific phenomena cannot be assumed and requires careful evaluation, with knowledge of which psychotropic agents are more likely to adversely affect specific cognitive domains at treatment initiation, or in certain high-vulnerability patients.

• Some psychotropic agents have been shown to exert neuroprotective or neurotrophic effects (e.g., lithium, divalproex), which may help to minimize potential neurotoxic effects that are thought to result from repeated affective episodes, although the extent to which neuroprotective agents may be of value to minimize or possibly reverse illness-related cognitive deficits in people with bipolar disorder remains speculative and largely unstudied.

Assessment

The degree to which individuals with bipolar disorder are able to recognize their own cognitive deficits, when present, often varies depending on factors such as insight and the ability to differentiate cognitive deficits from signs of depression, anxiety, or other forms of psychopathology. For example, our group found that about three-quarters of bipolar outpatients manifested signs of cognitive impairment (mainly in the domains of verbal learning and memory) on performance tasks, yet patients' subjectively reported cognitive complaints correlated poorly with objective cognitive deficits, and they tended toward overreporting of problems in domains where no objective deficits existed (Burdick et al. 2005). Similar findings were reported in adults by Martinez-Aran et al. (2005). Among euthymic late-adolescent outpatients with bipolar I disorder, Robertson et al. (2003) identified ongoing subjective attentional complaints in subjects with a suspected history of attention-deficit/hyperactivity disorder, despite the absence of frank deficits on objective, performance-based measures of attention. Findings such as these indicate that clinicians must critically and systematically evaluate patients' self-reported symptoms regarding cognitive or other mental processes and consider that patients may not always reliably interpret the clinical meaning of their own cognitive, perceptual, or emotional experiences.

Clinicians should be alert to the potential for cognitive deficits in patients with bipolar disorder when 1) symptom profiles appear complex or atypical; 2) responses to appropriate, traditional treatments for affective or psychotic symptoms appear suboptimal; 3) work, academic, or social functioning deficits persist despite the apparent remission of affective, anxiety, or psychotic symptoms; 4) patients or their significant others identify problems related to routine cognitive performance tasks (e.g., paying bills, following directions, remembering appointments) that are not commensurate with intellectual abilities; and 5) patients themselves report subjective cognitive problems.

The management of cognitive complaints hinges on careful evaluation, with particular attention to differentiating plausible iatrogenic effects from illness-specific problems. As noted above, patients who complain of subjective cognitive problems may or may not actually have objective neurocognitive deficits—as opposed to other types of symptoms that they construe as cognitive in nature; hence, clinicians must assess cognitive complaints beyond their face value. Clinicians sometimes might assume that subjective cognitive complaints necessarily reflect adverse iatrogenic effects of psychotropic medications, although, as noted in Chapter 7 of this volume, "Adverse Cognitive Effects of Psychotropic Medications," medication-induced cognitive problems are fairly rare, apart from those caused by anticholinergic drugs, benzodiazepines, lithium, or some anticonvulsants (notably topiramate). It is thus critical for practitioners to determine when patients' cognitive complaints might signal the presence of other problems that pertain more fundamentally to psychopathology, such as untreated depression, mania, anxiety, psychosis, or substance misuse. Table 12–1 summarizes differential etiologies for cognitive dysfunction before attributing deficits to bipolar disorder itself.

A medical or neurological workup for new, age-inappropriate cognitive deficits (as delineated in Chapter 11 of this volume, "Cognition Across the Life Span: Clinical Implications for Older Adults With Bipolar Disorder") should be considered as part of the overall evaluation for new cognitive complaints when accompanied by physical signs or symptoms suggestive of systemic illness (e.g., weight loss, headache) or histories suggestive of persistent or severe toxic exposures (including alcohol or other neurotoxic substances).

Psychiatric Etiologies of Cognitive Complaints

As noted throughout this book, patients can misinterpret cognitive deficits as being signs of affective illness (see Case Vignette 1 in Chapter 7 of this volume), and, likewise, psychopathology can be wrongly identified as reflecting cognitive impairment. It is of critical importance for clinicians to recognize the latter of these instances and to assess for the presence of affective, anxiety, or psychotic symptoms that patients may misconstrue as problems with memory or attention. Other sources of cognitive dysfunction, such as alcohol or substance abuse, may often become overlooked as likely contributors to psychiatric symptoms or to impaired memory and attention.

The concept of "pseudodementia" (Salzman and Shader 1978) was originally developed to describe the diffuse cognitive problems similar to

TABLE 12–1. Differential etiologies of cognitive complaints in patients with bipolar disorder

- Head trauma
- Initiation of new medications—particularly those with anticholinergic or sedative properties, or steroids; key psychotropic agents include lithium, divalproex, carbamazepine, topiramate, benzodiazepines, and possibly antipsychotics (see Chapter 7 of this volume)
- Toxin exposures (e.g., heavy metals)
- Alcohol or substance abuse/dependence, including acute intoxication or withdrawal states
- Minimal cognitive impairment as precursor to Alzheimer's dementia or other dementias (e.g., Pick's disease, Lewy body dementia, alcoholic dementia)
- Medical illness (e.g., infection, neoplasm, vasculitis) and cerebrovascular insufficiency unrelated to dementia (e.g., hypoxia secondary to pulmonary disease)
- Sleep deprivation
- Depression
- Anxiety
- Psychosis
- Stress and distress

subcortical dementias that may be associated with depression in older adults that could be mistaken for a primary dementia; more recently, there has been debate about whether older adults who manifest cognitive problems during depressive episodes may be at increased risk for the eventual development of frank dementia (Reifler 2000). Insofar as most patients with bipolar disorder display symptoms before age 30, and new cases after age 50 are relatively rare (Perlis et al. 2004), cognitive problems related to bipolar disorder would be expected to manifest themselves during the first few decades of life; hence, the presence of new cognitive problems in an older adult, with or without a history of bipolar disorder, warrants independent assessment for the possible onset of dementia.

The Approach to Clinical Assessment

Practitioners should be reasonably facile with conducting a basic assessment of cognitive domains, and they should understand the meaning of errors detected on standard questions that assess higher integrative functioning, including attention, memory, and executive planning. Clinicians should recognize the hierarchy of cognitive domains; there is little meaning, for example, in testing memory or executive function in patients with a depressed sensorium or impaired attention. Clinicians also must consider the ways in which the presence of affective, anxiety, or psychotic symptoms can influence cognitive performance during testing (as described in Chapter 5 of this volume, "Impact of Mood, Anxiety, and Psychotic Symptoms on Cognition in Patients With Bipolar Disorder"). In the presence of prominent depression, for example, cognitive test results may be biased by poor performance effort or low motivation. Significant psychomotor slowing in depressed patients can also result in poor performance on a number of timed tasks in higher domains (e.g., verbal fluency), yielding scores in the impaired range when pure fluency deficits are not truly present. Even intelligence quotient (IQ) testing may yield discrepant results dependent on mood state, particularly on measures of performance IQ, several of which require rapid response, and for which scoring depends on normal rates of response (e.g., the Wechsler Adult Intelligence Scale—Third Edition, Block Design subtest [Wechsler 1997] is timed, with bonus points given based on response time).

Clinicians should not be deterred from referring patients for neuropsychological assessment simply because of the presence of affective symptomatology. Rather, it is incumbent on the neuropsychologist to recognize patterns of performance that are or are not consistent with depressive mood states, and to make appropriate attributions based on a priori knowledge of differential diagnosis. It is, therefore, critical for practitioners to share any clinical information that might be of value to the neuropsychologist to ensure adequate assessment in the context of each specific case.

A frequent recommendation in cases evaluated during acute episodes, or when mood symptoms are believed to be causing at least some portion of impaired cognitive test performance, is to repeat cognitive testing at some later time interval (typically at least 6 months subsequent to initial testing) and/or when mood symptoms are in remission. These types of serial evaluations, when feasible, are ideal in that they capture mood-dependent impairments over time in the same individual. However, multiple assessments may become subject to bias from practice effects (i.e., improved performance due to familiarity with the test and the testing materials and environment). Formal neuropsychological evaluations should typically be conducted at least 6 months apart in a psychiatric population to allow for adequate interpretation of data. Furthermore, when serial testing is planned in advance, practice effects can be minimized by using tasks with available alternate forms (different but psychometrically equivalent versions).

Psychiatrists and other mental health professionals routinely conduct brief global assessments of gross cognitive function (e.g., the Mini-Mental State Examination [Folstein et al. 1975] in dementia patients) without the need for formal training in test administration. Typically, such mental status examinations provide a global estimate of cognition and can be used reliably to track significant changes in cognition over time (e.g., in the case of a dementia patient with progressive decline across multiple domains) or to screen for the possible need for more comprehensive neuropsychological evaluation. Importantly, however, individuals with bipolar disorder generally do not display the type of gross cognitive deficits measured by brief global measures such as the Mini-Mental State Examination or the Dementia Rating Scale–2 (Junica et al. 2001). More thorough assessment tools are often necessary to identify and quantify the nature of distinct neurocognitive deficits. The tests selected to screen for, or more comprehensively assess, cognitive deficits are of fundamental importance. In most cases, once a referral is made, the neuropsychologist will choose the appropriate instruments and measures that best suit the question at hand. This approach to assessment is common in clinical settings so that testing batteries can be made to accommodate any given setting and patient.

There has been recent progress in schizophrenia research to develop a uniform battery that is intended to be brief but comprehensive in its assessment across domains and that is tailored specifically for the needs of patients with schizophrenia (the Brief Assessment of Cognition in Schizophrenia by NeuroCog Trials; available at http://www.neurocogtrials.com/instrument.htm). A similar battery is being developed by the same group to be used in patients with affective disorders (the Brief Assessment of Cognition in Affective Disorders).

Some common self-report questionnaires that are designed to elicit patients' own perceptions of their cognitive function are summarized in Table 12–2. Such measures vary greatly in their sensitivity and specificity and can be difficult to interpret in the absence of contextual information and supportive material from direct clinical assessment, including interview probing to clarify responses. Therefore, they should not be regarded as a substitute for formal performance-based evaluations of cognitive function.

Formal Neurocognitive Testing

As described in Chapter 1 of this volume, "Overview and Introduction: Dimensions of Cognition and Measures of Cognitive Function," a neuropsychological evaluation consists of a series of tests and/or procedures originating in psychometric psychology, cognitive psychology, and behavioral neurology. They are designed to provide information about the brain's integrity by comprehensively sampling its behavioral products, especially the so-called higher functions (e.g., language, memory, intellect). A neuropsychological evaluation is in some respects a large, formalized cognitive status exam. Conventional cognitive status exams are useful but (due to brevity and the limited range of functions covered) are limited (e.g., they may have a 50% false-negative rate and provide little information about what a person specifically can and cannot do).

TABLE 12–2. Common self-report questionnaires for the assessment of cognitive functioning

Instrument	Description
Medical Outcomes Study Short Form 36 (Leidy et al. 1998)	Generic health status assessment that includes a subscale for cognition (by self-report). It has been used in multiple medical populations and has been shown to have good reliability and validity overall.
A-B Neuropsychological Assessment Schedule (Brooks et al. 2001)	Specifically developed to assess the patient's perception of cognitive side effects of antiepileptic drugs. Reliability and criterion validity have been established. It consists of 24 items with ratings from 0 (no problem) to 3 (serious problem) in multiple domains of cognitive function.
Cognitive Failures Questionnaire (Broadbent et al. 1982)	Identifies the frequency of making common types of cognitive mistakes (e.g., misplacing one's keys) over the preceding 6-month period. Previous studies suggest that it is unlikely to be sensitive to transient disruption of cognition but may be best used to detect a more stable change over time. Total score on the measure appears to be the most valid variable, as specific subscales have not been identified.
Patient's Assessment of Own Functioning (Chelune et al. 1986)	Self-report measure that includes five subcomponents assessing diverse cognitive domains, with total score being highly correlated with the five subscales.
Cognitive Difficulties Scale (McNair and Kahn 1983)	A 39-item Likert-type questionnaire that taps memory and general cognitive complaints. Based on use in head trauma patients, factor analytic studies derived seven validated subscales: Distraction, Activities of Daily Living, Prospective Memory, Long-Term Memory, Orientation, Language, and Fine Motor Control.

Neuropsychological evaluations are intended to assess brain-behavior relationships in the broadest sense, including changes that can occur in clinical populations, such as in the areas of intellectual/information processing, personality, emotions (feelings, motivation), and behavioral control/self-regulation. Thus, neuropsychological batteries typically assay a wide range of functions and domains in sufficient depth to have reasonable reliability, as described in detail in Chapter 1. Assessments of educational attainment are frequently included, along with evaluations of personality and emotional functioning. Not all neuropsychologists perform "psychological" testing in the context of a neuropsychological evaluation; however, it is rather common in psychiatric populations for a referral to include both "neurocognitive" and "psychological" testing due to the considerable impact that psychopathology can have on cognitive test performance. Psychological testing typically includes formalized personality profiling, using standardized measures such as the Minnesota Multiphasic Personality Inventory, and projective testing aimed at identifying subconscious thoughts/beliefs and intentions, using tests such as the Rorschach Inkblot Test or Thematic Apperception Test (Hilsenroth et al. 2003). In addition, combined neuropsychological and psychological testing can be helpful when it is difficult to discern in the context of regular treatment whether a patient is displaying specific affective/psychotic symptoms or frank cognitive impairment. Consider the following example.

Case Vignette 1

A 32-year-old woman with bipolar I disorder had been in remission from affective symptoms for 2 months while on a stable regimen of lamotrigine and risperidone. During a psychiatric follow-up appointment, her mood seemed euthymic and her affect was appropriate, but her psychiatrist noted unusual delays in her responses to questions. In light of a history of psychosis, her psychiatrist became concerned about the possible presence of a thought disorder, thought blocking, or distractibility due to preoccupation with internal stimuli. The patient denied any new or recurrent delusions or hallucinations and further denied depressed mood, anhedonia, and apathy. She also denied fatigue, sleep problems, and feeling sedated during the daytime. However, the patient was aware of feeling easily distracted, having trouble multitasking, and finding it difficult to maintain her concentration while reading or having a conversation. Neuropsychological and psychological tests were requested to help clarify the nature and extent of problems with information processing alongside the potential presence of unrecognized psychopathology.

In addition to the diagnostic utility of neurocognitive testing, there has been growing interest in the potential value of neuropsychological assessment as a means to help gauge a patient's adaptive status and functional capabilities, especially in psychiatric settings, where there are often multiple causes of functional capacity deficiencies. Hence, findings from neurocognitive batteries may help to identify a role for cognitive remediation or occupational therapy, or inform the nature and scope of psychotherapy. Generally, neuropsychological assessment should be viewed as complementary to procedures such as the neurological examination, electroencephalograms, and magnetic resonance imaging or computed tomography (e.g., any of which may be indicated based on the presence of focal neurological signs). However, it is entirely possible that neuropsychological tests may reveal cognitive deficits in the absence of clear neurological signs or neuroimaging findings. These indications may nevertheless have important treatment and management implications.

Neuropsychological test results entail summaries of performance on tests that assess specific cognitive domains (as outlined in Chapter 1 of this volume). They usually do not include raw scores on individual measures administered because raw score data in themselves are of limited value; neuropsychologists interpret findings within the context of other sources of patient data (history, interview, current circumstances, behavior during testing), and the validity of findings often depends on the integration of multifaceted information. A well-formulated neuropsychological report will include detailed interpretation of the results in the context of psychiatric, neurological, and family histories, as well as any findings from personality inventories or projective tests.

When a clinician refers a patient for neuropsychological evaluation, it is not necessary to request specific tests to be performed, because part of the tester's role is to make this determination based on the clinical information provided. Rather, it is more important that the referring clinician describe the clinical problems of interest in as much detail and as specifically as possible. Following are several examples of situations in which neurocognitive testing may be useful:

- A 32-year-old man with bipolar I disorder and mild depression has persistent difficulty maintaining jobs because of problems following complex instructions, and there is a suspicion of impaired executive function.

- A 41-year-old college-educated woman with bipolar II disorder and a remote history of head trauma with loss of consciousness is now euthymic and nonpsychotic, has had chronically poor work functioning, and seems perseverative during an initial interview; there is concern about frontal lobe disease.

- A 28-year-old man with bipolar II disorder denies current or recent affective symptoms but complains of chronic trouble concentrating and poor attention, describing himself as "the poster boy for ADD [attention-deficit disorder]." There is no clear history of childhood attention or behavior problems and no substance abuse, but the patient is concerned that he is inefficient at work due to undiagnosed and untreated ADD.

- A 59-year-old man with bipolar I disorder and comorbid generalized anxiety disorder complains of increasing forgetfulness in everyday matters, and his wife corroborates that he has seemed "increasingly absent-minded" for the past several months. There is a question of minimal cognitive impairment and early-onset dementia.

When to Make Referrals for Neuropsychological Testing

There are a number of instances in which neuropsychological testing may be especially useful, summarized as follows:

- When a patient's neurological exam reveals abnormal signs, and one wishes to know more about the cognitive, personality, and behavioral correlates of the condition
- When one wishes to better understand the neurobehavioral sequelae of known insults (e.g., head injury, surgery, stroke)
- When one suspects brain compromise due to chronic illness (e.g., diabetes, hypertension, HIV, epilepsy, alcoholism)
- When one suspects a neurodegenerative illness, dementia, or a chronic confusional state and one desires a comprehensive evaluation to facilitate differential diagnosis and monitoring
- When one is concerned about the effects of a particular treatment and wants data to facilitate monitoring (e.g., anticholinergic effects on memory)
- When one wants to rule out premorbid cognitive problems such as learning disabilities, attention-deficit/hyperactivity disorder, or mental retardation
- When there is a significant change in adaptive functioning, a sudden personality change, or acute memory complaints

Formal neurocognitive testing also establishes a benchmark against which potential future deterioration can be monitored. Assessment can thus be for purposes of establishing a baseline or for follow-up monitoring (of value either intraepisode or interepisode) and should be considered when possible for psychiatric patients experiencing a first episode of mania, depression, or psychosis.

Pharmacological Considerations

Pharmacological explanations for cognitive complaints warrant consideration after other medical or psychiatric etiologies have been assessed. As discussed in Chapter 7 of this volume, psychotropic agents used to treat bipolar disorder differ in their potential to cause cognitive problems. Clinicians should be particularly alert to the time course in which cognitive complaints arise relative to changes in existing treatment regimens, including recent dosage increases, coprescription of additional agents (e.g., anticholinergic drugs or benzodiazepines), and pharmacokinetic or pharmacodynamic factors that may effectively delay drug metabolism or cause neurotoxicities (e.g., use of thiazide diuretics or nonsteroidal anti-inflammatory agents in patients taking lithium). Cognitive testing ideally should be performed at least 8 hours after a most recent dose of benzodiazepines or similar sedative-hypnotics, anticholinergic drugs, or other agents known to adversely influence attention, reaction time, or overall performance.

As noted in Chapter 7, the potential for adverse effects associated with most psychotropic drugs is often related to rapidity of initial dosing and can be minimized by gradual titration with eventual habituation. Knowledge of predictable domains of cognitive impairment with specific agents also can help prescribers to assess the likelihood of iatrogenic effects and advise patients on the rationales for changing medications or dosages as opposed to pursuing alternative management strategies.

As described in Chapter 8 of this volume, "Pharmacological Strategies to Enhance Neurocognitive Function," there are limited data to support the use of adjunctive pharmacotherapies to counteract cognitive or sedating effects produced by psychotropics. No agents carry U.S. Food and Drug Administration approval for this purpose, but off-label use may be of value in select instances, particularly when supported in the literature by clinical trials. For example, psychostimulants such as amphetamine salts or novel agents such as modafinil are among the best studied in patients with bipolar disorder or schizophrenia; they appear safe provided there is an absence of current psychosis or mania; and risks for potential abuse have been carefully assessed. In general, suspected medication-induced problems with attention, memory, or related cognitive processes that do not remit with time or dosing adjustments merit a reassessment of therapeutic risks and benefits; efforts also should be made to refrain from prescribing additional pharmacologies with sedative properties to minimize further confounding of cause and effect until presumed adverse drug effects resolve.

Future Research Directions

Advances in cognitive neuroscience have begun to usher in an era of previously unimaginable studies that may eventually help elucidate the processes of attention, learning, memory, motivation, and the interplay of thought and emotion. Efforts to refine endophenotypes of bipolar disorder rely heavily on measures of cognitive activity in probands and their unaffected family members. Early molecular genetic studies suggest that neurocognitive impairment may indeed be a useful endophenotypic tool for detecting risk genes for bipolar disorder and for elucidating the underlying biological mechanism through which these genes may act to influence disease susceptibility. Brain imaging during the performance of cognitive tasks represents only one modality of assessment; more dynamic information will likely come from neuroimaging during repeated cognitive tasks, or during habituation to visual or auditory stimuli that engage limbic and prefrontal circuits or that engage limbic and hippocampal regions during learning paradigms that involve emotional processing (Hölzel et al. 2007) or mindfulness meditation (Ivanovski and Malhi 2007). Structural brain changes in corticolimbic circuitry from before to after specific forms of psychotherapy or pharmacotherapy lend further support to the potential for architectural remodeling of distinct cognitive pathways (Kennedy et al. 2007; Linden 2006; Roffman et al. 2005).

Cognitive remediation strategies—adapted from work originally conducted with traumatic brain injury patients and applied to patients with schizophrenia—also hold promise for adaptation to individuals with bipolar disorder whose cognitive problems differ from those of patients with schizophrenia in terms of global pervasiveness or severity (Burdick et al. 2006). Clinical research is needed to develop and adapt such techniques for the kinds of cognitive dysfunction seen in bipolar disorder. Such techniques might potentially involve rehabilitative strategies that incorporate context processing (Brambilla et al. 2007), performance monitoring and signal adjustment (MacDonald et al. 2000), or other therapeutic targets for corticolimbic dysregulation.

Clinical psychopharmacology trials have only fairly recently begun to measure influential dimensions of outcome other than primary psychopathology (i.e., affective symptoms), such as impediments to work and social functioning, including cognition. The few such studies conducted thus far have mainly assessed cognition by self-report measures, which may not reliably capture domains of interest and importance to the encoding and manipulation of information. By incorporating formal neurocognitive measures that assess attention, verbal memory, and executive function—those domains central to cognitive vulnerability in bipolar disorder—future therapeutic intervention trials may provide a more comprehensive and meaningful assessment of therapeutic drug targets for real-world problems affecting daily functioning in real-world patients with bipolar disorder.

References

Brambilla P, MacDonald AW III, Sassi RB, et al: Context processing performance in bipolar disorder patients. Bipolar Disord 9:230–237, 2007

Broadbent DE, Cooper PF, FitzGerald P, et al: The Cognitive Failures Questionnaire (CFQ) and its correlates. Br J Clin Psychol 21:1–16, 1982

Brooks J, Baker GA, Aldenkamp AP: The A-B Neuropsychological Assessment Schedule (ABNAS): the further refinement of a patient-based scale of patient-perceived cognitive functioning. Epilepsy Res 43:227–237, 2001

Burdick KE, Endick CJ, Goldberg JF: Assessing cognitive deficits in bipolar disorder: are self-reports valid? Psychiatry Res 136:43–50, 2005

Burdick KE, Goldberg JF, Harrow M, et al: Neurocognition as a stable endophenotype in bipolar disorder and schizophrenia. J Nerv Ment Dis 194:255–260, 2006

Chelune GJ, Heaton RK, Lechman RAW: Neuropsychological and personality correlates of patients' complaints of disability, in Advances in Clinical Neuropsychology, Vol 3. Edited by Goldstein G, Tarter RE. New York, Plenum Press, 1986, pp 95–126

Folstein MF, Folstein SE, McHugh PR: "Mini-Mental State." A practical method for grading the cognitive state of patients for the clinician. J Psychiatr Res 12:189–198, 1975

Hilsenroth MJ, Segal Dl, Hersen M (eds): Comprehensive Handbook of Psychological Assessment, Vol 2: Personality Assessment. New York, Wiley, 2003

Hölzel BK, Ott U, Hempel H, et al: Differential engagement of anterior cingulate and adjacent medial frontal cortex in adept meditators and non-meditators. Neurosci Lett 421:16–21, 2007

Ivanovski B, Malhi GS: The psychological and neurophysiological concomitants of mindfulness forms of meditation. Acta Neuropsychiatrica 19:76–91, 2007

Jurica PJ, Leitten CL, Mattis S: Dementia Rating Scale-2: Professional Manual. Lutz, FL, Psychological Assessment Resources, 2001

Kennedy SH, Konarski JZ, Segal ZV, et al: Differences in brain glucose metabolism between responders to CBT and venlafaxine in a 16-week randomized controlled trial. Am J Psychiatry 164:778–788, 2007

Leidy NK, Palmer C, Murray M, et al: Health-related quality of life assessment in euthymic and depressed patients with bipolar disorder: psychometric performance of four self-report measures. J Affect Disord 48:207–214, 1998

Linden DE: How psychotherapy changes the brain—the contribution of functional neuroimaging. Mol Psychiatry 11:528–538, 2006

MacDonald AW III, Cohen JD, Stenger VA, et al: Dissociating the role of the dorsolateral prefrontal and anterior cingulate cortex in cognitive control. Science 288:1835–1838, 2000

Martinez-Aran A, Vieta E, Colom F, et al: Do cognitive complaints in euthymic bipolar patients reflect objective cognitive impairment? Psychother Psychosom 74:295–302, 2005

McNair D, Kahn R: The Cognitive Difficulties Scale, in Assessment in Geriatric Psychopharmacology. Edited by Crook T, Ferris S, Bartus R. New Canaan, CT, Mark Powley and Associates, 1983, pp 137–143

Perlis RH, Miyahara S, Marangell LB, et al: Long-term implications of early onset in bipolar disorder: data from the first 1000 participants in the Systematic Treatment Enhancement Program for Bipolar Disorder (STEP-BD). Biol Psychiatry 55:875–881, 2004

Reifler BV: A case of mistaken identity: pseudodementia is really predementia. Am J Geriatr Soc 48:593–594, 2000

Robertson HA, Kutcher SP, Lagace DC: No evidence of attentional deficits in stabilized bipolar youth relative to unipolar and control comparators. Bipolar Disord 5:330–339, 2003

Roffman JL, Marci CD, Glick DM, et al: Neuroimaging and the functional neuroanatomy of psychotherapy. Psychol Med 35:1385–1398, 2005

Salzman C, Shader RI: Depression in the elderly, I: relationship between depression, psychologic defense mechanisms, and physical illness. J Am Geriatr Soc 26:253–260, 1978

Waddington JL, Brown K, O'Neill J, et al: Cognitive impairment, clinical course and treatment history in out-patients with bipolar affective disorder: relationship to tardive dyskinesia. Psychol Med 19:897–902, 1989

Wechsler D: Wechsler Adult Intelligence Scale, 3rd Edition. San Antonio, TX, Harcourt Assessment, 1997

Index

*Page numbers printed in **boldface** type refer to tables or figures.*